SMART MEDICINE FOR YOUR EYES

A GUIDE TO NATURAL, EFFECTIVE AND SAFE RELIEF OF COMMON EYE DISORDERS

SECOND EDITION

DR. JEFFREY ANSHEL

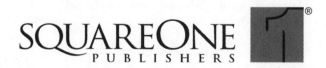

SQUAREONE
PUBLISHERS

The therapeutic procedures and suggested remedies in this book have been selected based on the training, personal experiences, and research of the author. Because each person and situation are unique, the author and publisher urge the reader to check with a qualified health professional before using any procedure when there is any question regarding appropriateness. The publisher does not advocate the use of any particular health program, but believes the information presented in this book should be available to the public.

Because there is always some risk involved, the author and publisher are not responsible for any adverse effects or consequences resulting from the use of any of the suggestions, preparations, or procedures described in this book. Please do not use this book if you are unwilling to assume the risk. It is always an intelligent decision to consult with a physician or other qualified health professional. Also, it is a sign of wisdom, not cowardice, to seek a second or third opinion.

TYPESETTER: Gary A. Rosenberg

Square One Publishers
115 Herricks Road • Garden City Park, NY • 11040
(516) 535-2010 • (877) 900-BOOK
www.squareonepublishers.com

Library of Congress Cataloging-in-Publication Data

Names: Anshel, Jeffrey, author.
Title: Smart medicine for your eyes : a guide to natural, effective, and
   safe relief of common eye disorders / Dr. Jeffrey Anshel.
Description: Second edition. | Garden City Park, NY : Square One
   Publishers, [2023] | Includes bibliographical references and index. |
 Identifiers: LCCN 2022023260 (print) | LCCN 2022023261 (ebook) | ISBN
   9780757005237 (paperback) | ISBN 9780757055232 (ebook)
Subjects: LCSH: Eye—Care and hygiene—Popular works. |
   Eye—Diseases—Popular works.
Classification: LCC RE51 .A633 2023 (print) | LCC RE51 (ebook) | DDC
   617.7/1—dc23/eng/20220629
LC record available at https://lccn.loc.gov/2022023260
LC ebook record available at https://lccn.loc.gov/2022023261

Printed in the Nutech Print Services - India

10   9   8   7   6   5   4   3   2   1

Contents

Part Three Therapies, Procedures, and Eyewear for Eye Care

This book is dedicated to my son, Casey.
He continues to be my inspiration,
and a great example from whom I continue to learn.

Acknowledgments

No book can be written to this depth by one person alone.

I would like to thank Nobu Asano, LAc, for his contribution on Chinese herbs; the late Brian Banks of Natural Ophthalmics, for his contribution on homeopathy; Carol Brown, herbalist, for her guidance on herb research; Dr. Stuart Richer, for his friendship and informative discussions on ocular wellness; and

Ellen Troyer, MT, MA, for her belief in my ideas and her extensive contribution to my nutrition education.

And a special thank you to the hundreds of eyecare professionals who have joined the Ocular Wellness and Nutrition Society, thereby showing their support for nutrition-oriented continuing education in the field of eye care.

Preface

"The eye is the window to the soul." "An eye for an eye." "We see eye to eye." "I see what you mean." These are just a few of the sayings we use that indicate how important our eyes and vision are to our everyday lives. Surveys have shown that of all of our senses, the one we find the most frightening to lose is our sight. We live in a visual world and, as the saying goes, "Seeing is believing."

For more than forty-five years, I have been helping people to see well. It has been a very rewarding experience. However, what I have found is that most people (including me, before I began to study optometry) know very little about their eyes. Parents don't know when they should have their children's eyes first examined. Parents and teachers don't realize that students' reading problems may be related to their eyes. The majority of people assume that getting cataracts is a normal part of the aging process. Moreover, most of us don't know the difference between cataracts and glaucoma. And many of us firmly believe that carrots are the best food for your eyes—something that's not particularly true.

Despite these misconceptions, however, many people are thirsty for knowledge about their eyes. They just don't know where to find it. If you are like the average person, unless you have a specific eye concern, you don't actively search for eyecare information. The fact is that most of us don't get eye examinations unless we notice a problem. And even if you go to an eye doctor, you may not get a complete picture of what your problem is and what alternatives are available in the way of treatment. Doctors in their office settings often just don't have the time to explain all of the various conditions and remedies. But if you go to your doctor already possessing some general knowledge of what your problem may be and what might be available in the form of treatment, you and your doctor together can make an informed decision about what will work best for your visual well-being.

Moreover, the eyecare industry, like the healthcare industry in general, is going through significant changes in the face of managed care. Because of managed care, you have less access to the doctor of your choice, and you are treated more like a statistic than a patient. One popular physician once said, "We don't have a healthcare system here in the US; we have a disease management system—and it's not working!"

The bulk of your health care, including your eye care, is dependent upon your own education rather than just the word of your doctor. And while the Internet might contain a wealth of information, studies show that most of the health-related sites have little or no accurate information. My goal in this book is to help you be as informed as possible when it comes to your eyes and your vision.

I designed this book to be a handy, yet comprehensive guide to any of the vision-related problems that may crop up in your life. The content of this book is easily accessible, thorough, and up-to-date, offering the latest information on a large variety of eye disorders and the possible treatments available for them. There are many things that you can do for yourself, not only to treat eye problems that may arise, but also to prevent them. This book is not intended to undermine eyecare professionals, since they play an essential role in the treatment of vision disorders, but to supplement their care. With the knowledge in this book and the care offered by your eye doctor, it is my hope that you will have clear vision and healthy eyes to last a lifetime.

A WORD ABOUT GENDER

In an effort to avoid lengthy and awkward phrasing within sentences, it is our publishing style to alternate the use of generic male and female pronouns according to section. Therefore, one section will employ the female "she" and "her" pronouns, while the next will apply the male "he" and "his" pronouns. Hopefully, this provides an unbiased and easy-to-read text.

Introduction

You may have never thought about how easy it is for you to read the words on this page. That's because your eyes are probably doing their job pretty well. In fact, you may be one of the 42 percent of Americans who don't wear corrective lenses. If so, congratulations! However, that doesn't mean you don't have a vision-related problem. And let me ask you a question: Are you one of the 90 million Americans who are overdue for an eye examination? Whatever your particular situation may be, consider the fact that over 80 percent of what you learn comes in through your eyes. That says a lot about the importance of good eye health and vision.

The act of seeing can seem automatic, so taking our eyes for granted is an easy thing to do. We are born with two eyes that, for the most part, are fully functional at birth. However, the complex function of vision, which involves the processing and understanding of visual input, also requires learning. This learning happens over the first decade of life, and if it doesn't occur, a child's development can be impaired. Humans are visually directed creatures; our eyes are our most important connection to our world.

Vision problems are not often painful and are usually slow to develop. Many of the problems that occur are preventable, not just by reading letters on an eye doctor's chart once per year or eating a lot of carrots, but by taking a little extra time to learn about the eyes and how they work. A vision problem may start with occasional blurriness or a dull headache after reading for a short period of time. Or you may have trouble seeing distant objects, such as road signs, at night. Your eyes may burn a little bit or feel dry occasionally. Or perhaps you have noticed recently in the mirror that your eyes look different than they used to. Fortunately, even if something does go wrong, you can usually correct the problem if you act quickly. But why wait until there is a problem? There is such a thing as preventive eye care, and it's easier than you may think.

This book, by itself, will not give you the knowledge or the ability to cure all eye problems or allow you to throw away your glasses. However, it will teach you about your eyes and how to interpret the messages they send. It may therefore help to keep you from being stuck behind glasses for the rest of your life— or at least from needing a stronger prescription every year. In addition, this guide will show you how to prevent serious eye damage and loss of vision. It is a lot easier to prevent eye problems than to reverse changes that have already taken place.

Do you already use corrective lenses? If you wear glasses, you should learn all you can about them. And you might as well get glasses that enhance, rather than detract from your appearance. In this book, I offer help concerning both of those tasks. Contact lenses are especially complicated and should be treated more like the medical devices that they are rather than an over-the-counter commodity. This is another subject I discuss, from options concerning the various types of contacts to proper lens care.

Whether you wear corrective lenses or not, you should have enough knowledge about vision to know when to see an eye doctor and what kind of eye doctor to see. Studies continue to show that many people don't know if their eyecare professional is an optometrist, an optician, or an ophthalmologist. I define all of these terms for you in the coming pages.

The purpose of this book is to introduce you to the eyes and visual system, give you basic information on the most common eye problems, provide an overview of what is available in traditional and alternative treatments for them, and guide you in finding more information. Part One discusses the various elements of eye care. Included are sections on the anatomy and function of the visual system, the development of vision, how to find the right eyecare professional for your needs, and the effects of nutrition on vision. Also offered are introductions to herbal therapy and homeopathy, as these approaches can be helpful in

maintaining and improving eye health. Ultimately, Part One serves as the foundation for the subsequent material presented in the book.

Part Two provides information on problems that commonly afflict the eyes. It begins with basic first-aid information for your eyes, and includes an important section on the ocular side effects of certain common medications. Next, there is a helpful "Troubleshooting Guide" for quick reference; it consists of a list of symptoms and identifies the conditions that might be causing them. Then, eye disorders are discussed in alphabetical order. Each entry starts with a description of the problem, its causes, and how to identify the signs and symptoms. Treatment options follow, including recommendations for conventional treatments, nutritional supplementation, herbal treatments, and homeopathic approaches. Many of the entries also have a section on self-treatment options. Such sections detail the most commonly helpful natural treatments. In the last part of each section, general tips are offered for preventing the disorder or easing the symptoms.

Part Three further explains a number of the treatment procedures mentioned in Part Two. Acupuncture and acupressure, eyeglasses and contact lenses, eye surgeries, and vision therapy are among the topics explored at length. When appropriate, helpful illustrations are included. The information in Part Three will aid you in conducting a more thorough and educated discussion with your eye doctor.

Equally important are the appendices at the back of this book. There is a helpful glossary, a directory that lists numerous organizations related to eye care and eye health, and a section that recommends suppliers so that you can have a jump-start on purchasing reputable, effective eye products.

The format of this book is simple, yet the facts presented are extremely significant and wide-ranging. The information is up-to-date and based on available research, my experiences, and common sense. This book should answer your most common questions about your eyes and the way you see. My hope is that it will open your eyes to the world of vision and teach you about your eyes so that you can talk intelligently with your doctor about your vision problems. I also hope to dispel some myths about what's good for your eyes and what isn't. Should you have any questions about a condition or the appropriate treatment, contact an eyecare professional. In the meantime, here's looking at you!

The Elements of Eye Care

The eyes are very small but complicated organs. It is not the purpose of this book to teach you how to become an eyecare professional, nor do I want you to think that you can bypass professional eye care. However, with the proper background and basic information, you can join your eye doctor in making intelligent decisions that will help you see clearly and comfortably. Part One sets you on that path.

The first section of Part One covers the basics of the eyes and the visual system. Remember that the eyes are directly connected to the brain, so studying the process of vision can get quite complex. However, I've attempted to put this information into accessible language that almost everyone can understand. I will cover the common "refractive" changes—nearsightedness, farsightedness, and astigmatism—so that you can identify the problem and learn what to do about it, if you have a vision problem that falls into one of those categories. I will also offer some basic visual skills tests so that you can tell how your eyes are functioning. Some of these tests aim to detect serious vision-threatening conditions, but others serve just to make sure that your eyes are working together well.

In the second section of Part One, I will review the process of visual development—how the human being learns to see as she grows up. This section contains good background information to assist you in following your young child's eye and vision development. It is a must for parents because every child thinks that everyone else sees the way that she does!

Third, I will provide guidance on how to find an eyecare professional. Given that there are three different types of professionals who can take care of your eyes, it can be very difficult to remember which doctor does what and who to go to. I'll help you select the most appropriate professional so that you can find and stick with someone who is capable of managing your eyecare needs.

Once you are familiar with the basics of eye care and the professionals involved, it's time to start educating yourself on specific ways to improve or maintain your eye health. Thus, Part One continues with a comprehensive section on nutrition. Many people think that the connection between nutrition and vision involves nothing more than eating a lot of carrots. However, this section will dispel that old wives' tale and show you how you can maintain the health of your eyes with the proper nutrition and/or supplementation. It is here that you'll learn how the eyes' connection to the rest of the body really works. We are not only what we eat, but we also "see as we eat." Moreover, including herbal therapies and homeopathic treatments in your eyecare regimen can be very effective. Therefore, sections on each of these approaches follow, as well.

By the end of Part One, you will have accumulated a lot of helpful information on the eyes. From understanding how your eyes work to taking pro-active measures to maintain ocular health, Part One starts you on a thorough exploration of the eyes and their precious role in your life. Let's get started.

The Eyes and the Visual System

I would like to introduce you to a part of your body that you don't see very much—your eyes. Because you are always seeing *with* them, you don't often get a chance to look *at* them. Yet your eyes are two fascinating organs with which you should become very familiar if you want to maintain their optimal health. So, get ready, we are about to embark on a tour of the wonderful world of vision.

This book is not meant to be a technical medical synopsis of the anatomy and physiology of the human visual system. Instead, it is intended to be the layperson's guide to conscientiously caring for the eyes. However, you still need a solid foundation of knowledge about the eyes so that you can make intelligent decisions regarding eye health and the treatment of eye diseases. Thus, this chapter offers general information on how the eye is put together and how it works. We'll start with some basic eye anatomy.

A CLOSER LOOK AT YOUR EYES

The eyeball is basically that—a ball. Its diameter is roughly 1 inch, and its circumference is about 3 inches. The part of the eyeball that is visible between the eyelids is actually only one-sixth of the eye's total surface area. The remaining five-sixths of the eyeball is hidden behind the eyelids.

Figure 1.1, "The Eye," clearly illustrates the elements of the eyeball. The outer surface of the eye is divided into two parts: the *sclera* (SKLER-ah), the white part that is the outer covering of the eye, and the *cornea* (KOR-nee-ah), the transparent membrane in front of the eye. The sclera is made of tough fibers that allow it to perform its function of supporting the contents of the eyeball. It has a white appearance because the fibers are light in color and because it contains very few blood vessels. The cornea, which is steeper in curvature than the sclera, may be difficult to see because it is transparent and backed by the colored *iris* (EYE-ris). You can see the cornea more easily if you look at a friend's eye from the side. It is a very sensitive membrane that serves to protect the eye and acts as a lens to begin the focusing of light. Also in this area is the *conjunctiva* (con-junk-TIE-vah), the mucous membrane that covers the front of the eye and lines the inside of the eyelids.

Just inside the sclera and covering all of the same area is the *choroid* (KOH-royd), which is a vascular membrane that provides the main blood supply to the inner eyeball. And just inside the choroid is the *retina* (RET-in-ah), the nerve membrane that receives the light. The small but important central area of the retina is called the *macula* (MAC-you-lah). It is used for sharp, detailed vision, such as threading a needle or spotting a distant object. The measurement of 20/20 is a measure of the focus at the macula. And the central part of the macula is called the *fovea* (FOE-vee-ah).

interpreted. We actually have a blind spot at the point where the optic nerve enters the eyeball, since there is no retina covering that area.

So far, the parts of the eye fulfill relatively basic roles. The eye needs protection and support, which is provided by the sclera. The eye needs a blood supply, which is provided by the choroid and through the optic nerve. Finally, the eye needs a mechanism for seeing, which is provided by the retina. But we're not done yet.

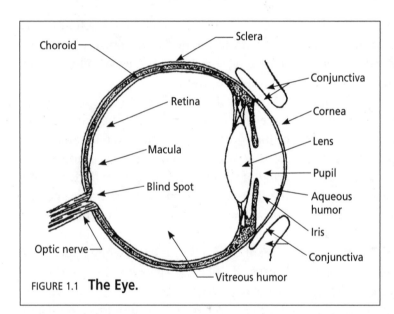

FIGURE 1.1 **The Eye.**

When you look at an eye, the first thing you'll notice is the iris, the colored area of the eye, as mentioned above. If you look closely, you'll see that the iris is actually enclosed in what is known as a *chamber*, which is the medical term for a closed space. The *pupil* (PEW-pill) is nothing more than a hole in the iris, which allows the light to enter the interior chamber of the eye. It expands and contracts to allow more or less light into the eye. The iris is also surrounded by a watery fluid called the *aqueous* (AY-kwee-us) *humor* or *aqueous fluid*. Here, the term "humor" doesn't have anything to do with being funny; it's the Latin word for "fluid." Just behind the iris is the *lens*, which facilitates focusing. The lens, also known as the *crystalline lens*, is transparent and can't really be seen from the outside unless special equipment is used. Behind the lens, and filling the main chamber within the eye, is the *vitreous* (VIT-ree-us) *humor*. This substance, which is more gelatinous and less watery than the aqueous humor, helps in the support of the retina and other structures.

Because these two areas are so small and close together, the terms fovea and macula are often used interchangeably.

In addition to the blood vessels of the choroid, there are also blood vessels that enter the eye through the *optic nerve* and lie on the front surface of the retina. These vessels supply nutrition to the retina and to other structures that are found inside the eye. The optic nerve is directly linked to the brain; that's how the images received by the eye travel into the brain to be

That's it! You have learned the basic anatomy of the eyeball and can follow further discussions on the eye without feeling intimidated or lost. We are now ready to delve into how the eye actually functions. You will soon understand just how all of these parts work in unison to produce vision.

HOW THE EYE WORKS

Let's examine the visual process from the beginning. Light enters the eye by passing through the tears, the cornea, the aqueous humor, and the pupil. It is focused by the lens and then travels across the vitreous humor, ultimately reaching the retina. The retina is an extension of the brain, since, as mentioned earlier, the nerve fibers from the retina directly enter the brain.

When the light strikes the retina, it first stimulates chemical changes in the light-sensitive cells of the retina known as the *photoreceptors.* There are actually two kinds of photoreceptors. *Rods,* which are long and slender cells, respond to light or dark stimuli and are important to our night vision. *Cones,* which are cone-shaped, respond to color stimuli and therefore are also called *color receptors.* There are about seventeen times as many rods as there are cones—about 120 million rods and 7 million cones—in the retina of each eye. These rods and cones interconnect and converge to form networks of nerve fibers. About 1 million nerve fibers make up each optic nerve.

When the rods and cones are struck by light, they convert the light energy to nerve energy. We'll call this nerve energy a *visual impulse.* The impulse travels out of the eye and into the brain via the optic nerve at a speed of 423 miles per hour. First it reaches the middle of the brain, where a pair of "relay stations" combines the visual information that the impulse is carrying with other sensory information. The impulse then travels to the very back part of the brain, the *visual cortex.* It is there that the brain interprets the shapes of objects and the spatial organization of scenes. It recognizes visual patterns as they belong to known objects—for example, it recognizes that a flower is a flower. Further visual processing is done at the sides of the brain, known as the *temporal lobes.* Once the brain has interpreted vital information about something the eyes have "seen," it instantaneously transfers the information to the different areas of the brain that must play a part in the response. For example, if the information is that a car is moving toward you, it is relayed to the *motor cortex,* which is the area that controls movement and enables you to get out of the car's way. The motor cortex is located in a band that goes over the top of your head, from just above one ear to just above the other ear.

So, vision is really the combination of the eyeball receiving the light and the brain interpreting the signals from the eye and initiating a reaction. We will discuss this process of vision (or "visual processing") in more detail in the next section of Part One, titled "The Development of Vision." But for now we should dig a little more deeply into what causes acute and not-so-acute vision.

Measuring Visual Acuity

The visual process I have described above is how the normal eye and visual system function when working perfectly well. The condition of the eye being optically normal is called *emmetropia* (em-e-TROH-pee-ah). Figure 1.2, "The

Emmetropic Eye," illustrates what occurs when light enters the normal eye. Unfortunately, not all eyes are emmetropic. Very often, there is something that goes wrong, and the visual process is disrupted. About 40 percent of the adults in the United States have difficulty seeing clearly at a distance, and about 60 percent have difficulty seeing up close with no corrective lenses. How do we measure visual acuity, and what are some of the problems that affect it?

Recall the last time you visited your eye doctor's office. You probably got a full exam-

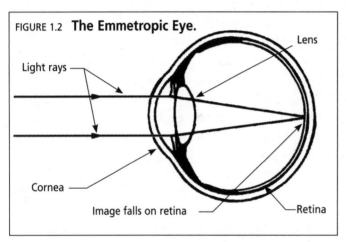

FIGURE 1.2 **The Emmetropic Eye.**

Lens

Light rays

Cornea

Image falls on retina — Retina

ination, had what seemed like 100 different tests, and finally asked, "How are my eyes?" Your doctor might have said, "You have 20/20 vision!" If that was the case, you probably walked out of the office satisfied that your eyes are in good shape. But are they? To what does "20/20" refer? What does it mean?

The term "20/20" is a notation that relates to the *resolving power* of the eye. An eye's resolving power is its sharpness of sight, which we can define as the ability to distinguish two points from each other and not see them as just one point. This resolution occurs at its maximum in

the foveal portion of the retina. If your vision is 20/20, it means that you are seeing at 20 feet what the optically normal—or emmetropic— eye can see at 20 feet. That is, your eyes can distinguish one point from another on a specific line of characters from a standard eye chart placed 20 feet away. The standard chart is called a Snellen chart, which is named after Hermann Snellen, a Dutch ophthalmologist who introduced the chart in 1862 to study visual acuity.

Now, if your vision is 20/40, it means that you can see at 20 feet what the emmetropic eye can see at 40 feet. You have to be closer to the object than normal in order to see it correctly. And if your vision is 20/100, you must be 20 feet away from an object to see it clearly, while the emmetropic eye can see it clearly from 100 feet away.

In short, the larger the bottom number is, the poorer your resolving power, which is also known as your *visual acuity.* Visual acuity is measured for distance and near vision. So now you know that 20/20 is something like a grading, or scaling, of eyesight. To assess your own, see the inset titled "Visual Acuity Tests" on page 11.

Understanding Refractive Errors

One of the more common eye problems—and one that disallows 20/20 vision—is the mis-focusing of the light as it is directed onto the retina. The light can be focused too soon or too late, or it can even be distorted. Because the bending of light is technically called "refraction," the mis-focusing of light in the eye is called a *refractive error.*

VISUAL ACUITY TESTS

While nothing can replace a full eye exam at a doctor's office, the tests below will help you get a sense of how acute your vision is. Follow the steps for a measurement of both your distance and near visual acuity.

DISTANCE VISUAL ACUITY

1. While you are sitting or standing comfortably, have a friend hold this book open to the Distance Visual Acuity chart on pages 12 and 13 (Figure 1.3) exactly 20 feet away from you. Very good light should be shining on the page. Cover (don't close) your left eye.

2. Read down to the lowest line that you can easily read. Then try the next line, even if it's difficult. Be sure to read the letters loudly enough for your friend to hear and check against the page.

3. Have your friend write down the line at which your visual acuity began being challenged and how many letters you saw incorrectly on that line.

4. Switch the cover to the other eye and repeat the test once again. You might try to read each line's letters from right to left this time, to avoid memorization.

To attain your score, you are going to note which line you had trouble reading and how many of the letters you misidentified. If you got several but not all of the letters correct, then you get credit for that line. For example, you missed just one letter on the 20/30 line (but you could not read down any further), then your score is 20/30-1. If you got all of the 20/30 line correct and could only get two letters on the 20/25 line, then your score is 20/30+2. Follow the procedure for each eye individually.

NEAR-POINT VISUAL ACUITY

The near visual acuity test is almost exactly the same as the distance visual acuity test, except that you use the Near-Point Visual Acuity Chart, which can be found on page 14. (Figure 1.4.) Hold the page 16 inches from your nose—a standard reading distance. With that exception, follow the steps given earlier for the distance visual acuity test, and score it the same way. Again, perform the test with one eye at a time. Make sure you are not squinting or straining to see the letters (I call that "cheating") because you should be seeing clearly and comfortably throughout the assessment. If you have to squint, then you're working too hard.

First, let's define a few necessary terms. *Nearsightedness*, also called *myopia* (my-OH-pee-ah), occurs when near vision is good but distance vision is poor. For the nearsighted person, a distant image—that is, an image at least 20 feet away—falls in front of the retina and looks blurred. Nearsightedness results when an eye is too long, when the cornea is too steeply curved, when the eye's lens is unable to relax enough to provide accurate distance vision, or from some combination of these and other factors. While many professionals feel that myopia is a benign refractive error, new research is discovering that it can

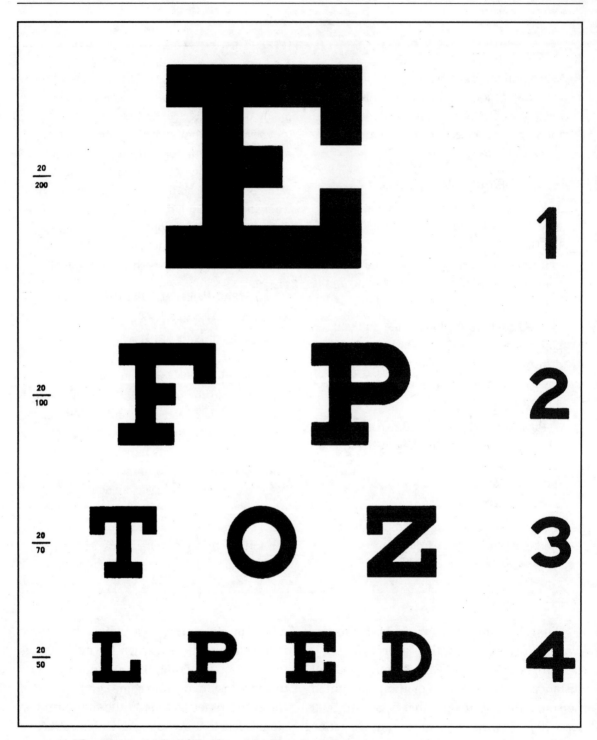

FIGURE 1.3 **The Distance Visual Acuity or Snellen Eye Chart.**

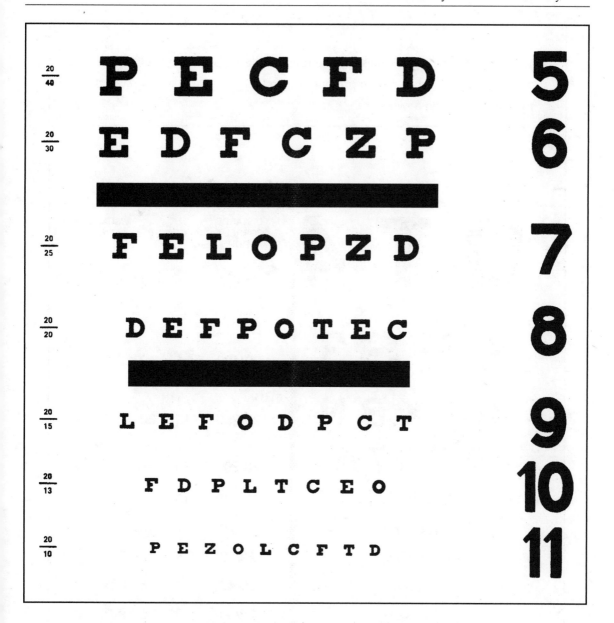

have long-term consequences. We will discuss myopia control in a later chapter. See Figure 1.5, "The Nearsighted Eye," for an illustration of what occurs in the myopic eye.

Farsightedness, also called *hyperopia* (hy-per-OH-pee-ah), is *not* exactly the opposite of myopia. For the farsighted person, the image of an object that is 20 feet or more away is directed past the retina, as shown in Figure 1.6, "The Farsighted Eye." It looks blurred because it hasn't yet been brought into focus. Farsightedness results when an eye is too short or a cornea is too flat, or from some combination of other factors. The main difference between

This card has been specially designed to test your near-point acuity. Hold the card approximately 16 inches away from your face and read each line, starting with the top line and moving downwards.

	DISTANCE CORRELA- TION	JAEGER	PT	VISUAL EFF%
# D T 4	20/800		72	5%
## L E S 3	20/400		42	10%
### R F X B N	20/250	18	30	15%
P O 5 7 A	20/200	16	26	20%
9 V M C L	20/100	10	14	50%
K S 3 Z 7	20/70	7	10	65%
N R E T X	20/50	5	8	75%
O R D F M P	20/40	3	6	85%
V J F X G H	20/30	2	5	90%
P 3 B E A R	20/20	1	4	100%

FIGURE 1.4 **The Near-Point Visual Acuity Chart.**

nearsightedness and farsightedness is that the relaxed eye can increase its focal power, to some degree, to compensate for farsightedness, but it cannot reduce its power to compensate for nearsightedness.

Theoretically, the surface of the cornea should be almost spherical in shape—like the surface of a basket-ball—so that when light passes through it, it can be focused at a single point. However, nature isn't always perfect, and the cornea is often warped, resembling a football more than a round ball. The lens, too, can be irregular in shape. These distortions can be significant enough so that the light that passes through the cornea and lens in the vertical orientation will focus at a different spot from the light that passes through in the horizontal orientation. When that occurs, you have two points of focus with a blur between them. This is known as *astigmatism* (ah-STIG-mah-tism) and is illustrated in Figure 1.7, "The Astigmatic Eye."

If the difference between these separate points of focus is great enough, the eye will strain as it tries to decide which point of focus it should use. You might then develop occasional blurring of vision, fatigue, or possibly headaches. Astigmatism in small amounts is very common and not of great concern. But about 23 million Americans have a significant amount of astigmatism that requires correction. Glasses correct astigmatism because the curvature of the eyeglass lens

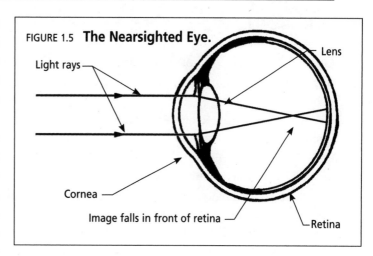

FIGURE 1.5 **The Nearsighted Eye.**

Light rays — Lens — Cornea — Image falls in front of retina — Retina

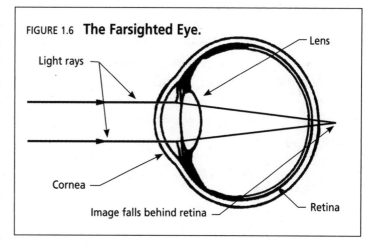

FIGURE 1.6 **The Farsighted Eye.**

Light rays — Lens — Cornea — Image falls behind retina — Retina

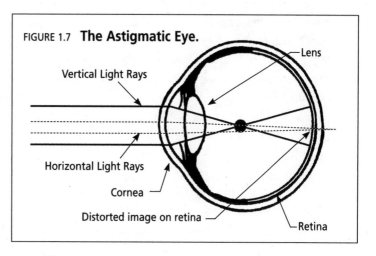

FIGURE 1.7 **The Astigmatic Eye.**

Vertical Light Rays — Lens — Horizontal Light Rays — Cornea — Distorted image on retina — Retina

compensates for the incompetent curvature of the eye. This is a simple optical correction. Glasses, however, will not change the amount of astigmatism—that is, they won't "cure" the problem.

You now know exactly what happens inside nearsighted, farsighted, and astigmatic eyes to cause blurring of vision. Again, these are very common problems due to the fact that the eyeball is not always perfectly shaped. And these anatomical dysfunctions not only are optically correctable but there are also surgical procedures that can change the way light is focused in the eye. We will cover that information later in the book, in Part Three.

It is not difficult to understand why people who experience refractive errors tend to strain their eyes in an attempt to clarify the images before them. Perhaps you have noticed yourself doing this. Of course, fatigue can also cause eyestrain. For a quick self-test on how much your eyes are straining to see, go to the inset titled "Cover Tests" on page 17.

Identifying Blind Spots

When you were in grade school, someone probably told you that everyone has blind spots in their eyes. I'm sure you looked and looked but, instead of locating missing pieces in your range of vision, you simply saw everything you looked at. It's actually hard to believe in blind spots if you don't know how to find them. See the inset titled "The Blind Spot Test" on page 18 for instructions on how to locate your blind spots.

You have learned that the back of the inside of your eye is covered with the retina, which receives light and transmits nerve impulses to the brain. The cells in the retina are connected to nerve fibers that collectively make up the optic nerve. The area where the optic nerve leaves the retina and heads toward the brain is not covered with retinal cells (the rods and cones) but serves solely as the exit for the nerve fibers. Since there are no cells to receive light, no visual perception occurs in that specific area. Thus, this area is actually blind and is called the *optic disc* (when viewed from the front of the eye, it is round and appears as a disc).

"Okay," you say skeptically, "if my eyes have blind spots, why don't I see any empty space in those areas?" Well, remember that you have two eyes. Each of your eyes has a visual field, or an area of visual perception. The fields of your two eyes overlap quite a bit, so you have a large area of binocular (two-eyed) vision. The seeing portion of one eye overlaps the blind spot of the other eye, so if both of your eyes are open and functioning, you will not have any gaps in your field of vision.

These "normal" blind spots are actually significant in the detection of eye diseases and other conditions, including brain tumors. For example, the eye disease *glaucoma* (glaw-KOH-mah), which involves an increase in pressure in the eye, will cause the blind spot to enlarge as the optic nerve begins to die off. (Glaucoma and many other eye diseases/disorders are discussed in detail in Part Two.) Tracking the changes in the size of the blind spot can give your doctor information about the progression of a disease. Moreover, if you ever perceive a blind area in your vision other than the normal one just discussed, be sure to have it checked immediately.

COVER TESTS

This is actually a two-part test that measures the tendency of your eye muscles to strain. The two parts are the Cover/Uncover Test and the Alternate Cover Test. To perform these tests, you'll need a single point target at a distance and the same at a near point, as well as a card (or your hand) to cover your eye. Follow the simple steps listed below.

1. Select a single point target at a distance of at least 20 feet away and fix your gaze on it.

2. Keeping both eyes open, cover the right eye and notice if the target appears to move. You should try this several times with the same eye, because the movement may be subtle.

3. Switch to the other eye. Cover the left eye and note if the target appears to move. This completes the "Cover/Uncover" portion of the cover tests.

4. Now, while maintaining your view of the target at a distance, just switch the cover (the card or your hand) from its location in front of one eye to the other, back and forth. Notice not only if the target moves, but also in which direction it moves. Does it move in the *same* direction as the cover moves, or does it move in the *opposite* direction? This completes the "Alternate Cover" part of the test.

5. Next, select a target at a reading distance. Repeat the steps above, viewing this nearer target.

Record your findings and report them to your doctor during your eye examination. The results will assist your doctor in finding subtle eye-muscle balance problems. In the Cover/Uncover portion of the test, you were testing to see if both eyes aligned properly when looking at a particular object. If you covered one eye and saw the image "jump" to a different position, then the previously uncovered eye was pointing to a different target. This indicates a loss of *binocular* (or two-eyed) *vision*. In the Alternate Cover portion of the test, you were testing to see if your eye muscles were in balance with each other—in other words, you were testing the tendency for your eyes to pull in one direction or the other but still maintain binocular vision when they are both open. If the image jumped when you moved the card back and forth, then your eyes do have a tendency to pull in one direction or another. Only your doctor can determine if your tendencies are significant for eyestrain or not.

Assessing Peripheral Vision

Right now, you are reading the words on this page with both eyes (I hope). You have your eyes pointed at these words, and all that you are really consciously aware of is the page you see. But if someone were to sneak up behind you and then slowly come around to your side, you'd probably see the person moving and know he was there (assuming the person didn't tip you off by knocking over a chair). Now, how would you see someone off to the side if your eyes were looking down here? You'd be using your *peripheral (side) vision,* which accounts for

THE BLIND SPOT TEST

Each of your eyes has a blind spot where the optic nerve meets the retina. It is easy to prove this using the following instructions and graphic.

1. Look at the illustration below. There is a plus sign on the left side and a large dot on the right side. To test your right eye, you are going to cover your left eye and look at the plus sign. To test your left eye, you are going to cover your right eye and look at the dot. (No, I didn't say that backwards!)

2. Hold the book 6 inches from your face, remembering to keep the eye that you are not testing covered. Now, slowly move the book back to about 12 inches from your face.

3. If you look directly at the plus sign with your right eye, the dot on the right side of the page will disappear from the corner of your vision at about 12 inches from your face. If you look directly at the dot with your left eye, the plus sign on the left side of the page will similarly disappear.

You may have to move the book slightly back and forth or left and right to get this effect because the blind spot is not very big. Remember to keep the uncovered eye still and directed straight ahead.

Try the other eye next. Remember to keep the eye that is not being tested covered.

a large percentage of your whole visual field. This visual field is all of what you can see at one time without turning your head or eyes. A normal visual field is about 170 degrees around, but certain medical conditions can narrow it. In fact, another definition of being *legally blind*, or suffering from *low vision*, is having a visual field of less than 20 degrees.

Over half of the inside of your eye is lined with the retina. When you look straight at an object, you line up that object with the macula—that tiny, 1 square-millimeter area of the retina that gives you the sharpest vision. So, there's a whole lot of retina that isn't completely "tuned in" to where you are looking. But when people come up beside you, they move enough to alert the rest of your retina that something is there. The peripheral retina area is very important. For example, think of how it factors in when you are driving a car. You catch glimpses of cars on either side of you without actually turning your head or eyes completely around. Besides motion detection, the peripheral retina is also important in balance, body movement ability, and light perception. See the inset titled "Peripheral Vision Test," on page 20, for instructions on how to assess your own visual field.

Further Defining Binocular Vision

Seeing a clear 20/20 is certainly a good indication that your eyes are doing their job well. However, sharp eyesight is just one of the functions that your eyes perform. Since there are two eyes, they must work in harmony with each other. One of the most fascinating abilities of the human visual system is the capacity to take images from two eyes and put them together into just one picture. As previously discussed, this complex process is called *binocular vision*. Because binocular vision normally prevents you from seeing two images, the idea of double vision might sound strange or even impossible to you. But double vision can occur and is one of the most dangerous manifestations of vision problems. Imagine seeing two cars coming toward you as you are driving down the road!

Here's how the healthy brain and eyes keep us from seeing double and going off the road. Let's assume that you have two eyes and they are both working about equally well. As you look at an object, each eye receives an individual image of that object. Both of these images are transmitted back to your brain where they are then "fused" together into one image. In order for that to happen, however, both eyes must be pointed at the same object, at the same spot, with the images approximately equal in size and clarity.

Now, if one eye does not aim at the same spot as the other, each eye will see a slightly different view of the object, and the two images won't match up. When these images are transmitted back to your brain, they will stimulate two different groups of brain cells and you will experience two pictures, otherwise known as

diplopia, or "seeing double." After a short period of time, your brain will decide to turn off or suppress the image from the eye that is pointed in the wrong (or less important) direction so that you can see one picture again. Although this *suppression* is necessary for our visual survival, it is certainly not the way we were meant to see.

When the eyes are not coordinated properly, suppression of an image is the brain's way of making our daily tasks easy and comfortable. While suppression of an image might *sound* devastating, it actually works pretty well in helping us function effectively. What is more serious is when there is a competition between the eyes—when the eyes struggle to work together. Lack of coordination between the eyes actually falls into the domain of brain function, for the brain is where coordination takes place. It is competition between the eyes that causes a person to grapple with reading tasks, and that can lead to poor reading comprehension, decreased job performance, and possible eyestrain.

Adequate binocular function is important for many common tasks, especially reading and, therefore, learning effectively. Thus, it is critical that children get *all* aspects of their vision checked—not just an exam for 20/20 eyesight. We will cover these issues in the next section of Part One, entitled "The Development of Vision," as well as under the specific disorders of double vision and suppression in Part Two. But for now, see the inset titled "Near Point of Convergence (NPC) Test" on page 21 for a quick way to assess your binocular muscle balance.

PERIPHERAL VISION TEST

To test your own peripheral vision, you'll need the help of a friend. You'll also need two chairs and an object that can be held at a slight distance from your hand, such as the eraser on a pencil.

1. Sit in a chair that is facing your friend, who should also be sitting in a chair. Your heads should be about 2 feet apart and at roughly the same eye level.

2. Have your friend cover one eye, and you cover the opposite one. For example, if your friend covers his right eye, you should cover your left eye. Look directly into each other's open eye without moving. (Blinking is allowed.)

3. Now, with the pencil in your right hand, extend the eraser all the way to the right as far as you can reach. Both of you must keep looking directly at each other's eye; avoid moving your heads or eyes. Slowly bring the eraser in toward you and your friend, but keep it on an imaginary line midway between the two of you. You'll need to bend your elbow to do this. (See Figure 1.8, "Testing Peripheral Vision," at right.)

4. Both you and your friend should each see the eraser come into view out of the corners of your eyes at about the same time. Be sure it's the eraser you see and not the pencil. If one person sees the eraser much sooner than the other, the

one who sees it last might have decreased peripheral vision and should contact an eye doctor. A difference of 4 inches may be significant.

5. Now do the technique again, but this time bring the eraser in from your left side.

6. Repeat the technique again, but bringing the eraser down from over your head.

7. Repeat the technique one more time, bringing the eraser up from your knees.

Each time, both you and your friend should see at the eraser about the same time. Remember, the procedure should *not* be done with both eyes at the same time. This home peripheral vision test will pick up only very significant problems. For more accurate testing to find more subtle defects in the visual field, see your eye doctor.

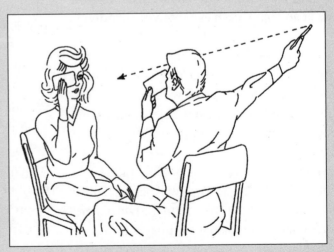

FIGURE 1.8 **Testing Peripheral Vision.**

Exploring Color Vision

Color vision is actually nothing more than the perception of different wavelengths of light. This perception is accomplished by the cones in the retina. Color vision is a hereditary trait, as is color deficiency, often referred to as *colorblindness.*

Before we can talk about color vision, we need to go over some basics about the nature of light. When light rays come from a source of light, they radiate from that source like the waves formed in water when a rock hits its surface. These light waves travel in varying lengths, some shorter than others. The unit of length used to measure waves of light is the *nanometer* (nan-AHM-iter), which is one-millionth of a millimeter, or one-billionth of a meter.

The range of light that we humans can see is called *visible light.* It is light with a wavelength of between 400 and 700 nanometers (nm). In order to put that into context, consider that ultraviolet light has a wavelength below 400 nanometers, and infrared light has a wavelength above 700 nanometers. What makes the

---

NEAR POINT OF CONVERGENCE (NPC) TEST

This test is intended to determine how well your eyes coordinate when looking at a near target. When you look closely at something, each eye's line of sight must turn in toward the other in order to maintain effective binocular vision. If your eyes have difficulty doing this, you are likely to be straining to see up close, and you most likely experience tiredness at the end of the day. Try these easy steps to test your NPC. For accuracy's sake, it is best to get a friend to help you.

1. Hold a pen or pencil at arm's length. Keep watching *just the tip* of the pen or pencil as you slowly bring it toward your eyes.

2. Stop bringing the pen or pencil closer to you as soon as you see two tips (or a double tip). At this point, it is important to record the distance—in inches—between your eyes and the tip of the writing device. A friend can easily do this for you with a tape measure, as long as you keep your hand steady.

3. Now gradually move the pen or pencil away from you until the "double tip" snaps back together and you once more see only one pen or pencil tip. Again, have your friend carefully measure and record the distance between your eyes and the tip of the writing device.

To attain your score, you should perform this test a number of times and take an average of your findings. If the tip of the pen or pencil split into two when it was 3 inches from your eyes, and then resumed its single image when it was 7 inches from your eyes, your NPC score would be 3/7. Substitute whatever numbers apply to your particular score. There are no hard and fast "normal" readings for this test. However, eye-health professionals do like to see a top number (the split) of less than 4 and a difference of only 2 inches or less between the top number and the bottom number (the recovery).

various colors we see? Let's use an example. When white light bounces off a red apple, the apple absorbs all of the light rays except for those with a wavelength of about 650 nanometers. In other words, the apple reflects rays of that particular wavelength. Humans have learned to call that wavelength of reflected light "red." Each color that humans can see has its own wavelength. Blue is about 460 nanometers, green is about 520 nanometers, and yellow is about 575 nanometers. When we perceive a colored object, what we see is that part of the light spectrum that is not absorbed by the object, but rather reflected back to our eyes.

In truth, we still don't know for sure what happens in the retina and brain to enable us to have color vision, but we do have some good theories on the subject. The most popular theory is called the *trichromatic* (try-kroh-MA-tik) *theory,* meaning "three-color theory," which says there are three different types of cones in the retina. There are cones that respond to red, cones that respond to blue, and cones that respond to green. When these cones receive a light stimulus, they send a message to the brain via nerve fibers. Color mixing is accomplished by these cones firing in varying proportions, so that the color we perceive is a combination of the signals coming from the three types of cones. White, for example, is perceived when the red, blue, and green cones fire together in equal proportions.

This is a pretty good working model for color vision, but it's probably not the whole story. Most likely, there are receptors that transmit light stimuli of particular wavelengths from the retina to the brain, and other receptors that inhibit light stimuli of particular wavelengths. The color we actually perceive is probably a result of some "yes" receptors and some "no" receptors sending messages to the brain. Ultimately, the eyes of humans can perceive about 7 million colors. The eye is truly a wonderful organ!

Over the course of a few pages, you have learned quite a bit. You have tackled everything from how to assess your visual acuity to why some people truly struggle with blurred vision. You have learned how your eyes merge two images into one, as well as how they bring color into your life. Congratulations, for you are now much closer to taking command of your eye health.

CONCLUSION

Now that you know the fundamentals of eye anatomy and function, we are ready to study the development of vision as it progresses over various life stages. But before we leave this section, I want to emphasize the importance of being pro-active about your eye health. The basic information and quick little vision tests presented in this section are intended to help you become more familiar with your eyes and how they work. The tests will also help you generally to assess whether or not your eyes are working properly. If you suspect that something is amiss with your eyes, consult your eye doctor and fully discuss your concerns. The more information you can take with you to your eye exam, the easier it will be for your doctor to detect any problems.

The Development of Vision

Since the vast majority of children are born with two eyes situated in the proper position in their heads, it is easy to understand why parents may assume that vision is just "there," and that their children see adequately from the very beginning of life. Yet, as children grow, their eyes must develop along with the rest of their bodies, or their maturation might be hindered. Moreover, young children most likely think that everyone sees the way they do. They may not realize that they are supposed to be able to see the leaves on a tree from across the street or the letters on a blackboard from the rear of a classroom. These children may not know they have a problem or may not think to say anything about their vision. But the estimates are that one out of every twenty preschool children in the United States has a vision problem that will eventually result in a needless loss of sight or a severe learning disability.

Vision is our most important sense. Between 80 and 85 percent of our learning comes through vision. Moreover, most vision problems can be corrected if detected early. Thus, it is the parents' job to talk with their child and find out what is happening with her vision. Most parents don't realize that a child's vision should be routinely checked as early as when the child is six months old. A child's vision is her parents' responsibility.

This section of Part One will discuss the development of vision that occurs throughout early life. It also will provide some techniques for testing your child's vision and for helping to improve her visual perception. If you do not have children, this section is still important to read. It discusses how our vision evolves over the course of various life stages, how certain learning and behavioral disorders might be linked to vision, how technology affects vision, and more.

NORMAL VISUAL-MOTOR DEVELOPMENT

By the time a child is three years old, the eyeball closely resembles an adult's eyeball in structure and size, with some growth and refinement continuing into adulthood. For example, the macula is not refined at birth and must develop as the child grows. However, there is much more to the visual system than the physical structure of the eyeball—that "more" being the difference between eyesight and vision.

Visual perception develops in an individualized manner; each person's way of seeing is just a little different from the next person's way. This is due to the variety of stimuli that children receive (or don't receive) as they grow up. An ancient proverb states, "We see things not as they are, but as we are." Yet there are also predictable stages of vision development, and they coincide with motor development—the development of the large and small muscle movements in a child's body.

At one time, people believed that the eyes were just two little balls that sat in the front of the face to catch light. But for many years now, we have known that the eyes are an integral part of the central nervous system and are very much influenced by the other parts of the body. As the body develops, so do the eyes. Vision is not a separate function; instead, it is integrated into the total "action system" of the child, which includes posture, manual skills and coordination, intelligence, and even personality traits. This is the total vision process, and the development of the muscular system and the visual system together is known as *visual-motor development.*

Although vision is one of the five senses, the actions surrounding the visual process are motor, or muscle, driven. When you are awake, your eyes constantly respond to shifts in your body posture, and they initiate shifts as well. Thus, vision influences and is influenced by the sensitive patterns of movement of the total person. An excellent way to illustrate this point is to stand on one foot and look straight ahead at a distant object. Once you feel stable and secure, close your eyes. Notice how quickly you lose your balance! And just as it's possible to have poor coordination between two body parts, it is also possible to have poor coordination between the eyes and another body part, or even between the two eyes. Thus, the relationship between vision and motor skills is quite complex.

Motor development begins in infancy and continues throughout childhood. In the following paragraphs, as we discuss normal motor and visual-motor development in children, any references to ages are only approximations. It is the sequence of development that is important.

At birth, infants have only reflexes with which to work. However, these reflexes shape the patterns of their motor development. The first basic motor patterns to develop are the *gross motor movements.* "Gross motor" refers to the movements of the large muscles, such as those in the arms and legs. The gross motor movements include crawling, standing, walking, leg and arm movements, head and neck movements, and other large-muscle actions. These movements are necessary for normal growth and development, enabling babies to move in space and use the perceptual tool that is the most developed during babyhood: touch.

Babies' explorations and touching experiments eventually lead to the second basic motor pattern, which is *fine motor movement.* Fine motor movements involve the smaller muscles and include finger bending, toe wiggling, wrist and ankle movements, and other subtle motor actions. These types of motor movements are necessary for fine manipulation and, in general, more detailed inspection of the environment by infants. Fine motor coordination is more difficult to achieve if the gross motor abilities did not develop on schedule.

The *oculomotor skills* develop simultaneously with the gross and fine motor skills. The eyes are controlled by the muscles that surround them and are directly connected to the brain. Oculomotor development refers to the gradual development of the eye-related muscles and their coordination. Efficient eye movement is essential for good eyesight. The six *extraocular* (outside the eye) muscles have to be able to align each eye with a visual target, and the *intraocular* (inside the eye) muscles must be able to focus the light on the retina in order for the person to see the visual target. In addition, the movements of both eyes have to be coordinated in order to avoid excess strain or double vision.

Once oculomotor development is underway, children can begin to *feel* with their eyes. The process starts slowly. At six to twelve months of age, touch is still a child's main avenue of perception. But once the eye muscles begin to coordinate with each other at about twelve to fifteen months of age, the majority of sensory input begins to be transferred to the eyes. Eventually, children don't have to crawl across a room to identify an object by touch. They can merely look at it and see what it is.

The next phase of development is called *hand-eye coordination*. This is the ability of the brain to take in information through the eyes and speedily transfer it to the hands and back again. This ability begins at around the age of two (although it is present to some degree well before that), but it really develops continually throughout life. For example, learning to play a sport at any age is a continuing process of developing hand-eye coordination.

As the visual system matures and oculomotor control increases, the first aspects of *form perception* begin to develop. Loosely defined, form perception is the perception of, first, the shapes of objects and, eventually, more abstract things, such as words on a page. Form perception starts as the perception of forms by oral investigation. That is why young babies try to put everything in their mouths. Then, once fine motor development has been established, form perception is transferred to the fingers. Eventually, it is transferred to the eyes, with children recognizing forms from a distance based on previous experiences. Advanced form perception includes figure-ground discrimination—that is, seeing the main form as being different from the background—as well as perception of general shapes, size differentiation, differentiation of the details of configuration, and directional orientation. Research has shown that when experienced readers read, they don't perceive individual letters or even individual words, but rather the "forms" of the words. That is why you can probably make sense of the following combinations of letters and successfully read the quoted phrase as though it is a regular sentence: "Raserceah has sowhn that when eripexeeicd raedres read, they don't prcieeve idiivnualdl letters or even wrdos, but rehratr the 'forms' of the wdors." Form perception is a complicated process for the brain and the visual system to master, and it is crucial for good reading.

One aspect of advanced form perception is called *laterality*. Laterality is the ability to perceive left and right in reference to your own body, and it begins to develop at about the age of five or six. After laterality comes *directionality*, which is the ability to make left-right distinctions for things other than yourself—say, for other people or objects in the room, or for letters on a piece of paper. This kind of perception usually develops around the age of six or seven. If children can't tell their left from their right or can't make left-right distinctions for other objects, then words and letters don't have any meaning. The letter "p" may look the same as the letter "q," and "b" may look the same as "d," for example. These confusions, called *reversals*, are common and expected up to when children are about seven or eight. After that, children who still reverse letters need some help in figuring out which way is up. Later in this chapter, I'll describe some methods to help them.

The next step in the development of visual-motor skills is *visual memory*, which is the ability to recall visual images including everything from a mother's face to last evening's dinner, and even to a list of spelling words. Visual memory begins to develop about six months of age and continues to develop as children mature. This ability is essential for the retention of written material and is, in fact, one measure of intelligence.

Children's eyes are closely influenced by their ever-changing muscle systems. Visual defects and deviations from the norm may not be apparent if all you look for is sharpness of vision such as can be measured using an eye chart. Vision problems in children may make themselves known as poor coordination, awkwardness, poor timing, hesitation, and sometimes lack of body movement. If you have any doubts about your child's visual-motor development, don't wait too long to alert your pediatrician and to have your child checked out by a developmental optometrist. See below for more information on that latter type of specialist.

MATURATION OF THE EYES THROUGHOUT EARLY LIFE

We have just reviewed the general progression of visual-motor development in young children. Now let's take a more in-depth look at how the eyes mature over various life stages. We will trace the development from the prenatal stage to adolescence.

As you learn about the development of vision, if you have any doubts about whether your child's vision is developing on schedule, I advise you to consult a *developmental optometrist*. While pediatricians might be well versed in the health and development of children in general, they do not have the background in visual development that optometric specialists do. Developmental optometrists have a specific interest in children's eyes and how they relate to the general maturation of children. They usually consider a non-surgical therapeutic approach in the resolving of visual development issues. Pediatric ophthalmologists are also a source of consult; however, their view tends to be more medically oriented for early diseases and surgery, which is fine if a surgical intervention is needed. But if surgery is not necessary, a developmental optometrist is the best professional to see. You can find information on developmental optometrist organizations in the Resource Organizations list, which starts on page 413.

Before Birth

The first rudiments of the eyes are evident in the fetus at about twenty days after conception. And the first trimester (first three months) of pregnancy is the most critical time for the eyes. Good nutrition, good prenatal care, and avoidance of medications and other chemicals (such as alcohol and tobacco) are all important for the development of the fetus's visual system.

There are some eye traits that are genetically determined, and eye color is one. All Caucasian babies are born with blue eyes—although there are many variations of that blue color—because very little pigment has accumulated in their irises by birth. As children grow, more pigment is deposited in the irises, and the eyes begin to look darker. The final eye color depends on how much pigment has accumulated. A blue eye simply has less pigment than a brown eye does, and a green or hazel eye is somewhere in between.

If both parents have blue eyes, then all of their children will have blue eyes. If both parents have brown eyes, there is a 25-percent chance that their child will have blue eyes and a 75-percent chance that the baby will have brown eyes. The brown eye form of the eye color gene is dominant, whereas the blue eye form of the gene is recessive.

Another hereditary trait is color deficiency. Females have two X chromosomes, and males have an X and a Y chromosome. The gene for color deficiency is carried on the mother's X chromosome. For a boy to develop color deficiency, he needs to have inherited only one defective X chromosome from his mother. For a girl to develop color deficiency, she must have two defective X chromosomes—one from her mother and one from her father. This is the reason why color deficiency is so much more common in boys than girls. In fact, 8 percent of males are color deficient, compared to only .5 percent (or one-half percent) of females.

Are some babies programmed to have certain eye problems from the moment of conception? Well, nearsightedness, lazy eye, and strabismus (crossed eyes and wall eyes) do seem to "run in families," but I'm not convinced that genes are entirely to blame for these conditions. Children's genetic makeup may make them more or less likely to develop certain eye problems in any given environment, but it's becoming more apparent with genetic research that the way children use their eyes in that environment can affect their vision. So, if you are nearsighted, don't throw up your hands and say, "I guess Jenny will be nearsighted, too." Start Jenny off right with regular eye examinations and good visual habits. Don't wait until it's too late. We will review the development of nearsightedness in a later chapter.

Newborns

You might think that there is nothing that can be tested regarding the vision of newborn children. However, it is possible to do some eye testing on newborn babies. No, you can't hold an eye chart in front of an infant! However, there are certain visual reflexes that are present at birth. If you have children, you should know what these reflexes are and how to test for them, or ask your optometrist or pediatrician to test for them.

The *pupil reflex* to light is present at birth and can easily be tested by shining a small light into either eye. When the light enters the pupil, the pupil should become smaller. Of course, this should happen for the pupils of both eyes. In fact, both pupils should get smaller when light is shined into either eye.

The pupils also should be approximately the same size and should stay small as long as the light is shined into the eyes. (Adult eyes react the same way.)

To test for the *doll's-eye reflex,* gently nod your child's head back and forth as you look into her eyes. Notice whether the baby tries to compensate and keep looking at you, which is what the baby should do. The doll's-eye reflex was named after old-fashioned dolls of the more expensive type, which had eyes that swiveled as if to keep looking at you as you turned the doll's head.

The *blink reflex* is the fastest reflex in the body. This is a good indication of the importance of preserving our eyesight. Very carefully blow a tiny puff of air at your baby's eyes. (Do this very gently!) The eyes should blink immediately.

Our vision is dependent on these reflexes being present at birth, and visual development builds on these abilities. That is why it is important to confirm that your infant's reflexes are developing as they should be. And given the fact that these reflexes are so simple to test, there is no reason not to conduct these quick checks. If you are unsure if your infant is adequately responding to the reflex tests, please contact your developmental optometrist or pediatrician immediately so that you can make arrangements to have your newborn baby's eye development assessed.

Infants

During the first year of life, babies make the greatest leaps in development. They turn from helpless beings who sleep through most of the day into active toddlers interested in exploring all of the sights and sounds filling their worlds. Following are some rough guidelines you can use in evaluating your child's developing vision.

At one month old, babies usually stare blankly around the room, although a bright light or window light should attract their attention. Occasionally, they will follow an object brought in front of their face for a little bit. Contrary to popular belief, babies are not born blind. However, the retina is not completely developed at birth, so their visual acuity is not as sharp as it will be. They gradually develop visual discrimination, and that may take as long as five or six years—at the latest. Also, the cornea (front dome of the eye) is almost adult size, which is why babies appear to have huge eyes.

At the two-month mark, babies display a few additional eye movements, although these movements are still limited. At this age, children generally start to realize what their parents' faces look like and may be able to distinguish them from other faces. This is the first indication of visual memory. Some authorities believe that babies are "programmed" to recognize faces better than other kinds of visual patterns. In terms of evolution and infant survival, this makes good sense.

At three months of age, babies are able to follow a dangling object from one end of their visual gaze to the other, although their eye movements may be unsteady. If they hold a rattle, they may look at it occasionally. At this stage, babies prefer using the mouth over the eyes for investigational purposes. Since any kind of investigation that babies do is important to their developing vision, be sure to keep plenty of clean, harmless toys close by. Gross motor development at this point usually consists of lifting the head and chest when lying prone, as well as kicking the legs in random movements.

Babies stop occasionally to visually inspect things, such as their hands or a toy, when they reach the four-month stage. Their head movements are more pronounced and should be more independent of their eye movements. This is the early stage of oculomotor development.

At five months old, babies may try to keep an object in sight as it is brought to their mouth. However, they lose their fixation easily and can be distracted. Also, at this age babies can most likely differentiate between their mother's face and a stranger's face.

Around six months of age, babies are able to follow an object for a few seconds, although they might lose it to follow another object. Their eye movements are more fluid now, and any interest in an object across the room should be encouraged to help them learn about size and distance. Six-month-old children need plenty of room to crawl and explore. Their gross motor development is much more apparent as their repertoire of movements expands. They generally roll around and attempt to lift themselves upright. As their fine motor development also progresses, they may attempt to manipulate toys, and their hands become more independent. Their movements are beginning to integrate all the parts of their body, and therefore they match their sense of sight with other kinds of perception, such as touch and hearing.

At seven months old, babies have much-improved eye movements—specifically, *convergence*. In other words, they are now able to coordinate their eyes to inspect a toy at a close range, although they may momentarily lose this fixation and then regain it. Their hand-eye coordination begins to become refined as they feel more comfortable with fine motor movements, such as lifting a toy to inspect it. Their large muscles allow them to sit up and start creeping.

Babies begin to manipulate objects with more sophistication by the time that they are eight months old, turning the objects about in their hands to explore them visually. They might hold one toy while manipulating another. At this age, babies become more aware of the space outside their reach and will watch other people across the room. They should be well into crawling now.

Actually, during the second six months of life, in general, infants need plenty of crawling opportunities. Crawling is an important stage of development that allows children to fully integrate all of their major muscle groups with their perceptual abilities—at ground level. Unfortunately, many parents are too anxious for their little Johnny or Mary to walk and therefore try to hurry their child through the crawling stage. Don't rush your child. I've seen many learning-disabled children with behavior problems who walked at an early age without the benefit of crawling.

At the ten-month mark, babies are able to more easily move their heads and trunks. Vertical surfaces become intriguing as they prepare to stand. Their eye muscles and large muscles work together in this process. Children now start to see the "whole" of objects, which is a rudimentary form of perception.

Finally, at twelve months, babies usually have mastered their vertical orientation. Walking with assistance and temporarily standing alone indicate that gross motor development is proceeding on schedule. Visually, eye movements are more refined, and children may at times display unusual facial expressions as part of this process. Smooth, easy visual pursuit of objects and increased mobility of the eyes become apparent. Eye movements should be more independent and not necessarily associated with head movements.

Preschoolers

Between the ages of two and five years old, children make great strides toward adult visual capabilities. Their vision, as well as their bodies and brains, get ready for the challenges of school and formal learning, including reading and writing. The guidelines

---

A CHILD'S-EYE VIEW

Let's say that right now you are sitting on a chair at a desk, reading. You are well aware of the distance from yourself to the desk, from the desk to the wall, and from the room to the rest of the house. If you shift your attention from this book to the refrigerator in your kitchen, you remain aware of the book's location so that you can return to it after eating instead of spending ten minutes looking for it around the house.

Now think of how preschool-aged children relate to these things. Each time they shift their attention from one object to another, they forget where the original object is. It's not just poor memory; it's actually an inability to relate to spatial locations in their visual world until the age of about five or six years. If, for some reason, children are a little late at comprehending these spatial relationships and can't keep them straight in their heads, they can't progress in their development. Every new experience builds on the previous ones, and if a previous problem isn't conquered, a tool is missing for tackling the next.

What does all of this have to do with children's vision and achievement? Just this: If children have a perceptual lag that persists into the school years, they may have trouble with arithmetic and spelling. They won't understand that "two plus two equals four," because that is a relationship among three different objects. They may have trouble remembering that the letters "g" and "o" spell "go," because these letters do this only if they are arranged in a particular order. A child who can't tell left from right (a spatial relationship) might come out with "og." This may be the basis of the reversals commonly seen in poor achievers and children with learning disabilities. Moreover, adults may find these problems difficult to understand unless they have experienced such problems themselves.

It's important to be aware of perception from a child's point of view. If you are, it will be easier to find ways to help your child catch on to what should be accomplished. This can easily be achieved by giving your child rich experiences with shapes, movements, and distances, and by scheduling regular eye examinations starting at the age of one year (earlier, if you suspect a problem). Once you address any ocular development concerns, you can spend more time on the fun stuff, like hugs and kisses.

presented here will help you to evaluate your preschooler's visual development. But again, the information provides a rough guide, so don't hold your child to these milestones too closely. However, if your child's abilities deviate considerably from the norm, contact your pediatrician or developmental optometrist. Most problems are easier to correct before children enter school; once the child is in school, one problem can lead to another in a domino effect. See "A Child's-Eye View" on page 30, for more on how preschoolers' developmental problems in vision can severely affect school performance several years down the road.

At two years old, children generally have good footing—good enough to be able to run without falling (well, at least some of the time). They use their eyes more responsively, watching what they do as they do it. The eyes and hands are less closely associated now than they were earlier, so children usually look and then act, instead of doing both simultaneously. Whirling disks and brightly colored objects are quite a source of fascination at this age. Small objects might be studied with more intensity than before, which is a sure sign of increased visual discrimination. The attention span is about seven minutes.

At three years of age, children are definitely more organized in their actions than they were at two. Their hand-eye activities are more unified. Thus, they will color within the lines of pictures, and they can use their hands more freely without having their eyes riveted to them. Their eyes may take a more directive role, often not accompanied by head movements anymore, leading where they had previously been following. An increase in space orientation is evident; children know

where they are and know more about where other objects are in relation to themselves. *Eye teaming,* in which the two eyes function as one unit, continues to develop. To test one aspect of your child's ability to use both eyes together, see the inset titled "Eye Teaming Test" on page 32. (Actually, it is very similar to the Cover Test provided in the previous section of Part One.) The attention span is about nine minutes now.

Children experience a definite leap in motor development at the age of four. Enjoying bursts of racing, hopping, jumping, skipping, and climbing, they seem to be saying, "Look out, world, here I come!" Motor patterns show a tendency for symmetry, with children using both hands and also being able to recognize two halves as a whole picture. Eye teaming becomes more obvious. There is now a loose organization of the visual system that allows children's eyes to work together and to accommodate (adapt) better. At this stage, the attention span is about twelve to fifteen minutes.

Children reach a new maturity in terms of coordination when they reach about five years of age. They enjoy a greater ease and control of general body activity. Their movements are more refined, and so is their hand-eye coordination. Children move with more deliberation and finer synchronization. Their eyes can fix on things more easily, and their mechanical ability to focus is developed to the point at which focusing is more accurate. The attention span should be up to thirty minutes now.

School-Aged Children

School and vision—the two are practically synonymous. School is for learning, and at least 80 percent of learning is mediated by vision. All the skills and abilities that children develop during the preschool years come into play during the school years. And there is not a more demanding test of visual abilities than school.

Unfortunately, 25 percent of students in kindergarten through sixth grade have visual problems that are serious enough to impede learning. Visual handicaps include not only seeing a blur when looking at a blackboard, but also poor oculomotor coordination, strabismus (crossed eyes or wall eyes), lazy eye, focusing insufficiency, perceptual problems, and developmental lags. The following is a list of a few of the visual skills children need in school:

• Near vision—the ability to see things that are 12 to 16 inches away (in other words, at reading distance) clearly with both eyes.

• Distance vision—the ability to see things that are at least 20 feet away with sharpness and very little effort.

• Accommodation—the ability of the eyes to adjust for near-point (or hand-held) tasks easily—that is, with no effort. This process must be done with comfort and must be maintained for long periods of time.

• Focusing flexibility—the ability to alternate between distance and near vision quickly and effortlessly.

• Binocular coordination—the ability of both eyes to work together as a team using either distance or near vision. Tiring, double vision, poor reading ability, and headache are a few signs of inadequate binocular coordination.

EYE TEAMING TEST

As soon as your child is able to focus on objects for several seconds at a time (usually at about three years of age), you can try this test to see if she can use both eyes together properly.

1. Have your child look at one particular object that will hold her attention. A good choice is a finger puppet with a small flashlight inserted inside.

2. While making sure your child stays focused on the object and not on your hand, cover one of her eyes and closely observe the uncovered one. Did the uncovered eye move when the cover was put in place?

3. Repeat this step a few times to confirm the results. If your child has both eyes focused on the object to begin with, refocusing when one eye is covered should be unnecessary. In other words, your child shouldn't display any movement of the uncovered eye.

4. Remove the cover and let the child focus on the object with both eyes again.

5. Repeat steps 2 and 3 with the other eye.

This test evaluates your child's ability to use both eyes together properly. It is the same as the "Cover/Uncover" test described in Chapter 1 (see page 17) except that it is taken by your child rather than by you. If you saw any movement of the uncovered eye when the cover was put into position, consult your eye doctor. At this early age, any binocular dysfunction is much easier to rectify.

• Adequate field of vision (or peripheral vision)—the ability to see up, down, left, and right while focusing on one spot. This saves unnecessary head and eye movements and is crucial for reading.

These are only some of the visual abilities that are needed for good performance in school. Please keep in mind that a vision "screening" done in school does *not* substitute for a complete eye examination. Most schools do just the standard eye-chart test that is required by state law in many locations.

Vision problems can develop at any age, but there do seem to be certain times during a child's school career when those problems are more likely to occur. Second grade, fourth grade, seventh grade, and ninth grade are key years to pay special attention to your child's vision development.

In second grade, there is often a sudden increase in nearsightedness among students. That is understandable, since second grade is the time when heavy emphasis is placed on the final stages of learning to read. In addition, the demand for close work is greatly increased over the previous school years.

When they reach fourth grade, instead of learning to read, children begin reading to learn. This means that a possibly un-mastered skill must now be used to investigate new areas of knowledge. Imagine if you had just begun to learn French and then suddenly had to study nuclear physics in the new language. The result of this kind of stress, and of the even more intense close work, is often nearsightedness. Sometimes a child will just quit trying and become an "underachiever."

In seventh grade, children are in the heart of middle school. The physical growth spurt that they experience, combined with the tremendously increased demand for near-point work, is a recipe for nearsightedness. And speaking of recipes, the foods that are consumed at this age can actually contribute to the development of nearsightedness. Refer to the section on myopia for more details about this concern.

As ninth grade progresses, the reading assignments pile up and the pressures to achieve increase. Teenagers may adapt to the stress by developing nearsightedness (if they haven't done so already). If vision problems go uncorrected, teenagers may give up on schoolwork and show declining achievement.

All of these periods of high stress require a good vision examination, which should be done every year anyway. So, when September rolls around and you buy new clothes and school supplies for your child and make appointments for medical examinations and dental checkups, don't forget about the one school supply that needs to be in the best working order—your child's vision. In fact, it is a great idea to make a complete vision examination a part of your child's back-to-school routine. In addition, if at any time your child has vision problems or is in the lower third of the class in terms of grades, take your child to the eye doctor for another complete vision examination. For a list of signs and symptoms of vision trouble, see "Know Your ABC's," on page 34. And again, please remember that school vision screenings are *not* a substitute for a complete visual examination.

We have now traced visual development through the early years. Moreover, we have confirmed how important it is to detect and

KNOW YOUR ABC'S

Here are the ABC's of signs and symptoms that may signal vision trouble during the school years. Make it a point to observe whether or not your child suffers from any of these markers. Also, directly ask your child if she is having any vision difficulties.

A. APPEARANCE OF EYES

- crossed eyes or eyes pointing out (wall eyes), up, or down
- red eyes
- watery eyes
- encrusted lids
- frequent styes

B. BEHAVIOR

- squinting or closing one eye
- rigid body posture
- avoidance of close work
- rocking back and forth
- head-turning

- excessive head movement
- sitting too close to the work
- using a finger to read
- blinking much and with effort
- rubbing the eyes during or after short periods of reading

C. COMPLAINTS

- blurred vision
- headaches
- nausea or dizziness
- burning or itching eyes
- double vision
- tiring quickly while reading

If your child has any of these signs or symptoms, contact her eye doctor for a complete eye examination. Through testing and questioning, the doctor will be able to trace the problems to their source and hopefully correct the issues so that your child no longer struggles.

---

diagnose any vision problems as early in life as possible. By now, you are well aware that there are many vision problems that can arise. Often, by the time a child's distance vision starts to decline enough to show up with the Snellen test, the problem is well on its way to becoming a permanent handicap. Distance vision is usually the *last* thing to go wrong. The next section will offer an in-depth look at more specific vision and learning problems that warrant detailed discussion.

SPECIFIC DISORDERS AND THEIR RELATIONSHIPS TO VISION

There are a number of vision problems, as well as conditions that affect vision, that tend to occur in children. Among them are dyslexia and attention deficit/hyperactive disorder (ADHD). These problems can severely and negatively affect a child's experience in school. It is important to understand what these disorders are and how they can be managed.

Dyslexia

The term *dyslexia* (dis-LEX-ee-ah) was coined years ago to describe a set of symptoms relating to the inability of some people to read and understand written language despite normal intelligence and educational opportunities. In the United States, researchers estimate the prevalence of dyslexia to range from 5 to 9 percent of school-aged children, though some have put the figure as high as 17 percent. There are several subtypes of the condition, usually relating to the cause of the problem.

Many individuals with dyslexic symptoms involving reading, writing, and spelling also exhibit symptoms in other domains, such as poor short-term memory skills, poor personal organizational skills, and problems processing spoken language. Most often, the symptoms manifest in *reversals:* "was" is "saw"; "b" is "d"; "eye" is "eye" (ha, fooled ya!). While reversals and other reading difficulties are common with dyslexia, they do not define the condition. And while most often dyslexia is acquired and incurable, it can be dealt with successfully. Many individuals with this condition go on to achieve success in their lives.

Early research in dyslexia looked for a single factor to explain the disorder. Some experts thought the problem had to do with visual acuity or binocular coordination, while others felt it was related to anything from an inner-ear condition to psychological difficulties, faulty educational methods, or brain damage. As with most complex problems, it is now apparent that there is no simple answer to the puzzle of dyslexia. There are probably different causes for the symptoms in different children, although researchers have now uncovered some pretty hard evidence that certain areas of the brain develop more slowly in dyslexic children than they do in non-dyslexic children.

Researchers continue to investigate the role of the visual system in dyslexia. The visual system is almost certainly involved in some way with the problem, although exactly how it is involved is not clear. Dyslexic children usually have good visual acuity, although they seem to have difficulty focusing their eyes. Interestingly, children with severe strabismus (crossed eyes or wall eyes) usually do not have difficulty reading because they manage to suppress the image from the severely affected eye and read with the good eye. Children with mild strabismus, on the other hand, may *seem* to be dyslexic because they struggle to fuse the two different images from their two eyes. This is not true dyslexia, but rather a binocular vision problem that may mimic dyslexic symptoms.

In the 1980s, psychologist Helen Irlen found another problem related to dyslexia. Her findings suggest that at least some dyslexics are extremely sensitive to light. She named this disorder *scotopic sensitivity syndrome (SSS)*. To assist persons with SSS, Irlen developed a treatment using special light-filtering lenses, now called *Irlen lenses*. While not widely accepted in the eyecare community, Irlen's theory is an interesting concept that is discussed more fully in the inset titled "Light Sensitivity and Irlen Lenses" on page 36.

Again, while there is no cure for dyslexia, dyslexic individuals can learn to read and write with appropriate education or treatment. Some research evidence indicates that specialized phonics instruction can help remediate

LIGHT SENSITIVITY AND IRLEN LENSES

In the 1980s, psychologist Helen Irlen, PhD, developed a theory that at least some dyslexic people have an unusual sensitivity to light that interferes with their reading ability. According to Dr. Irlen's theory, these people use their night vision all the time, which creates some visual distortion when they try to read black letters on a white background. Irlen named this problem *scotopic sensitivity syndrome* (SSS). Like dyslexia, SSS can be broadly categorized as a reading disorder.

In an effort to find a way to help people with SSS, Irlen experimented with colored light-filtering lenses to use while reading. These lenses are now called *Irlen lenses.* The approach used by the Irlen Institute is to first give the patient a complete vision examination to rule out any refractive problem—that is, to make sure the patient can see clearly. Next, an evaluation determines the exact visual distortions experienced relating to light sensitivity, visual resolution (blurring), span of focus, and sustained focus during the reading process. Lastly, lenses are designed to minimize or eliminate the distortions using the appropriate tint from among 150 different color possibilities.

Dr. Irlen's process has created some controversy in the medical community. A few studies have looked at the concept and methods of Irlen lenses, and most have concluded that there is no consistent evidence that Irlen therapy improves reading comprehension in dyslexic persons. It is likely that a motivational or placebo effect is present in some studies that support Irlen therapy. There are probably underlying vision problems that are responsible for the symptoms experienced by candidates for Irlen filters.

That being said, some research has suggested the blue filter lenses do improve reading skills, although these results do not confirm the Irlen philosophy. Clinical research has confirmed that blue filters have a significantly positive impact on reading comprehension in reading-disabled children but not in normal readers. The study was conducted with children in fourth, fifth, and sixth grades. One result showed that 87 percent of the reading disabled children showed an improvement in comprehension when using the blue filter. In fact, their improvement averaged 45 percent!

While the above-discussed study was limited to blue filters, it might lend some rationale to the work done by Dr. Irlen and suggests a visual-processing component to the SSS condition. Some doctors also use the therapeutic technique of syntonics (color therapy) to treat these types of reading problems. For a complete discussion of syntonics, see page 383.

For more information on the Irlen method and lenses, see *Reading by the Colors: Overcoming Dyslexia and Other Reading Disabilities Through the Irlen Method* by Helen Irlen, or write to the Irlen Institute. The current address and phone number of the Irlen Institute are given in the Resource Organizations section of this book. (See page 413.)

the reading deficits. The fundamental aim is to make children aware of the relationships between what they see on the page and the sound of the language, and to relate these to reading and spelling. It has been found that training which is focused towards both visual language and oral expression yields longer-lasting gains than mere oral training. The key in this context is to realize that the symptoms of dyslexia are often similar to the symptoms of a visual disorder, so ruling out the visual component is critical to avoid a life-long label that may not be appropriate for the child.

Attention Deficit/Hyperactivity Disorder (ADHD)

Many underachieving children actually have *attention deficit/hyperactive disorder (ADHD)*. This is a medical term that describes children who are chronically inattentive, impulsive, and hyperactive. Such children often have problems both at home and at school. As they grow up, they are more likely to drop out of high school and experience patterns of anti-social behavior. Because ADHD has become a buzzword in learning today, vision problems are often masked and labeled as ADHD.

If children cannot pay visual attention to close work, they will look far away and possibly daydream or even try to stir up other children in the immediate area. Paying attention to near-point work requires a sophisticated visual system that must be controlled carefully and for long periods of time. The most common symptoms of ADHD are distractibility, difficulty with concentration, and inability to "focus." But that sounds like a possible *vision*

problem to me! Ultimately, many children with vision problems that cause distractibility are being misdiagnosed with ADHD.

For years, the standard prescription treatment for ADHD has been Ritalin (methylphenidate), which is a stimulant. It does not cure ADHD but can improve attention, reduce restlessness, and foster better relations with peers, parents, and teachers. There are, however, a number of possible side effects of Ritalin, including allergies, eczema, asthma, stomachaches, ear infections, dry skin, agitation/irritability, insomnia, dry mouth, headache, nausea, and weight loss. Other possible side effects are reduced stature, ticks, "zombie" demeanor, and moodiness.

Recent research shows that nutrition can strongly affect ADHD as well; improper nutrition is believed to exacerbate ADHD. It has now been well established that artificial food dyes and flavors are responsible for much hyperactivity in children. In addition, it is almost certain that the same substances will cause other disabilities. Food dyes and colorings, convenience foods, food additives of all kinds, and all artificial flavors should be prime suspects when a child has learning and/or behavioral disabilities. Studies have demonstrated a number of cases in which hyperactivity is completely absent when the diet strictly avoids all such additives. In such studies, the disorder reappears within twenty-four to forty-eight hours if just a tiny amount of food color or flavoring is ingested. Eliminating these substances should be the first act in a program of biological rehabilitation for learning-disabled children.

Most ADHD children do not have good habits of eating. They eat a poor diet, they chew poorly, they eat too quickly, and they don't pause for digestion. Typically, they do not eat healthy foods but will gobble down sweet, highly processed foods. It is important that parents not stop working on the problem if Ritalin, Dexedrine, or other energizers relieve the children's symptoms. All such children should be tested for allergies, should have sugar taken as thoroughly out of their lives as possible, and should be evaluated for thyroid imbalance. As they reach adolescence, their fat and insulin metabolism should be evaluated. Moreover, their urine should be tested at least twice per year, particularly after loading the night before with a rich meal that was high in sweets. If sugar or acetone is found in the urine, a physician should order a study of blood glucose and insulin.

Omega-3 fatty acids, zinc, and magnesium may have benefits with regard to ADHD symptoms. Many children have difficulty getting enough omega-3 essential fatty acids; the omega-6 fatty acids are more readily available in the American diet. Since as early as 1981, researchers have found a correlation between children with ADHD and a reduced nutritional status of essential fatty acids. While all children with ADHD are not deficient in omega-3 fatty acids, it is likely an important factor for at least a portion of these children. Thus, it is a good idea to carefully examine the diet of any child diagnosed with ADHD to see if any of the food issues discussed here might be contributory to the disorder.

But let's return to the connection with vision. Because vision and learning are intimately connected, a vision problem can be easily mistaken for a learning problem. Children who have learning-related visual problems often cannot sustain their close work at school. They may be misdiagnosed as having ADHD because children with ADHD also can't sustain attention on their work. Same behaviors, different diagnoses.

A study released at the University of California San Diego's (UCSD's) Shiley Eye Center showed that ophthalmologists and researchers have uncovered a relationship between ADHD and a vision imbalance characterized by an inability to focus on a target. In looking at the ADHD population, they found that almost 16 percent of all children analyzed were diagnosed with *convergence insufficiency*, a vision imbalance. (See page 195 for details on this disorder.) Psychiatrists and pediatricians need to become aware of the connection between vision and attention so that those experts dealing with ADHD can refer to the appropriate doctors instead of just medicating children with stimulants.

If you suspect that your child may have dyslexia, ADHD, or any other type of learning problem, it's best to get a thorough vision examination *first*, to rule out a visual problem that may mimic a learning disability. It is also important to have educational and perceptual testing done, including an assessment of the child's visual-motor development. Contact your pediatrician or school nurse for referrals to appropriate specialists. Also, many optometrists who specialize in vision development can also perform appropriate tests to rule out any visual components that may be contributing to a learning disability. To find an optometrist, contact the College of Optometrists in Vision Development (COVD) or the Optometric Extension Program (OEP). For contact information, see page 415 of Resource Organizations.

Of course, a nutrition profile is a key investigative tool as well. It's important to remember that just giving a child some extra vitamins will not reverse the negative effects of a poor diet. Of course, balancing out a child's nutritional intake will be beneficial, but it will not automatically increase her scores in school testing. On the other hand, it will increase her mental and visual abilities so that she can produce better results as she continues to learn.

Autism

Autism spectrum disorder is a condition related to brain development that impacts how a person perceives and socializes with others, causing problems in social interaction and communication. Autism spectrum disorder begins in early childhood and eventually causes problems functioning in society— socially, in school and at work, for example. Often children show symptoms of autism within their first year.

One reason that this discussion is included here is that the most significant early signs of autism are reduced eye contact and a lack of response to being called or an indifference to caregivers. Other children may develop normally for the first few months or years of life but then suddenly become withdrawn or aggressive or lose language skills they've already acquired. Signs usually are seen by age two.

Some children with autism spectrum disorder have difficulty learning, and some have signs of lower than normal intelligence. Other children with the disorder have normal to high intelligence—they learn quickly yet have trouble communicating and applying what they know in everyday life and adjusting to social situations.

A child or adult with autism spectrum disorder may have problems with social interaction and communication skills, including any of these symptoms:

• Has poor eye contact and lacks facial expression

• Fails to respond to his or her name or appears not to hear you at times

• Resists cuddling and holding, and seems to prefer playing alone, retreating into his or her own world

• Doesn't express emotions or feelings and appears unaware of others' feelings

• Doesn't speak or has delayed speech, or loses previous ability to say words or sentences

• Can't start a conversation or keep one going, or only starts one to make requests or label items

• Repeats words or phrases verbatim, but doesn't understand how to use them

• Doesn't appear to understand simple questions or directions

• Doesn't point at or bring objects to share interest

• Speaks with an abnormal tone or rhythm and may use a singsong voice or robot-like speech

• Inappropriately approaches a social interaction by being passive, aggressive, or disruptive

• Has difficulty recognizing nonverbal cues, such as interpreting other people's facial expressions, body postures, or tone of voice

Many individuals with autism have problems with sensory integration that affect the visual system and other sensory-processing abilities. Vision therapy enhances the neurological connections between the eyes and brain to help people with autism better perceive what their eyes see and make better sense of their environments. Your pediatrician or pediatric optometrist should be able to counsel you on the possibility of your child having any of these symptoms. Again, a proper diet can help young children to manage these types of problems with more control. Thus, a consultation with a nutritionist should be among the first visits.

TECHNOLOGY AND YOUNG EYES

In the previous section, we discussed the internal environment—the brain and the body—and some of what affects it. Now let's turn to the external environment and learn about the effects of common technology on the eyes of children. It's no surprise to anyone that some children want to spend as much time watching television as they spend at school. Television has been a powerful influence on children (and adults) for several generations. And now computers have taken over as the technology-of-choice for most children. Since watching a television or computer screen involves intensive use of the eyes, many people have become concerned about the effects of extended viewing on the eyes.

Several studies have been done in this area, and some interesting conclusions have been reached. One study found that 30 percent of school-aged computer users were at risk for *computer vision syndrome*. This is a designation by the American Optometric Association for a complex of eye and vision problems that occur during or related to computer use. (See page 189 for a detailed explanation.) For now, here are answers to some of the most frequently asked questions about television, computers, and vision.

General Effects on Vision

How does watching television affect the eyes? And which is worse for the eyes—television or computers? Close concentration on and staring at the television screen at too close of a distance over an extended period of time may result in general fatigue, eyestrain, and tired eyes. As for comparing the two activities, the eyes suffer less focus strain from viewing television than they do from performing close work such as reading or operating a computer. However, while television requires less visual concentration than do computers, too much of either can be stressful on the eyes.

Risk of Radiation

Do televisions and computers emit radiation? Some radiation is emitted by television sets. At this time, however, it does not seem to pose a health hazard, although many experts still think you should not sit too close to the screen. Stick with the distance recommended—four times the diagonal dimension of the screen—for safety as well as comfort.

No studies to date have shown any negative radiation effects from sitting in front of a computer. So someone sitting a reasonable distance (arm's length) from a monitor should have no fear of radiation exposure. And the newer flat-panel monitors emit almost no radiation to speak of, so this is a non-issue regarding the newer computers.

Proper Lighting in the Room

Can a room be too bright for comfortable television viewing or computer use? Yes. Excessively bright room lighting tends to reduce the contrast on the screen and to wash out the picture. Lamps and other lights should be positioned so that no glare or reflections will be seen on or near the screen.

What is the best way to adjust the lighting when watching television or working on a computer? It is better to first turn on the desired room lighting and then to adjust the brightness and contrast of the television picture or computer screen. Note that all computer screens have brightness and contrast controls, usually in the form of buttons on the front or side of the monitor.

Should television or computers be viewed in a totally darkened room? No! The contrast between the screen and the surrounding area is too great for comfortable and efficient vision. When the room is softly illuminated, this undesirable high contrast is kept to a minimum.

Proper Distance from the Screen

What's the best distance to sit from the screen? A television picture appears much sharper and more defined if viewed from a distance that is at least four times the diagonal dimension of the screen. For example, if you have a 19-inch screen, measured from the lower-left to the upper-right corner of the screen, you should sit at least 6 feet away from it. Nearsighted children are the ones most likely to persist in sitting 2 or 3 feet from the screen. This should be strongly discouraged. If you notice a child's tendency to sit up against the screen, that child needs to have an eye exam. There is really no such thing as sitting too far from the television.

Now with the new plasma and LCD televisions, things have changed a bit. The screen size is enormous compared to the "old days." The basics still apply, so don't purchase a screen that is too large for your room. And it's still prudent to keep the kids back from the TV for more comfortable viewing.

When working at a computer, a child should sit at least 20 inches or more from the screen (farther for adults). One easy way to determine this is to have the child sit back in her chair and then reach for the computer screen. If she can touch the screen, she is too close! This rule-of-thumb can also apply to adults who use computers on a moderate basis. Further recommendations will be discussed in the section on Computer Vision Syndrome in Part Two.

Proper Physical Placement/Posture During Screen Time

Does body posture affect viewing comfort? Yes. Watching television in a twisted or leaning position will cause one eye to work more than the other eye. This will lead to eyestrain because the vision is not balanced equally between the eyes. An erect, straight-ahead position is the best for television watching. But in the world of reality, sitting back on the couch is fine as long as your face is relatively parallel to the screen.

A computer screen, which is usually situated more closely to you than a television set, should be in a lowered position, enabling you to look straight ahead and see over its top. This is obviously more difficult to set up for children, who are usually much shorter when sitting in a chair. Special considerations for comfort should be addressed when children use computers.

Cell Phones

Cell phones have taken over as the "display of choice" for the younger generation. Children are viewing these displays more frequently and for longer periods of time without taking breaks at sensible intervals. Data from the DQ Institute's Child Online Safety Index reported that children in the eight- to twelve-year-old age bracket spend approximately thirty-two hours a week looking at screens. Further analysis showed that adolescents thirteen to nineteen years old spend more than forty-nine hours a week on their mobile devices. These numbers have skyrocketed since the 2020 pandemic.

Obviously, a display screen has many variables associated with its use. Several studies review some of the features that might influence the viewing distance of smartphones in people of different ages. In one study comparing under-forty-year-olds and presbyopic users, smartphone viewing distances were measured in two natural positions, sitting and standing. Results showed that the average viewing distance can vary significantly, and the same person can hold the smartphone at different distances while sitting or standing. Thus, it is imperative that an eye examination include inquiries regarding smartphone or tablet use.

Another study of young adults looked at viewing distance and visual discomfort while using handheld displays. The subjects were filmed as they viewed five different handheld displays and hardcopy in five different font sizes. The study also asked about visual discomfort via a questionnaire. The results showed that when reading hardcopy viewing distance decreased for smaller text sizes. When using handheld devices, viewing distance was even closer. Minor visual and body stresses were observed in only ten minutes of handheld use. This confirms that handheld devices tend to be viewed at a closer viewing distance than hardcopy of comparable size. This closer viewing distance could be the source of the visual and body stresses exhibited by the subjects.

We will further discuss cell phone display usage in the chapter on Computer Vision Syndrome in Part Two.

Proper Age for Use

What is the earliest age for a child to view a television or use a computer? For television, moderate viewing times are usually fine for any age, if the optimal viewing distance is maintained. But use your judgment and remember that televisions are not babysitters!

Have you noticed that parenting magazines often have ads for computer software designed for children as young as eighteen months old? But most experts suggest no computer use before the age of three. Regarding older children, forty-five to sixty minutes per day is the suggested amount of computer time for those under ten years of age. For those who are ten to thirteen years old, the suggestion is one to two hours per day, while for fourteen- to fifteen-year-olds, it's three hours per day. Just use common sense when it comes to young people who are sixteen and older. Be sure they include regular breaks and good general ergonomics during their computer use. And, by the way, computer games count as computer usage!

Clearly, television viewing and computer use are here to stay. Plus, many school districts are increasing their typing requirements so that students perform more and more of their work on computers. This can have a devastating effect on the visual performance of children and the visual stress that goes along with this highly intensive visual task. So children must be properly prepared and instructed concerning computer use. The jury is still out when it comes to the long-term effects of computer use on developing eyes. However, with a little common sense, a few facts, and pro-active eye exams, you and your child can learn to live with television and computers and make the most of the experiences. Junk-food commercials and pop-up ads aside, television and computers have much to offer children and are a big part of modern life. Since these venues are becoming unavoidable, the real issue is how to healthfully manage television and computer time.

MORE ON A PARENT'S ROLE IN GOOD VISION

If you've read this section thus far, you know that children's vision is an integral part of their whole development. Good vision goes hand-in-hand with the maturation of the large and small muscles and the brain. As discussed earlier, for some children, the development of vision is delayed or deficient, which usually means that the parents will need to seek help from an eyecare specialist, a pediatrician, and/or a school-associated professional. But for most children, vision, like the rest of the body, develops properly and on schedule. Even when vision does seem to be developing properly, there are things that you, as a parent, can do to ensure that it stays on track.

What to Look for When Your Child Reads and Writes

Vision problems can be subtle and develop very slowly. So even if your child seems to be doing well in school and is not sitting too close to the television at home, you still want to be observant—especially during your child's reading and writing times. To evaluate your child for vision problems that may affect these fundamental activities, look for the following signs while watching her write and listening to her read:

- poor reading comprehension
- frequent loss of place during reading
- short attention span for reading
- frequent omission of words
- re-reading or skipping lines unknowingly

- failure to recognize the same word in the next sentence

- confusing two or more words with the same or similar beginnings

- failure to visualize what is read

- writing uphill or downhill on paper

- repeated confusion over left-right directions

- poor orientation of drawings on the page

- quick loss of interest

You now have a list of "symptoms" when it comes to reading and writing problems. But it's also important to remember that children develop at their own paces. So if you suspect problems with reading, writing, and vision in your child, be sure to take her to an eyecare professional for a thorough vision examination. A professional assessment will ensure that she gets off to a good educational start.

What to Do at Your Child's Eye Examination

When you take your child for an eye examination, the doctor should be able to explain, *in a way that you can understand*, any visual difficulties that your child may have. If you don't understand something, don't hesitate to ask questions until the situation is clear to you. And be sure that you don't leave the exam without fully understanding the following aspects of your child's vision:

- Visual acuity—although 20/20 is only an arbitrary figure, it will still give you an idea of how close to "normal" your child's vision is.

- Refractive errors—you should understand your child's nearsightedness, farsightedness, or astigmatism, if any of these is present, and how the condition can be corrected.

- Eye health—the external and internal health of the eyes is a very basic and necessary finding, since the eyes must be healthy to see well.

- Eye-brain coordination—you should know about any special eye-brain coordination problems, such as strabismus and lazy eye, and the possible treatment plans.

- Focusing ability and flexibility—it should be determined whether or not your child can maintain her focus for near and for distance vision, and whether or not she can switch easily from near to far and back again.

- Binocular efficiency—it is extremely important to determine if your child can maintain binocular fixation on a certain point for a sustained period of time, as well as the quality of her depth perception. This is a critical area in children's vision.

- Color vision—if your child is a boy, his color vision should be tested, and particular color deficiencies, if any, should be determined.

- Perception and development—if your child is having some difficulty in school, a series of tests may be recommended to determine if the problems are due to perceptual difficulties or a developmental lag. Make sure you understand the purpose and results of each test. If vision therapy is prescribed, it, too, should be thoroughly explained to you.

In addition to understanding the different aspects of the examination, make sure you understand all of the instructions the doctor gives you if glasses or contact lenses are prescribed. If glasses are prescribed, be sure you and your child know exactly for which activities to wear the glasses and how to care for them. If contacts are prescribed, be sure you and your child know how to insert them, remove them, and take care of them.

How to Further Encourage Healthy Vision in Your Child

Can you pro-actively work with your child to maintain her good vision? Absolutely, you can. If you have a young child, try some of the following activities for good fun and good vision.

To Enhance Coordination

Coordination is the ability to move your body in a controlled manner. Remember that good body coordination translates into eye-muscle coordination. To assist your child's development of coordination, do the following:

• Let your child crawl around, over, and under furniture. (Watch for sharp corners.)

• Play "Mother, May I?" with your child. Use running, hopping, crawling, and jumping skills in the game.

• Ask your child to walk backwards or sideways when you go for walks together.

• Have your child hop first on one foot for ten seconds, and then on the other foot for ten seconds. Then have her hop on both feet or run in place to music while you count to ten.

• Have your child jump forward or backward over a line or a crack in the sidewalk.

• Have your child run on tiptoes, and then stand on tiptoes, for ten seconds.

• Play "Simon Says" with your child. Use directions that include the terms "right" and "left." In fact, encourage any activity that requires and reinforces the concept of "left and right."

• Practice naming parts of the body while touching them.

• Bounce a ball to your child and have your child catch it. Then tell her to bounce the ball back.

• Have your child hop forward on the right foot, and then walk the left foot up to the right.

• If you have a 2-by-4-inch balance beam available, have your child walk along it with arms outstretched or clasped behind the body. Also, have your child try different techniques and games on the beam, including walking back and forth with the eyes closed. (Do not allow your child to do these things without a spotter.)

To Enhance Visual-Motor Control

Visual-motor control is the ability to control the movements of the small-muscle groups in conjunction with the eye muscles. To assist your child's development of visual-motor control, do the following:

• Have your child make pictures using scrap materials such as string, buttons, beads, and shells.

• Draw a line pattern on a piece of paper. Have your child trace the pattern with a finger.

• Have your child practice turning the pages of a book or magazine.

• Have your child string pieces of macaroni like beads.

• Fold a piece of paper into many parts. Open the paper up, and have your child draw along the crease lines.

• Help your child practice tying knots and bows in shoelaces and pieces of string.

• Put some cornmeal or sand on a tray. Have your child draw shapes and letters in it.

• Make dotted letters. Have your child trace over them with a pencil, pen, or crayon.

• Have your child color in the "O's" in a newspaper article. (Watch her body posture—not too close, now!)

To Enhance Visual Perception

Visual perception is the ability to perceive such things as colors, shapes, sizes, letter forms, and words. To assist your child's development of visual perception, do the following:

• Place some objects on the floor. Have your child arrange them according to size or color.

• Play "smaller-larger." For example, ask your child to "find something smaller than your head, but larger than your hand."

• Talk about colors.

• Have your child separate teaspoons and tablespoons into two stacks.

• Have your child measure the sizes of things such as furniture, paper, and rooms.

• Have your child take a piece of string and find five things longer and five things shorter than it.

• Draw arrows in different directions on one index card, and one arrow on a second index card. Hold the second card so that the single arrow faces in different directions, and have your child match the arrow to the correct arrow on the first index card.

To Enhance Visual Memory

Visual memory is the ability to reproduce letters and other objects and images from memory. To assist your child's development of visual memory, do the following:

• Have your child circle all the words in a newspaper article that begin with a certain letter.

• Play "What's Missing?" For example, set out a few articles of clothing, and have your child look at them. Then have the child close her eyes while you remove one article. Next, ask her to open her eyes and tell you which article is missing.

• Touch several objects on a table. Have your child try to touch the same objects in the same order.

• Arrange three different shapes in a certain sequence. Then mix them up, and instruct your child to rearrange the objects so that the original sequence is restored.

• Open a storybook to a certain page. Let your child look at the page for a moment, then close the book and have your child find the page again.

• Write three numbers, then quickly cover them. Have your child write the numbers from memory.

To Enhance Reading and Writing Abilities

Has your child already begun to read and write? If so, here are some activities that will encourage the continued development of her abilities.

• Correct the mistakes your child makes when reading to you—but first have her continue reading to the end of the sentence or paragraph in order to avoid loss of concentration.

• When your child reads a page, ask her questions about it.

• Have your child look for words on a page that start or end with a certain letter.

• Have your child look at a picture in a storybook and then guess what the story is about before reading it.

• Encourage your child to write stories.

• Let your child see you reading often. Imitation is a strong teacher.

The various games and exercises that have been suggested prove that supporting your child's vision can be fun and easy. Most children would love to take part in these activities. They won't even know they're doing something healthy and constructive!

Being a conscientious parent is important to the healthy development of vision in your child. However, do not feel overwhelmed by the suggestions and instructions offered in this chapter. Simply by reading the information provided, you have taken wonderful steps toward helping your child make the most of her visual contact with the world around her. And, most likely, you will naturally accomplish the recommendations made in this section of the book as you become more comfortable with assessing your child's vision and talking with eyecare professionals.

CONCLUSION

After reading this chapter, you should have a solid understanding of the development of vision during the early years. And, hopefully, you are convinced of the importance of annual eye exams. As stated, most children's vision develops on schedule and with few problems. But for some children it does not. When a child has vision problems, it falls to the child's parents and teachers to pick up the clues that vision or visual-motor skills may be lacking, and to get the child the help that she needs. Of course, different children develop at different rates, and what looks like a major problem could simply be a delay. But only an eyecare specialist can provide you with the answers that are right for your child. While we're on the subject, the next chapter will familiarize you with the various types of eyecare professionals and the tasks they accomplish.

Your Eye Exam

Okay, it's time for your eye examination. But how do you find an eye doctor? Which type of eye doctor should you see? Are there really different types of eye doctors? How do you know you are making the right choice? And once you decide on a practitioner, what should you ask him? What will he ask you?

There seems to be an endless series of questions surrounding eye doctors and their services. Let's consider the different types of eyecare professionals and see if we can figure out who does what and which one is appropriate for you. Then we'll review what you can expect to happen at a routine eye exam.

THE THREE O'S

There are three general kinds of professionals involved with the care of the eyes. Thus, it may not come as a surprise to you that there is some confusion on the part of the general public over what each one does. What are the differences between an ophthalmologist, an optometrist, and an optician? Time and again, studies show that most people don't know the differences, and so it's likely the majority never will. But in this section, we can explore the responsibilities

of each of these practitioners, ultimately defining their roles in simple and straightforward terms. Therefore, when it comes to your eye examinations, you will at least be an educated patient.

Ophthalmologists

An *ophthalmologist* (of-thal-MAHL-oh-jist) is a medical doctor (MD) who specializes in eye health and eye diseases. After graduating from college and medical school, an ophthalmologist spends three more years learning about the diseases and surgeries of the eye. All ophthalmologists are surgeons. In order to become what is known as a board-certified ophthalmologist, the MD must pass a written, oral, and practical certifying examination in the specialty of ophthalmology.

Clearly, an ophthalmologist has a lot of training. However, that doesn't mean an ophthalmologist is the correct professional for every eye problem. Ophthalmologists are the people to see when you have a serious eye injury or an eye disease requiring surgery. Most ophthalmologists also prescribe glasses or contact lenses for healthy eyes, but many refer all or part of this work to someone else. For example, in a recent survey of about 600 ophthalmologists, 75 percent indicated that someone in their practice fitted contact lenses, but only 40 percent said that they did fittings themselves.

Ophthalmologists sometimes specialize within the specialty of ophthalmology. Some are retinal specialists, while others specialize in the problems of the cornea or the lens. Some are pediatric ophthalmologists, specializing in children's eye problems. And some confine themselves to surgery or even specific kinds of surgery, such as cataract surgery. There are also refractive surgeons, who perform only prescription-changing procedures. You should choose a specialist according to your specific needs and reliable recommendations.

Optometrists

An *optometrist* (op-TAHM-e-trist) is a doctor of optometry (OD). Optometrists complete pre-professional undergraduate education at a college or university, and then four years of professional education at a college of optometry. Most optometrists also complete residencies, so that makes it a five-year program. There is a national board examination for licensing in optometry, and most states accept passage of this examination along with passage of an additional practical or oral examination given by the particular state.

Optometrists are further defined as healthcare professionals trained and state licensed to provide primary eyecare services. These services include performing comprehensive eye-health and vision examinations; diagnosing and treating eye diseases and vision disorders; detecting general health problems; prescribing glasses, contact lenses, low-vision rehabilitation, vision therapy, and medication; performing certain limited surgical procedures; and counseling patients regarding their surgical alternatives and vision needs as related to their occupations, avocations, and lifestyles. Over 70 percent of the eye exams in the country are performed by optometrists.

It is true that optometrists also have their areas of specialization. Some of these are contact lenses, low-vision treatment, vision therapy, and occupational vision. There is a board certification for optometrists, which is not "specialty specific." Board certification is a voluntary credential that goes above and beyond licensing requirements for practicing optometry. However, there are well-qualified optometrists who are not board certified.

Some optometrists choose to work for commercial organizations, such as Walmart or Costco. They are most often self-employed and must maintain legitimate licensing requirements. There is rarely a requirement that they have a quota to write a certain number of prescriptions in a given amount of time. However, in some cases their ability to follow up with unusual or complicated conditions is hindered by their lack of equipment or training.

Opticians

An *optician* (op-TISH-an) is a technician trained to fill lens prescriptions written by optometrists and ophthalmologists. Opticians generally have an associate college degree, which is normally awarded for completing a two-year undergraduate program. Most states license opticians and require continuing education.

There is also an American Board of Opticianry, which certifies opticians. However, not all states accept this certification as qualifying an optician to practice. At this time, the requirements vary a great deal from state to state.

More specifically, opticians are trained to make glasses, fit eyeglass lenses into frames, and adjust eyeglass frames to people's faces. In some states, they are also allowed to do fittings of contact lenses. Some opticians work for store chains, while others maintain their own businesses.

Hopefully, this discussion has clearly defined the services of various eyecare professionals. Do you now know which type of practitioner you would like to see, or are you still a little confused over which one you should make an appointment with? If you need a little more guidance, read on.

THE CORRECT PROFESSIONAL FOR YOUR NEEDS

Let's assume you have an eye problem and decide you need some professional help. Whom do you see? Well, there are no hard-and-fast rules to help you make the decision of which eyecare specialist to see because, if you are like most people, you are unsure of exactly what your problem is and what treatment it requires. I can, however, make a few generalizations that should at least facilitate your decision.

Selecting the Type of Eyecare Professional

It is probably most helpful for me to give you a few examples of common eye concerns and then recommend a type of eyecare professional for each of those particular needs. Perhaps you will fit into one of these categories. If so, your decision will become a lot easier to make.

If you are having trouble seeing clearly, either at a distance or up close, or if you suffer from eyestrain, you probably need the services of an optometrist. If you have a family history of glaucoma and have been noticing some halos around lights at night, an optometrist who treats eye diseases is the correct choice. If your child is having difficulty reading in school or is a "problem" student, then a developmental/behavioral optometrist is appropriate. If all you want to do is trade in your glasses for contact lenses or update your contact lens prescription, an optometrist who fits contacts is your answer.

Now how about for more serious health conditions? If you believe you might have a condition that could require surgery, then start with an ophthalmologist for an opinion. And for less serious needs? If you had an eye exam recently and simply broke your glasses and need them repaired, visit an optician. I hope this simplifies the decision-making process.

From the above information, it seems that optometrists have the biggest range of services, right? You might be reading this and saying, "Well, the author is an optometrist, so of course he'll say that they do everything!" Yes and no. I am an optometrist, and we do have an expanded range of services to offer the public, but we don't do it all. It is acknowledged, though, that the optometrist is the "general practitioner" of eye care who can determine if a problem needs further attention from another specialist. And since optometrists are licensed to treat eye diseases and prescribe medications, this is now truer than ever.

Let me give you one more example. A patient of mine, whom I had treated previously, called the office and said he had "floaters," or dark spots in front of his eyes. He'd had them before, but this time he saw a large one over an entire segment of his vision. Without hesitation I sent him to a retinal specialist because it did not sound like a "traditional" floater complaint. Sure enough, he was seen immediately and was diagnosed with a retinal detachment. The detachment was repaired and his vision was saved. It's not often that we can diagnose correctly over the phone, but in this particular situation, the patient was fortunate and we did the right thing in time.

In many states, optometrists are capable of treating just about every eye disease; they refer to ophthalmologists for surgical intervention. If, for example, you visit an optometrist for a routine examination and a cataract is diagnosed, the optometrist may want to follow you for some time before recommending a surgical procedure. The optometrist may make nutritional recommendations or other environmental suggestions first, thus delaying surgery. However, if it is determined that surgery is the best route for you, an ophthalmologist will perform the procedure. Following the surgery, you should return to your optometrist for continued follow-up care. This is referred to as *co-management* and is the norm for dealing with specific eye conditions.

Selecting the Individual Doctor

Let's say that you've now decided which kind of professional you should see, but you still have to select the individual doctor. Since we are discussing an eye exam here, you will be choosing an ophthalmologist or an optometrist. How do you know whether you've found the right person? This is a tough one! There are as many different types of doctors as there are types of people.

In the selection process, you can always turn to reliable people whom you trust for recommendations. One of the best sources of good doctors is word of mouth. If you have a friend who wears glasses or contacts and has been with a capable doctor for several years, there's a good chance that this doctor will be good for you, too.

Of course, you can always start from scratch and consult the Internet for practitioners in your area. However, I don't advise browsing through the Internet for a doctor. It still amazes me how many people choose an eye doctor based simply on the size of the display ad or the cost of the examination. I often wonder if these people would shop around for a bargain-priced brain surgeon as well!

That being said, you *can* safely use the Internet in one way. Consider starting a search for an optometrist by contacting your local or county chapter of the Optometric Society. The society can help you find a reliable, licensed practitioner in your area. Most local optometric and medical societies have listings of the doctors according to the counties where they practice, and most of the societies have websites that can be accessed for a quick referral. You can do your own search, too; use key words such as "eye exam," "optometrist," and "ophthalmologist." There is usually a "near me" option to choose. Most doctors also have websites, so you can review particular doctors, their locations, and their qualifications right on their web pages.

When looking for a doctor, don't necessarily bypass an experienced practitioner for a young professional fresh out of school. Although recent graduates may possess the latest technical knowledge, there's something to be said for experience in any field. And some new doctors are so cautious that they may keep you in the chair for what seems like hours doing every test in the book instead of just the ones related to your problem.

Now allow me to play the devil's advocate. On the other hand, you should also be cautious of experienced doctors who, nonetheless, have been doing the same routine since prehistoric times. If they have been keeping up with the advancements in eyecare technology and knowledge, they are perfectly fine doctors to see. But things change quickly, so be observant when it comes to the doctor's facility and his patient reviews. Is the office updated? Does it offer the latest tests? Since all states require continuing education as part of the re-licensing process for all eye doctors, checking to make sure that the doctor has a valid license should give you some comfort that he has kept abreast of at least the most important developments in the field.

Of course, technical knowledge is only one part of the doctor-patient relationship. The personal interaction between the doctor and his patients is equally important. You want a doctor who will listen to your problem and offer as many options as possible. After all, everyone wants to be heard and cared for. Moreover, you might be particularly interested in finding a doctor who takes natural approaches when possible and knows the latest research on the effects of nutrition on eye care. If this is of

interest to you, see the inset titled "Integrative Optometry: A New Approach to Consider," on page 54.

All in all, when deciding upon an eye-health practitioner, it is best to get a few names and then do some good research. To become familiar with the doctors on your list of possibilities and to make an intelligent choice from among them, you should inquire about those doctors' educational and professional backgrounds. You could ask each doctor for a resume and any office promotional materials that he has developed. Most likely, most of the contact will be through the receptionist at the office. Here are a few questions to ask the receptionist when searching (or calling) an office for the first time:

- How long has the doctor been in practice?

- How long does the examination take?

- Will my eyes be dilated for the examination?

- How much does the examination cost?

- Does the doctor specialize in (or have experience with) the particular condition or service I am interested in?

- Does the doctor offer treatment alternatives (for example, contact lenses, glasses, or vision therapy) according to the patient's preferences?

- Does the doctor work with a number of different contact lens companies? (If you want contact lenses, it's important to have a doctor who is not tied to one manufacturer. There are many different kinds of contacts available now.)

- Does the doctor offer alternatives in addition to surgery? (This question applies to ophthalmologists.)

Research and key questions are very important. But much of what you determine about a doctor will be based just on plain old gut feelings about the office in general. Sometimes it takes a little faith, a bit of time, and a lot of trust to find a good eyecare professional. It's true that a good doc might be hard to find, so once you find one, stay with him and appreciate the good vision care.

We have covered the pre-exam necessities—considering options and selecting an eyecare practitioner. Whether you decide to visit an optometrist or an ophthalmologist, and whether you find him through a friend's recommendation or through research on the Internet, at least you've conducted an intelligent search and maintained high standards. At this point, we are ready to talk about the actual eye exam itself.

THE BASIC EYE EXAMINATION

There are several topics to cover when it comes to the eye exam itself. First, I would like to suggest certain questions to ask before the exam gets underway. Then I feel it is important to identify the general components of the exam. Finally, there is the cost of the

INTEGRATIVE OPTOMETRY: A NEW APPROACH TO CONSIDER

I'd like to introduce a concept called *integrative medicine*. As defined by the US National Center for Complementary and Alternative Medicine (NCCAM), integrative medicine "combines conventional medical treatments and alternative treatments for which there is some high-quality scientific evidence of their safety and effectiveness." The term is used for a new movement that is being driven by the desires of consumers. It is not synonymous with complementary and alternative medicine (CAM), but it has a far larger meaning and mission in that it calls for the focus of medicine on health and healing and emphasizes the importance of the patient-physician relationship.

In addition to providing the best conventional care, integrative medicine focuses on preventive maintenance of health by paying attention to diet, exercise, stress management, and emotional well-being. It insists on patients being active participants in their health care, as well as on physicians viewing patients as whole people—minds, community members, and spiritual beings, as well as physical bodies. Finally, it asks physicians not only to be dispensers of therapeutic aids, but also to serve as guides, role models, and mentors.

Integrative optometry follows many of these same principles. It includes the development of a partnership between patient and practitioner in the healing process of the eye(s). The doctor uses an appropriate mix of conventional and alternative methods to facilitate the body's innate healing response. It is a philosophy that neither rejects conventional medicine nor accepts alternative therapies uncritically, and it uses natural, effective, less-invasive interventions whenever possible.

exam to consider. By learning about these three areas, you will be much better prepared and informed, which ultimately means that you will be much more confident and relaxed about your eye care.

The Questions to Ask

It is so important to share an open, serious conversation with your eye doctor. The best way to make sure that happens is to come prepared with a list of questions. The following questions are ones I advise you to ask the doctor or assistant *before* the examination. If

you do so, you will feel ready for the exam and not fear any surprises along the way. Just as important, your doctor will then know what you expect and (hopefully) will be more likely to provide the services for which you are looking.

• Will a case history be taken?

• How extensive is the examination form? (Although the form will probably look mysterious, see how big it is and how much of it should be filled out by the end of the examination. Be suspicious of an examination form that is the size of an index card.) Yes, this is more

---

The eye maintains inherently natural healing abilities. For example, there is an enzyme in the tears that is a natural antibiotic. If the doctor can balance the tear film with the proper nutrition and flush the eye with lubricating drops, this will allow the tears to fight off a potential infection. This is the type of approach that an integrative optometrist would seek to take.

Then there is the opportunity to treat chronic eye disease, as well as to prevent disease, with nutritional support. Extensive research is currently being conducted to determine exactly what nutrients, or combination of nutrients, work to support eye health and function. This brings up the concept of using natural substances to heal the body. The term "nutraceutical" has been used in the literature to label such natural substances. A *nutraceutical* can be defined as a supplement that provides medical or health benefits, including

the prevention and/or treatment of a disease.

However, the term, as it is commonly used in marketing, has no regulatory definition (that is, no insurance billing code). Ultimately, integrative optometry strives to make use of this natural approach whenever possible and reasonable.

Integrative practitioners are difficult to find because this is a relatively new field of medicine. Regarding integrative eyecare practitioners, we now have the Ocular Wellness and Nutrition Society. The mission of the society is to promote excellent patient care through nutritional support for eye diseases and disorders. Alongside that aim is the goal to do so through professional education and scientific investigation. The doctors who belong to this organization are learning more about nutrition and how to effectively use this mode of treatment for eye disorders. See the listing for the Ocular Wellness and Nutrition Society on page 417.

challenging if the doctor uses a computerized system, but that is a good thing!

• Is a full range of distance- and near-vision tests included in the examination?

• Is glaucoma testing a regular part of the examination?

• Will the doctor describe the different tests while performing them?

• Will the doctor refer me to other doctors when appropriate or necessary?

Here, what is important to realize is that you should feel in control of your eye care. You are entitled to ask questions and hold high expectations. If you feel you aren't getting high-quality, personalized service from your eye doctor, go elsewhere.

The Components of the Exam

Let's assume the doctor has answered all of your questions satisfactorily and you are ready to begin the vision assessment. A complete eye exam should be so thorough that it tires you out. There are some basic procedures that are included in every complete examination. The additional procedures will vary depending upon your doctor and your visual condition.

Every examination should begin with a case history. Be sure the doctor sits down and gives you his undivided attention. Your doctor should ask you questions about your health and lifestyle, starting with, "Why are you here?" You should also be questioned about the date of your last exam, your history with glasses and contact lenses, the quality of your distance and near vision, any headaches you may be having, any medications you are taking, your job-related visual tasks, and your personal and family history of eye disease. Beware of a doctor who doesn't ask many questions before beginning the testing.

Next, the examination should include visual acuity testing. This is when the doctor assesses the sharpness of your vision using the Snellen chart (see page 12). Each eye should be tested individually for distance vision and then again for near vision. This will give the doctor an idea of how well you see the world.

Also included in every examination should be a check of your external eye health. This involves checking the outer area of each of the eyes, including the pupil, iris, cornea, sclera, conjunctiva, lids, eyelashes, eyebrows, and surrounding skin area. The doctor usually uses a flashlight to do this assessment, although occasionally more sophisticated instruments are used to magnify the eye.

Your internal eye health is also important. Using an *ophthalmoscope* (of-THAL-moh-scope), the doctor should look into the back of each eye to see the retina, optic nerve, blood vessels, and surrounding tissue to rule out any diseases in those areas. Some doctors prefer to take pictures of the retina, which is good since it gives them a good reference for future changes, should they occur. This examination will often be done after your eyes have been dilated so that the doctor can see the entire retina more easily. Not all doctors dilate the eyes, but as long as they get a good view of the retina, this is the most important factor. For a discussion of eye dilation, see the inset titled "Eyes Wide Open: Dilation During an Exam" on page 57.

Refraction, used in the context of an eye examination, is the determination of refractive errors in vision. Refraction is done using a machine called a *refractor*, which contains all the different lens combinations. Using the refractor, the doctor can determine both your distance prescription and your near prescription. The refractor will also be used to provide information about your eye-muscle balance, focusing strength, and focusing flexibility.

This is usually the most time-consuming portion of the examination. Some practices use an "auto-refractor" to objectively measure the power of the eye. This is a good test but should not replace the "subjective" aspect (asking the patient which lens is sharper). Oh, and you should know that it's OK to say that both lenses look the same—that's actually the answer we are looking for!

Glaucoma testing should be part of the

EYES WIDE OPEN: DILATION DURING AN EXAM

Many patients wonder whether eye drops that dilate (widen) the pupil will be used during their eye examination, why those drops are necessary, and how long it will take the drops to wear off. Dilation drops are used for two main purposes: to enable the doctor to get a better view of the inner eye for the detection of eye diseases and retinal problems, and to paralyze the focusing muscle of the eye. The paralyzing is done so that you cannot inadvertently focus your eyes to affect the outcome of the refraction. However, most doctors just use lenses to relax the focusing. If there is a "spasm" of the eye muscle (which often happens with uncooperative kids), then the drops can paralyze the muscle so an accurate refraction can be done.

Some doctors dilate the eyes routinely, and, in fact, the practice is becoming the "standard of care." It may be especially necessary to use dilating drops in older patients with very small pupils, particularly if eye disease is suspected, and paralyzing drops in children, who often have trouble focusing at the required distances for the examination. Finally, doctors may also use the paralyzing drops if they suspect an unusual refractive problem.

If your eyes are dilated as part of your eye examination, they will most likely return to normal by the next morning. In the meantime, they will be extremely sensitive to light, and it may be difficult to read or to focus for any near-point activities. Your doctor will probably offer you disposable sunglasses to help with any excessive glare that you experience after your eyes have been dilated. Since the dilation drops may affect your distance vision, it's advisable to have someone drive you to the exam. If that is not possible, reschedule for a dilation at a future date when you can get this assistance.

It's true that dilation can be disruptive and uncomfortable for a while after the exam. However, that is mild compared to the possible eye disease that the doctor might miss if he does not get a good view of the inside of your eye! So the temporary inconvenience is worth the trouble.

eye examination. As previously touched upon, glaucoma is a condition in which the optic nerve is damaged, usually caused by increased pressure within the eye. The pressure of each eye is measured with an instrument called a *tonometer* (toe-NAH-met-er). Many of today's tonometers blow a puff of air at the eye, but the doctor may use a different technique. Although glaucoma testing, because of this puff of air, can be the most irritating part of the complete eye examination, it is also the most crucial, since there are usually no symptoms of high eye pressure.

In addition, many doctors perform visual field testing to determine whether your peripheral vision is intact. Visual field testing is most often performed if glaucoma or another disorder is suspected, but it can be done at any time, and some doctors do it routinely. Modern visual field testing employs a computerized system. The patient's head is positioned in a shell-like machine, and the patient is instructed to look straight ahead. Then small lights are flashed all around. The patient indicates when the flashes appear in his peripheral vision.

Every complete eye examination should end with a consultation. The doctor should spend some time explaining the results of all of the tests and the recommendations for your eyes. Be certain that you understand the test results and the options that you are given to remedy or treat any problems that were found. Be cautious of a doctor who pushes one option, especially one with which you may not be comfortable.

The Cost

It's difficult to put a price tag on eye care, but you should have some idea of what to expect when you walk into a doctor's office for an examination. The prices of examinations, contact lenses, and other services vary around the country. Yet you will probably find it helpful to consider a few averages.

A 2018 survey of optometrists around the nation found that the average cost of a complete eye examination was $100. A similar survey of ophthalmologists found that the average cost of a comprehensive examination was $175. The cost of a contact lens examination is always additional. Most medical doctors charge for various lab tests, and eye doctors are no exception. Depending on what your condition is, this might dictate additional charges, especially if diagnosis of a problem is difficult. And again, regional differences can vary these amounts greatly.

Sometimes you'll see "specials" offered for eye examinations. These are popular in shopping malls, and they are designed to entice you into the store, where you will hopefully purchase other services, such as ordering contact lenses or glasses. In other words, the examination is a "loss leader" technique used by some large chain operations. (Think of a megastore in your area. They sell stuff at a loss in order to get you into the store to buy more.) The emphasis in these stores is usually on *eyewear* rather than *eye care*. So be wary. As well, be very cautious where the exam is "free with purchase." This is a sure sign that every person who walks through the door gets glasses!

My personal belief is that you shouldn't do much shopping around when it comes to your vision. Find a professional whom you can trust and stick with. Quality rarely comes cheaply, but most people find that competent eye care is worth the cost.

Reading this section has put you at an advantage when it comes to getting the most out of your eye examination. You know about the process of vision and what can go wrong. And you know the best questions to ask your eye-care professional. Hopefully, you will leave the exam with the confidence that the doctor did a thorough job, as well as with several alternatives to consider for your eyecare needs. Together, you and your doctor can deal with any problems that may arise.

CONCLUSION

You are now much more aware of the types of eyecare practitioners available to you and the best ways to select the type that's right for your particular situation. You know the questions to ask and the tests you can expect when you go for an eye exam. And through an important inset, you have been introduced to a cutting-edge approach to eye health—integrative optometry. Meanwhile, you may have noticed that, throughout Part One thus far, the subjects of nutrition and natural ways to enhance your eye health have arisen on several occasions. Now, we are ready to turn to those topics in more detail. The following section will help you identify the many nutrients and supplements that not only enhance overall well-being but also put you in the best position for optimal eye health.

Nutrition and Vision

By now you should be getting the idea that the eyes and the visual system are an integral part of the body. It makes sense, therefore, that they require proper nutrition to maintain their optimal function. You might be surprised to find out that the brain and visual system, while composing only about 2 percent of your body weight, use up about 25 percent of your nutritional intake.

This chapter is designed to give you an overview of nutrition, explaining how it works and how it generally affects the body. In addition, we'll discuss the macronutrients (water, carbohydrates, protein, and fats) and some selected micronutrients (vitamins and minerals) that are especially important to vision. We'll even spend some time answering important questions such as, "If I eat well, do I need to take supplements?" and "How much of my health profile is simply inherited?" So, let's take a look at what your eyes—and your body—need for optimal performance.

THE PROCESS OF NUTRITION

Nutrition is the process by which the body digests food to obtain the nutrients it needs for growth and repair purposes. Proper nutrition involves consuming foods and supplements that supply the correct nutrients in adequate amounts for optimal health. In this section, we will examine what actually happens inside the body as it makes use of the nutrients.

The foods eaten by humans are chemically complex and must be broken down by the body into simpler chemical forms so that they can be taken in through the intestinal walls and transported by the blood to the cells. In the cells, they provide energy and building materials to maintain human life. The processes that work together to complete this job are digestion, absorption, and metabolism.

Digestion

Digestion is a series of physical and chemical processes that break down food in preparation for the absorption of its nutrients from the intestinal tract into the bloodstream. These processes take place in the digestive tract, which includes the mouth, pharynx, esophagus, stomach, small intestine, and large intestine. Digestive juices play an important role in this system.

The active materials in the digestive juices that cause the chemical breakdown of food are called *enzymes.* Enzymes are complex proteins that are capable of inducing chemical changes in other substances without being changed themselves. Each enzyme is capable of breaking down only a specific substance. For example, an enzyme capable of breaking down fats cannot also break down proteins or carbohydrates.

Digestion actually begins in the mouth, where the large pieces of food are broken down into smaller pieces via chewing. The salivary glands in the mouth produce *saliva,* a fluid that moistens the food for swallowing and contains an enzyme necessary for carbohydrate breakdown. But active chemical digestion begins in the middle portion of the stomach, where the food is mixed with gastric juices containing hydrochloric acid, water, and enzymes that break up protein and other substances. After one to four hours, muscle action pushes the food, now in a liquid form, out of the stomach and into the small intestine.

When the liquid food enters the small intestine, the pancreas secretes digestive juices that are added to the mixture. If fats are present in the food, *bile,* an enzyme produced by the liver and stored in the gallbladder, is secreted. The pancreas also secretes a substance that neutralizes the digestive acids in the food, as well as additional enzymes that continue the breakdown of the proteins and carbohydrates. At this point, nutrients are ready for absorption, as discussed in the following section. Finally, the undigested portions of the food enter the large intestine for eventual excretion. No digestive enzymes are secreted in the large intestine, and little occurs there aside from the absorption of water.

Absorption

Absorption is the process by which nutrients—in the form of glucose from carbohydrates, amino acids from protein, and fatty acids and glycerol from fats—are taken up by the intestine and passed into the bloodstream to function in cell metabolism. Absorption takes place primarily in the small intestine. The lining of the small intestine is covered with minute fingerlike projections called *villi* (VIL-eye). These villi contain lymph channels called *lacteals* and tiny blood vessels called *capillaries,* which are the principal channels of absorption. About 60 to 70 percent of fats and fat-soluble vitamins are absorbed by the lacteals into the lymphatic system and transported to the liver. The remaining nutrients are absorbed by the capillaries into the bloodstream and then also transported to the liver.

In the liver, many different enzymes help to change the nutrient molecules into new forms for specific purposes. Unlike the earlier changes, which prepared the nutrients for absorption and transport, the reactions in the liver produce the actual products needed by the cells. Some of these products are used by the liver itself, but the rest are held in storage by the liver, to be released as needed into the bloodstream. From the blood, they are picked up by the individual cells and put to work. This "work" is the beginning of the process of metabolism.

Metabolism

Metabolism is the final stage of "food handling." It includes all of the chemical changes that nutrients undergo from the time they are absorbed until they either become a part of the body or are excreted from the body. Metabolism is the conversion of digested nutrients into building materials for living tissues or energy to meet the body's needs.

Metabolism occurs in two general phases, *anabolism* and *catabolism*, which take place simultaneously. Anabolism involves all of the chemical reactions that nutrients undergo in the construction, or building up, of body chemicals and tissues such as blood, enzymes, hormones, and glycogen. Catabolism involves all the reactions that break down various compounds and tissues to supply energy. Energy for the cells is derived primarily from the metabolism of glucose, which combines with oxygen in a series of chemical reactions to form carbon dioxide, water, and cellular energy. The carbon dioxide and water are waste products, carried away from the cells by the bloodstream. Energy is also derived from the metabolism of essential fatty acids and amino acids, although the major purpose of amino acid metabolism is to provide material for the growth, maintenance, and repair of tissues. The waste products of essential fatty acid and amino acid metabolism are also carried away from the cells.

The process of metabolism requires that the body maintain extensive systems of enzymes to facilitate the thousands of different chemical reactions that take place and to regulate the rate at which these reactions occur. These enzymes often require the presence of specific vitamins and minerals to perform their functions. That is why a healthy diet and an effective supplementation plan are so important.

Nutrition is certainly a complex system. For proper nutrition, and therefore proper growth, the body needs the four basic nutrients of water, carbohydrates, protein, and fat, which are all referred to as *macronutrients*. It also needs vitamins and minerals, which are called *micronutrients*. In the remainder of this chapter, we will describe these various nutrients and explore how they interact to supply the body, including the eyes, with the materials needed to function well.

THE MACRONUTRIENTS

The macronutrients are the essential ingredients among the building blocks of nutrition. As mentioned above, they are water, carbohydrates, protein, and fat, all of which are necessary for the process of metabolism—the conversion of food to useable nutrients. All of the macronutrients are required, to some degree, by the body, and all of them are available from the foods we eat. Although the macronutrients are critical for life itself, there are no detailed Federal guidelines regarding their intake such as there are for the vitamins and minerals. Let's review the macronutrients, and see how they interact with our bodies to supply the fuel for life.

Water

Water is an essential nutrient, involved in every function of the body. It helps to transport other nutrients and waste products in and out of the cells. Water is necessary for all of the digestive, absorptive, circulatory, and excretory functions of the body, as well as for the body's utilization of the water-soluble vitamins. It is also needed for the maintenance of proper body temperature. Actually, the human body is two-thirds water.

Replenishing your body's supply of water, which is continually drained through sweating and elimination, is very important. To keep your body functioning properly, you must drink a substantial amount of quality water each day. The general consensus of eight glasses per day is a common recommendation, but recent studies dispute any exact number. While the body can survive without food for about five weeks, it cannot survive without water for more than five days.

How does your intake of water affect the eyes? Let's consider a few examples. Recall that the aqueous humor in the eye is a very watery substance that contains nutrients for the cornea and the lens. A decrease in water could create an imbalance that could reduce the infusion of nutrition to these structures. In contrast, if too much water dilutes the system, then the amount of nutrient/water balance is upset, potentially causing a malnutrition condition.

The tears of the eyes also require the proper water/salt balance to maintain their integrity. If enough water is not retained, then the salt concentration of the tears goes up and the eyes dry out. The opposite condition—too much water in the tears—is rare, but if your tears are overflowing on a regular basis, a nutritional review might be considered.

Carbohydrates

Carbohydrates supply the body with the energy it needs to function. They are found almost exclusively in plant foods, such as fruits, vegetables, grains, and legumes. Milk and products made from milk are the only animal foods that contain a significant amount of carbohydrates.

Carbohydrates are divided into two groups: simple and complex. The simple carbohydrates, sometimes called simple sugars, include fructose (fruit sugar), sucrose (table sugar), and lactose (milk sugar). Fruits are among the richest natural sources of simple carbohydrates. Complex carbohydrates are also made of sugars, but the sugar molecules form longer, more complex chains. The complex carbohydrates include fiber and starches. Foods rich in complex carbohydrates are vegetables, whole grains, and legumes.

Carbohydrates are the main source of blood glucose, which is a major fuel for all of the body's cells and the only source of energy for the brain and red blood cells. Except for fiber, which cannot be digested, both simple and complex carbohydrates are converted into glucose. The glucose is then either used directly to provide energy for the body or stored in the liver for future use. When a person consumes more calories than the body needs, a portion of the carbohydrates consumed may also be stored in the body as fat. Thus, when too many carbohydrates are consumed or not processed properly, excess fatty tissue accumulates and stresses the body. We'll discuss this process in more detail in Part Two's section on diabetes, tying in links to eye health at that point. But if you presently want to know a little more about the presence of glucose in the blood, read the inset titled "The Glycemic Index," on page 65.

Protein

Protein is essential for growth and development. It provides the body with energy and is needed for the manufacture of hormones, antibodies, enzymes, and tissues. It also helps

THE GLYCEMIC INDEX

When we eat carbohydrates, our bodies break them down to produce glucose. Our cells use this glucose as their main energy source. The glycemic index (GI) describes how carbohydrate-containing food affects blood-glucose levels.

For glucose to move from the blood into the body's cells, it needs insulin produced by the pancreas. Generally, in the healthy body, insulin production is stimulated whenever there is glucose in the blood. If there is insufficient insulin, glucose levels will rise. Insulin is not only involved in regulating blood-glucose levels, but it also plays a key role in determining whether our body burns fat or carbohydrates for energy. A high level of insulin means the body is forced to burn carbohydrates, rather than fats. By controlling the rate of glucose being absorbed, we can also control the amount of insulin secreted. This is where the glycemic index comes into play.

The GI is a way to rank carbohydrates on a scale from 0 to 100, according to the extent to which they raise blood-sugar levels after eating. Foods with a high GI are those which are rapidly digested and absorbed and therefore result in marked fluctuations in blood-sugar levels. Low-GI foods, by virtue of their slow digestion and absorption, produce gradual rises in blood-sugar and insulin levels, and they have proven benefits for health. Low-GI diets have been shown to improve both glucose and lipid levels in people with diabetes (type 1 and type 2). They have benefits for weight control because they help control appetite and delay hunger. Low-GI diets also reduce insulin levels and insulin resistance.

Foods and drinks that carry a high glycemic index trigger an undesirable insulin response. This reaction results in an excess of insulin in the bloodstream. Monitoring the glycemic index of foods and drinks allows for control over food-driven insulin stimulation and reactive *hypoglycemia* (low blood sugar). Understanding the GI of foods may have important implications for the prevention and treatment of the major causes of sickness and death in Western countries, including obesity, cardiovascular disease, and type 2 diabetes. Furthermore, considerable evidence exists supporting the value of a low-GI (below 55) diet for individuals with *hyperlipidemia* (high cholesterol) and for prolonging endurance during physical activity, improving insulin sensitivity, reducing food intake, and increasing colonic fermentation (something that is important for people who have digestive troubles).

More information can be found on websites such as www.glycemicindex.com. It is constructive to look up the glycemic index of your favorite and most often consumed foods, as well as the GI of healthful foods that you don't eat as frequently. Once you begin to understand how you can control your glucose levels, you will be able to better take charge of your health.

to maintain the proper acid-alkaline balance, known as "pH," in the body. When protein is consumed, the body breaks it down into *amino acids*; in fact, amino acids are referred to as the building blocks of protein. Some amino acids are considered *nonessential*. This does not mean that they are unnecessary, but rather that they do not have to come from the diet because they are manufactured by the body from other amino acids. The remaining amino acids are considered *essential*, meaning that they are not synthesized by the body and must be obtained from the diet.

Because of the importance of consuming proteins that provide all of the essential amino acids, dietary proteins are divided into two groups according to the amino acids they contain. Complete proteins, which constitute the first group, contain ample amounts of all of the essential amino acids. These proteins are found in meat, fish, poultry, cheese, eggs, and milk. Incomplete proteins, which constitute the second group, contain only some of the essential amino acids. These proteins are found in foods such as grains, legumes, and leafy green vegetables.

Although it is important to maintain the full range of amino acids, both essential and nonessential, it is not necessary to get them from meat, fish, poultry, and the other complete-protein foods. In fact, because of their high fat content, most of those foods should be eaten in moderation. It is possible to create complete proteins by combining various incomplete-protein foods. This is called *food combining*. For instance, although beans and rice are both quite rich in protein, each lacks one or more of the essential amino acids. However, when you combine beans and rice with each other, or when you combine either one with any of a number of other protein-rich foods, you form a complete protein that is a high-quality substitute for meat.

As proteins are the building blocks for the body structures, they are also critical for the eyes. The sclera (the white part of the eye) is made of *collagen*—the main protein of connective tissue. If the collagen is not strong and durable, it might tend to distort, which can cause an elongation of the eye. That's what we normally see in nearsighted eyes. We will review this process in the section on myopia in Part Two. Thus, an adequate supply of protein can directly lead to good eyesight!

Fats

Although much attention has been focused on the need to reduce the amount of fat in the diet, the body does need some fat. During infancy and childhood, fat is necessary for normal brain development. Throughout life, it provides energy and supports growth. Fat is, in fact, the most concentrated source of energy available to the body. However, after the age of two, the body requires only small amounts of fat—much less than what is provided by the Standard American Diet (appropriately called SAD).

Fats are composed of building blocks called *fatty acids*. There are three major categories of fatty acids: saturated, polyunsaturated, and monounsaturated. Saturated fatty acids, also referred to as saturates, are found primarily in animal products, including dairy items such as whole milk, cream, and cheese, as well as fatty meats such as beef, veal, lamb, pork, and ham. The fat marbling that you see in beef and pork is composed of saturated fat. Some vegetable products—including coconut oil, palm kernel oil, and vegetable shortening—are also high in saturates. The liver uses saturated fats to manufacture cholesterol. Excessive dietary intake of saturated fats can significantly raise the blood-cholesterol level, especially the level of low-density lipoproteins (LDLs), or what is commonly called "bad" cholesterol, because of its link to coronary heart disease. It's not really "bad"; we will discuss this issue a little later.

Polyunsaturated fatty acids are found in the greatest abundance in corn, soybean, safflower, and sunflower oils. Certain fish oils are also high in the polyunsaturates. Unlike the saturated fats, the polyunsaturates may actually lower your total blood-cholesterol level. In doing so, however, they also have a tendency, when present in large amounts, to reduce your high-density lipoproteins (HDLs), known as "good" cholesterol. For this reason, Federal guidelines state that the intake of polyunsaturated fats should not exceed 10 percent of the total caloric intake.

Monounsaturated fatty acids are found mostly in vegetable and nut oils such as olive, peanut, and canola oils. These fats appear to reduce the LDL level without affecting the HDL level in any way. However, this positive impact upon LDL cholesterol is relatively modest. Guidelines recommend that the intake of monounsaturated fats be kept between 10 and 15 percent of the total caloric intake.

Although most foods contain a combination of all three types of fatty acids, one of the types is usually predominant. Thus, a fat or oil is considered saturated, or high in saturates, when it is composed primarily of saturated fatty acids. Saturated fats are usually solid at

room temperature. Likewise, a fat or oil composed mostly of polyunsaturated fatty acids is called polyunsaturated, while a fat or oil composed mostly of monounsaturated fatty acids is referred to as monounsaturated. The latter two are liquid at room temperature.

We have recently begun to increase our awareness of *trans fats*. Basically, trans fats are produced when manufacturers add hydrogen to vegetable oil—in a complicated process called *hydrogenation.* Hydrogenation increases the shelf life and flavor stability of foods. Partial hydrogenation is a similar process; the action of hydrogenation is halted partially through the process so that all of the fat is not converted to trans fats, thus leaving the texture softer and more desirable. So unlike other fats, the majority of trans fat is formed when food manufacturers turn liquid oils into solid fats like shortening and hard margarine. A small amount of trans fat is found naturally, primarily in dairy products, some meat, and other animal-based foods. In general, trans fat can be found in vegetable shortenings, some margarines, crackers, cookies, snack foods, and other foods made with or fried in partially hydrogenated oils.

Trans fat, like saturated fat and dietary cholesterol, raises the LDL cholesterol that increases your risk for coronary heart disease. It is true that Americans consume, on average, four to five times as much saturated fat as trans fat in their diets. Yet although saturated fat is the main dietary culprit that raises LDL, trans fat and dietary cholesterol also contribute significantly.

At this point, I'd like to say something about the LDL, or "bad" cholesterol. I feel that this is a misnomer. If LDL cholesterol was really "bad" then the body would not produce it! In fact, both the HDLs and LDLs are very important in the transport of nutrients around the body. However, it is when the LDLs become *oxidized*—that is, when they turn into *free radicals*—that they become dangerous. This will cause a smooth lipoprotein to become "spiked" or sharp-edged. These sharp edges can cut the inside of blood vessels, which in turn creates an inflammatory reaction. The reaction will bring in various cells that the body uses to fight inflammation but that eventually get caught in the artery. This is where a clot can form. So, it's not the LDL by itself that is the problem, but it's the oxidation of that particle that creates health issues.

Now, while we're still on the subject of fats, let's talk about a term that has recently gotten a lot of attention in the press: *essential fatty acids (EFAs)*. These are the building blocks for fats and are considered necessary for a healthy life. The most widely discussed EFAs are the omega-3 and the omega-6 essential fatty acids. Omega-6 fatty acids are the most plentiful in our diet but can lead to inflammation if not balanced properly with the omega-3 fatty acids. They are in almost everything we eat that contains fat, including meat, most seed oils, dairy products, and eggs. Omega-3 fatty acids are also available in many seed oils and in most cold-water fatty fish.

A proper balance of fatty acids is essential to good health. The Institute of Medicine's daily intake recommendation is 4:1—four times as many omega-6 fatty acids as omega-3 fatty acids. It is widely believed that the standard American diet provides *twenty* times as much omega-6 as omega-3, which is a great cause for concern!

Fats are used in every cell membrane of our body. They have two primary functions. First, they ensure cellular fluidity, acting as sentinel gatekeepers for every cell, allowing vital nutrients to enter the cell and forcing destructive free-radical debris out of the cells. Secondly, both omega-6 and omega-3 fatty acids can be converted into three different types of active molecules called *prostaglandins* (PGEs). Without going into a great deal of detail, prostaglandins achieve three processes: PGE1 reduces inflammation and inhibits blood clotting; PGE2 allows for the constriction of blood vessels, increase of body temperature, and encouragement of blood clotting; and PGE3 also fulfills an anti-inflammatory role. All three types of prostaglandins are important for the body to maintain its health and balance.

Two products of the metabolism of essential fatty acids are *docosahexaenoic acid* (DHA), from omega-3s, and *arachidonic acid* (ARA), from omega-6s. DHA, a long-chain omega-3 fatty acid, is found in tissues throughout the body. It is a major structural and functional element of all membranes in the gray matter of the brain and the retina of the eye. It is also a key component of heart tissue. This EFA is important for optimal brain and eye development in infants and has been shown to support brain, eye, and cardiovascular health in adults. Studies have shown that a lack of DHA in pregnancy leads to some forms of visual defects in infants.

ARA, a long-chain omega-6 fatty acid, is the principal omega-6 in the brain, and it is abundant in other cells throughout the body. ARA is equally important for proper brain development in infants and is a precursor to a group of hormone-like substances called *eicosanoids.* Eicosanoids are important for immunity, blood clotting, and other vital functions in the body.

Humans obtain ARA by eating foods such as meat, eggs, and milk, whereas DHA is found in a limited selection of foods such as fatty fish and organ meats. The body can also synthesize DHA from its precursor, *alpha-lino-lenic acid* (ALA), but this process is inefficient. Both DHA and ARA occur naturally in breast milk and support the mental and visual development of infants. The health benefits of DHA extend from prenatal development through adult life. However, the need for ARA diminishes as we age. In fact, consuming too much ARA as adults leads to chronic inflammation and chronic disease.

Congratulations! You've just about finished your lesson on fats and fatty acids. The fats we've discussed are not only important in the development of vision but also in the maintenance of vision. The metabolism of essential fatty acids can affect the incidence of dry eyes, especially as we age. Moreover, the PGE1 that is created via the omega-6 metabolism pathway is directly responsible for creating a tear-specific anti-inflammatory. (This is effective only if enough omega-3 fatty acids are present to prevent the omega-6 from creating too much ARA!) While all of this seems rather confusing, it supports the concept of proper nutritional balance. And that's the main point that you should take from this section on fats.

So, what is a good dietary balance of the macronutrients? Most experts agree that a healthy diet consists of approximately 2,000 calories per day. And a proper balance of macronutrients consists of about 30 percent (600 calories) from fat, mostly monounsaturated oils and only 7 percent of which should be saturated fat; 50 to 60 percent (1,000 to 1,200 calories) from carbohydrates, mostly low-GI complex carbohydrates (see the inset titled "The Glycemic Index" on page 65; and about 10 to 20 percent (200 to 400 calories) from protein. These amounts could certainly vary from one individual to another, but they are generally considered a good starting point for a healthy diet in a healthy person.

THE MICRONUTRIENTS

Just like the macronutrients, vitamins and minerals are essential to life. They are therefore also considered nutrients. However, they are called *micro*nutrients because compared with macro-nutrients such as protein and carbohydrates, they are needed in small amounts.

Again, adequate intake of vitamins and minerals is necessary to sustain life. The Food and Nutrition Board of the Institute of Medicine of the National Academies establishes recommended vitamin and mineral intake levels called the Recommended Daily Allowances (RDAs). If there is no consensus from a panel of experts for an RDA, then an Adequate Intake (AI) is suggested. The amounts cited in these recommendations are adequate for disease prevention, but usually not for optimal health. Therefore, most adults should aim for a daily intake of more than the RDAs of vitamins and minerals through food and/or supplement sources. People who are active or exercise, are under great stress, are on restricted diets, are mentally or physically ill, take prescription drugs, are recovering from surgery, or smoke or consume excessive alcoholic beverages all need more than the recommended amounts. Women who take oral contraceptives also need increased amounts. Where applicable, the RDAs and general intake recommendations for specific micronutrients are provided in the discussions below.

Vitamins

Vitamins contribute to good health by regulating the metabolism and assisting the biochemical processes that release energy from digested food. Some vitamins are water-soluble, while others are fat-soluble. The water-soluble vitamins must be taken into the body daily, as they cannot be stored and are excreted within one to four days. These include the B vitamins and vitamin C. The fat-soluble vitamins can be stored for longer periods of time in the body, in fatty tissues and the liver. These include vitamins A, D, E, and K. The body needs both the water-soluble and fat-soluble vitamins for proper functioning.

Vitamin A and Beta-Carotene

Of all the micronutrients that are important to visual function, vitamin A is probably the most well known. Vitamin A is a fat-soluble vitamin that occurs in nature in a variety of chemical forms. It is found as *retinol* in animal tissues and as *beta-carotene* in plants. Interestingly, while retinol is readily absorbed just as it is by the body, beta-carotene must be broken down before it can function as a vitamin. High amounts of beta-carotene are present in fruits such as apricots and cantaloupes, and in vegetables such as carrots, pumpkins, sweet potatoes, spinach, squash, and broccoli.

Actually, beta-carotene is a *carotenoid* (ka-ROT-en-oyd), a class of compounds related to vitamin A. Some carotenoids, including beta-carotene, can act as precursors of vitamin A. When a food or supplement containing beta-carotene is consumed, the beta-carotene is converted into vitamin A in the liver. According to recent reports, beta-carotene appears to aid in cancer prevention by scavenging, or neutralizing, free radicals. However, this conversion does not readily occur if the body has adequate stores of vitamin A. Most people in developed nations have adequate vitamin A stores in their livers.

So now you can see why the concept of "eat carrots to see better" came to be. Carrots are flush with beta-carotene, which converts to vitamin A, which is the molecule in the retina that allows us to see. However, this is a flawed concept. Aside the poor conversion of beta-carotene to vitamin A and the competition with lutein and zeaxanthin, as long as the body has adequate stores of vitamin A in the liver, there is no need to convert more beta-carotene to vitamin A. Additionally, the molecule will not affect the "refractive status" of the eye. A nearsighted eye likely has as much vitamin A in the retina that a farsighted eye does. So, go ahead and eat your carrots, but still get those eyes examined yearly!

The upper intestinal tract is the primary area of absorption of vitamin A, since it's there that fat-splitting enzymes and bile salts convert beta-carotene into a usable nutrient. This conversion is stimulated by *thyroxine*, an amino acid obtained from the thyroid gland. Once converted into vitamin A, beta-carotene is absorbed in the same way that pre-formed vitamin A is absorbed. Yet the conversion of beta-carotene into vitamin A is never 100-percent complete. Approximately one-third of the beta-carotene in food is converted into vitamin A. More specifically, less than one-fourth of the beta-carotene in carrots and root vegetables undergoes conversion, and about one-half of the beta-carotene in leafy green vegetables does. Some unchanged beta-carotene is stored in the liver, and some is absorbed into the circulatory system and stored in the fat tissues. Unabsorbed beta-carotene is excreted.

In general, approximately 90 percent of the body's vitamin A is stored in the liver, with small amounts deposited in the fat tissues, lungs, kidneys, and retinas of the eyes. Under stressful conditions, the body uses this reserve supply if it doesn't receive enough vitamin A from the diet.

The degree to which beta-carotene is utilized by the body varies with the food source and the way the food is prepared. Cooking, pureeing, and mashing of a vegetable rupture the cell membranes and therefore make the beta-carotene more available for absorption. Factors interfering with the absorption of vitamin A and beta-carotene include strenuous physical activity performed within four hours of consumption of the nutrient, intake of mineral oil, excessive consumption of alcohol, excessive consumption of iron, and the use of cortisone and other medications. Also, the intake of polyunsaturated fatty acids with beta-carotene results in rapid destruction of the beta-carotene unless antioxidants also are present. Even cold weather can hinder the transport and metabolism of vitamin A and beta-carotene. Moreover, diabetics have difficulty converting beta-carotene to vitamin A.

Gastrointestinal and liver disorders, infections of any kind, and any condition in which the bile duct is obstructed can limit the body's capacity to retain and use vitamin A. Additional factors affecting the absorption of vitamin A include the amount of the nutrient consumed, the influence of other substances present in the intestines, and the amount of the vitamin stored in the body. For these reasons, the intake needs of vitamin A vary for each individual.

The RDAs for vitamin A are 500 international units (IU) for infants and children up to four years old, 1,000 IU for children from four to twelve years old, 2,300 IU for women, and 3,000 IU for men. These amounts increase during disease, trauma, pregnancy, and lactation. The requirements vary for people who smoke, who live in highly polluted areas, who easily absorb vitamin A, and who have pneumonia or nephritis (inflammation of the kidneys). Increased intakes of vitamins C and E will help to prevent excessive oxidation (free-radical damage) of stored vitamin A.

A deficiency of vitamin A may cause night blindness, dry hair or skin, dry eyes, or poor growth. Other possible results of a vitamin-A deficiency are abscesses in the ears; insomnia; fatigue; reproductive difficulties; sinusitis; pneumonia, frequent colds, and other respiratory infections; skin disorders, including acne; and weight loss. However, do not take an excess of vitamin A without first consulting your physician or healthcare practitioner. Taking large amounts of vitamin A over long periods of time can be toxic to the body, mainly the liver. Research indicates that no more than 50,000 IU per day of vitamin A can be utilized by the body except in therapeutic cases.

Toxic levels of vitamin A are associated with abdominal pain, amenorrhea (halt of menstruation), enlargement of the liver and/or spleen, gastrointestinal disturbances, hair loss, itching, joint pain, nausea and vomiting, water on the brain, and small cracks and scales on the lips. Vitamin C can help prevent the harmful effects of vitamin A toxicity. Overdose is unlikely with beta-carotene, although if you take too much your skin may turn slightly yellow-orange in color. It is important to take only natural beta-carotene or a natural carotenoid complex.

Supplemental beta-carotene was shown to increase the risk of lung cancer in smokers in the Alpha-Tocopherol, Beta-Carotene Cancer Prevention (ATBC) study, conducted in Finland. A second study, the Carotenoid and Retinol Efficacy Trial (CARET), also found a higher incidence of lung cancer in those people taking a whopping 30 milligrams (mg) of synthetic beta-carotene, plus 25,000 IU of pre-formed vitamin A retinol. The amount of supplemental vitamin A and beta-carotene included in both the ATBC and CARET studies was far beyond the safe upper limits (UL) for daily consumption established by the Food and Nutrition Board at the Institute of Medicine. Unfortunately, many misinformed people associate vitamin A retinol with the outdated ATBC and CARET studies and now refuse to take or recommend multivitamins that contain efficacious amounts of either pre-formed retinol or pro-formed beta-carotene. This decision can quickly lead to a dramatic decrease in night vision and a host of wound healing and other immune system maladies in vitamin A deficient older people.

At about the same time that the studies mentioned above were published, the twelve-year-long Physicians' Health Study (PHS), involving more than 22,000 physician volunteers, showed no statistical increase in lung cancer rates in doctors who were taking a full-spectrum multivitamin and 50 mg of synthetic beta-carotene—even in the 11 percent of physician volunteers who were heavy smokers. And the American Journal of Epidemiology's recent data clearly suggests that, in fact, smokers who consume small amounts of natural supplemental beta-carotene in combination with a wide variety of supplemental antioxidants actually have an overall 16 percent lower risk of developing lung and other cancers.

At this point, it is important to keep in mind that beta-carotene is not vitamin A. It is a fat-soluble carotenoid that can convert to vitamin A. It competes with the carotenoids lutein and zeaxanthin (see below) for cellular transport space. Lutein and zeaxanthin can effectively contribute to eye health. Therefore, excessive amounts of supplemental beta-carotene are not recommended to vision patients, especially those over fifty years of age.

The body's need for vitamin A is so critical that it will convert beta-carotene to vitamin A retinol, if and when the retinol liver stores are deficient. If there is no vitamin A retinol deficiency, beta-carotene functions as a powerhouse antioxidant, most particularly against retina-damaging free radicals, and does not convert to retinol. However, as people get older, the beta-carotene/retinol conversion becomes less efficient. So, several years ago, research-focused nutritional biochemists stopped recommending beta-carotene as a sole source of supplemental vitamin A for older men and women.

What about the benefits of vitamin A, in general? It enhances immunity, may heal gastrointestinal ulcers, protects against pollution and cancer formation, and assists in the maintenance and repair of mucous tissue. It is important in the formation of bones and teeth, aids in fat storage, and protects against colds, influenza, and infections of the kidneys, bladder, lungs, and mucous membranes. This powerful vitamin also acts as an antioxidant. (For a discussion of antioxidants, see page 97.)

Concerning the eyes, vitamin A is the molecule in the retina that is responsible for the transformation of light energy into nerve impulses. It is therefore critical in the function of the eye. A lack of vitamin A can cause some forms of night blindness. Since vitamin A is also necessary for the maintenance of the mucous lining of various tissues, including some of the tissues of the eye, it is important to the support of a proper tear level and the prevention of dry eye disease.

However, the issue of vitamin A is a controversial topic in the eyecare industry. In spite of recently published scientific findings, a few ophthalmic vitamin manufacturers continue to produce special macular degeneration formulations for smokers that include no, or miniscule, amounts of vitamin A retinol and no beta-carotene. Some of these companies even go so far as to suggest that the substitution of lutein for beta-carotene is appropriate. This can be compared to substituting apples for oranges. Lutein is, in fact, a very important player in the outer edges of the macula pigment and should be included in eye-specific multivitamins for that reason. But the carotenoids lutein and zeaxanthin have virtually no ability to convert to vitamin A, nor do they perform the same

antioxidant functions as beta-carotene. Therefore, to suggest that the inclusion of lutein in a multiple is a good substitution for a vitamin as important to the eye and body as vitamin A / beta-carotene is not scientifically sound. These marketing-based formulations do not serve science or the smoking macular degeneration patient well. And the bottom line for eye health in general is quite clear: Stop smoking!

Finally, vitamin A has been successfully used in treating several eye disorders, including Bitot's (BEE-totes) spots, which are white, elevated, sharply outlined patches on the sclera, as well as blurred vision, night blindness, and cataracts. Therapeutic dosages of vitamin A are necessary for the treatment of glaucoma, dry eye disease, and pinkeye. This is a powerful vitamin, but it is best to be assessed by a healthcare practitioner to identify your optimal dose.

Vitamin B Complex

All of the B vitamins are water-soluble substances that can be cultivated from bacteria, yeasts, fungi, or molds. The known B-complex vitamins are B_1 (thiamine), B_2 (riboflavin), B_3 (niacin), B_5 (pantothenic acid), B_6 (pyridoxine), B_{12} (cyanocobalamin), biotin, choline, folic acid, inositol, and para-aminobenzoic acid (PABA). The grouping of these compounds under the term "B complex" is based upon their common sources, their close relationship in vegetable and animal tissues, and their functional relationships.

The B-complex vitamins are active in providing the body with energy, basically by converting carbohydrates into glucose, which the body burns to produce energy. They are vital in the metabolism of fats and protein. In addition, the B vitamins are necessary for the normal functioning of the nervous system, and they may be the single most important factor in the health of the nerves. They are essential for the maintenance of muscle tone in the gastrointestinal tract, and for the health of the skin, hair, eyes, mouth, and liver.

All of the B vitamins are natural constituents of brewer's yeast, liver, and whole-grain cereals. Brewer's yeast is actually the richest natural source of the B-complex group. Another important source of the B vitamins is intestinal bacteria. These bacteria grow best on milk sugar and small amounts of fat in the diet. We can also take supplements of such bacteria, referred to as *probiotics.*

Because of the water-solubility of the B-complex vitamins, any excess of these vitamins is excreted rather than stored. Therefore, the B vitamins must be continually replaced. All of the B vitamins, when mixed with saliva, are readily absorbed. Sulfa drugs, barbiturates (sleeping pills), insecticides, and estrogen can create a condition in the digestive tract that can destroy the B vitamins. Sugar and alcohol also destroy them. And certain B vitamins are lost through perspiration.

The B vitamins have been used in the treatment of barbiturate overdose, alcoholic psychosis, and drug-induced delirium. An adequate dose has been found to control migraine headaches and attacks of Ménière's syndrome (a disease of the inner ear). Some heart abnormalities have responded to the use of the B complex because the nerves affecting the heart need the B-complex vitamins for smooth, quiet functioning. Massive doses of the B-complex vitamins have been used

to treat polio, to improve the condition of hypersensitive children who fail to respond favorably to medications such as Ritalin, and to improve cases of shingles. Nervous individuals and people working under tension can greatly benefit from taking larger-than-normal doses of the B vitamins. The B vitamins may also help reduce the incidence of beriberi (caused by a vitamin B_1 deficiency); pellagra (caused by a deficiency of vitamin B_3, specifically niacin or nicotinic acid); constipation; burning feet; tender gums; eyelid twitching; double vision; fatigue; lack of appetite; skin disorders; cracks at the corners of the mouth; anemia; and dry, burning eyes.

Then there are additional factors that weigh in on the way the body manages the B vitamins. Coffee uses up the B vitamins. The need for the B-complex vitamins increases during infection and stress. Alcoholics and individuals who consume excessive amounts of carbohydrates require higher intakes of the B vitamins for proper metabolism. Finally, children and pregnant women need extra B vitamins for normal growth.

The most important thing to remember is that all of the B vitamins should be taken together. In nature, we find the B-complex vitamins present in yeast and green vegetables, but nowhere do we find a single B vitamin isolated from the rest. There's a reason for that; the B vitamins are so interrelated in function that a large dose of just one of them may be therapeutically valueless or may cause a deficiency of other B vitamins. For example, if you take extra B_6, you must take a complete B complex along with it.

The B vitamins are so meagerly supplied in the American diet that almost every person in this country lacks some of them. If you are tired, irritable, nervous, depressed, or even suicidal, suspect a vitamin-B deficiency. Premature gray hair, baldness, acne and other skin problems, poor appetite, insomnia, neuritis (disease of the peripheral nerves), anemia, constipation, and a high cholesterol level are also indicators of a vitamin-B deficiency.

One reason there is such a great vitamin-B deficiency in the American population is that we eat so much processed food from which the B vitamins have been depleted. Another reason for the widespread deficiency is the high amount of sugar we consume. As mentioned above, sugar and alcohol destroy the B-complex vitamins.

Vitamin B$_1$ (Thiamine). Vitamin B$_1$, also known as thiamine, combines with pyruvic acid to form a particular coenzyme. That coenzyme is necessary for the breakdown of carbohydrates into glucose, which is then oxidized by the body to produce energy. Thiamine is vulnerable to heat, air, and water in cooking. It is a component of the germ and bran of wheat, the husk of rice, and that portion of all grains which is commercially milled away to give the grain a lighter color and finer texture.

Thiamine enhances circulation, assists in the formation of blood, and aids in the production of hydrochloric acid, which is important for proper digestion. It also optimizes cognitive activity and brain function. Thiamine has a positive effect on energy, growth, appetite, and learning capacity, and it is needed for muscle tone in the intestines, stomach, and heart. This vitamin also acts as an antioxidant, protecting the body from the degenerative effects of aging, alcohol consumption, and smoking.

The richest food sources of thiamine include brown rice, egg yolks, fish, legumes, liver, pork, poultry, rice bran, wheat germ, and whole grains. Other sources are asparagus, brewer's yeast, broccoli, Brussels sprouts, dulse, kelp, oatmeal, plums, dried prunes, raisins, spirulina, watercress, and most nuts. Herbs that contain this vitamin include alfalfa, bladderwrack, burdock, catnip, cayenne, chamomile, chickweed, eyebright, fennel, fenugreek, hops, nettle, oat straw, parsley, peppermint, raspberry, red clover, rose hips, sage, yarrow, and yellow dock.

The RDA for thiamine is 1.1 to 1.4 mg per day. A thiamine intake of 1.4 mg daily is recommended during pregnancy and lactation. The need for thiamine increases during severe diarrhea, fever, stress, and surgery. Thiamine has no known toxic side effects.

A deficiency of thiamine can lead to inflammation of the optic nerve, called *optic neuritis,* as well as to impairment of the central nervous system. The first signs of thiamine deficiency include easy fatigue, loss of appetite, irritability, and emotional instability. If the deficiency is not addressed, confusion and loss of memory appear, followed closely by gastric distress, abdominal pain, and constipation.

Vitamin B$_2$ (Riboflavin). Vitamin B$_2$, commonly known as riboflavin, occurs naturally in the same foods containing the other B vitamins. See the foods identified above. Riboflavin is stable in the presence of heat, oxidation, and acid, but it disintegrates in the presence of alkalis (high pH) and light, especially ultraviolet (UV) light.

Riboflavin functions as part of a group of enzymes involved in the breakdown and utilization of carbohydrates, fats, and protein. It is necessary for cell respiration because it works with enzymes in the utilization of cell oxygen. Riboflavin supports mitochondrial energy production by stimulating metabolism of fats, carbohydrates, and proteins. By the way, the *mitochondria* are the "energy producers" of the cell. Vitamin B_2 is required for red blood cell formation and respiration, antibody production, growth, and reproduction. It also helps in the prevention of many types of eye disorders, including bloodshot, itching, and burning eyes; cataracts; and abnormal sensitivity to light. This vitamin is necessary for the maintenance of good vision, skin, nails, and hair.

The RDA for riboflavin is 1.6 mg for adult males and 1.2 mg for adult females. During pregnancy and lactation, the requirement goes up to 1.5 mg and 1.7 mg, respectively. There are no known toxic side effects of the use of riboflavin. However, excessive amounts of vitamin B_2 make the retina extremely sensitive to light, and prolonged ingestion of large doses of any one of the B-complex vitamins, including riboflavin, may result in high urinary losses of the other B vitamins. Therefore, as mentioned previously, it is important to take a complete B complex along with any single B vitamin.

Riboflavin deficiency is the most common vitamin deficiency in the United States. This deficiency can result from long-established faulty dietary habits, food idiosyncrasies, alcoholism, arbitrarily selected diets used for the relief of digestive problems, and/or prolonged dietary restriction. Interestingly, undernourished women at the end of pregnancy often suffer from conditions such as visual disturbances, burning eyes, excessive tearing, and failing vision. Vitamin-B_2 deficiency is among those deficiencies often involved. The most common symptoms of a lack of B_2 are cracks and sores in the corners of the mouth; a red, sore tongue; a feeling of grit and sand on the insides of the eyelids; burning of the eyes; eye fatigue; dilation of the pupils; corneal changes; light sensitivity; lesions on the lips; scaling around the nose, mouth, or forehead; trembling; sluggishness; dizziness; and vaginal itching.

Riboflavin has found a new use in medicine as well for the condition known as keratoconus. Briefly, the eye is soaked with riboflavin and a UV light is emitted onto its surface. This interaction "stiffens" the cornea, therefore reducing the continued protrusion of the cornea. We will discuss this more in the section on keratoconus in Part Two.

Vitamin B_3 (Niacin). The next B vitamin on the list, vitamin B_3 or niacin, is more stable than either thiamine or riboflavin and is remarkably resistant to heat, light, air, acids, and alkalis. As a coenzyme, niacin assists enzymes in the breakdown and utilization of protein, fats, and carbohydrates. Niacin is effective at improving circulation and reducing the blood-cholesterol level. It is vital to the proper function of the nervous system and for the formation and maintenance of healthy tongue and digestive system tissues, as well as healthy skin.

Relatively small amounts of pure niacin are present in most foods. The niacin "equivalent" listed in some dietary tables refers either to pure niacin or to tryptophan, an amino acid that can be converted into niacin by the body. Lean meats, poultry, fish, and peanuts are rich sources of both niacin and tryptophan, as are such dietary supplements as brewer's yeast, wheat germ, and desiccated liver. Other than via the foods mentioned, niacin is difficult to obtain. Therefore, supplementation is recommended.

The RDA suggests that the daily allowance of niacin should be based on caloric intake, with 6.6 mg of niacin recommended for every 1,000 calories. There have been no toxic side effects reported for niacin, but taking extremely large doses can cause tingling and itching sensations, intense flushing of the skin, and throbbing in the head. There is also a possibility of a condition called *cystoid maculopathy,* where the macula of the retina swells, causing visual distortions. This condition is reversible when the overdose is stopped.

Excessive consumption of sugar and starches depletes the body's supply of niacin, as does taking certain antibiotics. The symptoms of niacin deficiency are numerous. In the early stages, they include weakness of the muscles, general fatigue, loss of appetite, indigestion, and various types of skin eruptions. Niacin deficiency may also cause bad breath, small ulcers, canker sores, chronic sleeplessness, irritability, nausea, vomiting, recurring headaches, tender gums, strain, tension, and deep depression.

Vitamin B$_5$ (Pantothenic Acid). Pantothenic acid, also known as vitamin B$_5$, is required for the conversion of carbohydrates, fats, and protein into usable energy for the body. It is necessary for the synthesis of red blood cells, the metabolism of steroids, and the synthesis of fatty acids, cholesterol, and other biological compounds. Pantothenic acid is the precursor of coenzyme A (CoA), which is necessary for mitochondrial energy production.

There are numerous foods that contain vitamin B$_5$. Among the best food sources of pantothenic acid are meat, poultry, free range eggs, nuts, molasses, oats, barley, green vegetables, cereal, yeast extract, dried brewer's yeast, wheat bran, and wheat germ.

The RDAs for pantothenic acid vary with age. In fact, the RDAs change frequently for the early years of life. Infants who are six months or younger should receive 1.7 mg of vitamin B$_5$ per day. The RDA climbs up to 1.8 mg for seven- to twelve-month olds. For children one to three years of age, 2 mg are recommended, and four- to eight-year-olds should have 3 mg of this vitamin. The RDA for young people aged nine to thirteen is 4 mg. Once an individual turns fourteen years of age, the RDA levels off at 5 mg and stays there, except during pregnancy and lactation, when it rises to 6 mg and 7 mg, respectively.

Pantothenic acid deficiency results in diminished adrenal gland function. A variety of metabolic problems will also manifest themselves. Fatigue is common, along with depression and problems associated with the digestive system. There will be loss of nerve function and problems with blood-sugar metabolism, with hypoglycemia being the most common. Pantothenic acid deficiency can reduce immune system responses, increasing the risk of infection. Other symptoms include skin problems, insomnia, lack of coordination, muscle cramps, and worsening of allergy symptoms.

Vitamin B$_6$ (Pyridoxine). Vitamin B$_6$ consists of three related compounds—pyridoxine, pyridoxal, and pyridoxamine. However, it is often simply referred to as pyridoxine. This member of the B-complex is required for the proper absorption of vitamin B_{12} and for the production of hydrochloric acid and magnesium. Pyridoxine plays an important role as a coenzyme in the breakdown and utilization of carbohydrates, fats, and protein. It is required for the production of antibodies and red blood cells. In addition, vitamin B_6 facilitates the body's release of glycogen, which is essentially a type of sugar used for energy. It is converted to pryidoxal-5 phosphate, which is directly involved in the creation of mitochondria. We lose mitochondria (energy producers in the cell) as we age, so increasing this vitamin with age is essential. And it helps to maintain the balance between sodium and potassium, which regulate the body's fluids and promote the normal functioning of the nervous and musculoskeletal systems.

The best sources of vitamin B_6 are meats and whole grains, specifically desiccated liver, and brewer's yeast. Regarding supplementation, according to the RDAs, the daily allowance of vitamin B_6 is based on protein intake. Adults need 2 mg of pyridoxine for every 100 grams (g) of protein they consume per day. Children need 0.6 to 1.2 mg for every 100 g of protein they consume. The need for vitamin B_6 doubles during pregnancy, lactation, exposure to radiation, cardiac failure, aging, and use of oral contraceptives.

Approximately 10 percent of the United States' population consumes less than half of the B_6 RDA. Recent epidemiological studies have indicated an association between B_6 deficiency and increased cancer. In cases of vitamin B_6 deficiency, there is low blood sugar and low glucose tolerance, resulting in sensitivity to insulin. Deficiency may also cause loss of hair, water retention during pregnancy, cracks around the mouth and eyes, numbness and cramps in the arms and legs, slow learning, visual disturbances, neuritis, arthritis, heart disorders, and increased urination.

Vitamin B_{12} (Cyanocobalamin). B-complex member vitamin B_{12} is unique in that it is the first cobalt-containing substance found to be essential for longevity. (*Cobalt* is an essential trace element for all multicellular organisms.) In addition, vitamin B_{12} is the only vitamin that contains essential mineral elements. It cannot be made synthetically, but must be grown, like penicillin, in bacteria or molds. One of the only foods in which B_{12} occurs naturally in substantial amounts is animal protein. Therefore, vegetarians frequently are low in vitamin B_{12}. At the same time, high blood levels of folic acid (discussed on page 80), also common in vegetarians, can mask a vitamin-B_{12} deficiency.

Vitamin B_{12} is necessary for the normal metabolism of nerve tissue. It is involved in protein, fat, and carbohydrate metabolism. And vitamin B_{12} is taken into the cells' mitochondria and plays an important role in amino acid metabolism. The actions of B_{12} are closely related to those of four amino acids, as well as vitamin B_5, and vitamin C. Vitamin B_{12} also helps iron to function better in the body, and it aids folic acid in the synthesis of choline.

Liver is the best source of vitamin B_{12}. Kidney, muscle meats, fish, and dairy products are other good sources. The human requirement for vitamin B_{12} is minute, but the vitamin is essential to health.

The RDA for vitamin B_{12} is 3 micrograms (mcg) for adults and 4 mcg for pregnant and lactating women. Infants require a daily intake of 3 mcg, and growing children need 1 to 2 mcg. No cases of vitamin-B_{12} toxicity have ever been reported.

Deficiency of the vitamin is usually due to a lack of the *intrinsic factor,* a glycoprotein necessary for the absorption of B_{12}. The symptoms of a vitamin-B_{12} deficiency may take five or six years to appear. Deficiency begins with changes in the nervous system, such as soreness and weakness in the legs and arms, diminished reflex response and sensory perception, difficulty walking and speaking, and jerking of the limbs. A B_{12} deficiency has been shown to affect 10 to 15 percent of individuals over the age of sixty in the United States. Patients with B_{12} deficiency exhibit *megaloblastic anemia,* a type of anemia in which the red blood cells are larger than normal and don't have contents that are fully developed. This problem causes the bone marrow to manufacture fewer red blood cells. Moreover, the ones produced might not live for the full life expectancy of 120 days. Vitamin B_{12}-deficient people also often suffer from *hyperhomocysteinemia,* or increased levels of homocysteine—an amino acid that causes blood-vessel destruction if it is found in large amounts. In regard to the eyes, hyperhomocysteinemia has been associated with increasing the risk of dry macular degeneration progressing to wet macular degeneration.

Interestingly, the condition known as *tobacco amblyopia,* a loss of vision due to tobacco poisoning, has been improved with injections of vitamin B_{12}. This was found to be true whether or not the patient stopped smoking. The symptoms of tobacco amblyopia are blackouts, headaches, and farsightedness.

Vitamin H (Biotin). Vitamin H, or biotin, is used in cell growth, the production of fatty acids, and in the metabolism of fats and proteins. It plays a role in the *Krebs cycle,* which is the process in which energy is released from food. Biotin is also indicated for healthy hair and skin, sweat glands, nerve tissue, and bone marrow, and it takes part in alleviating muscle pain. Vitamin H not only assists in various metabolic chemical conversions, but it also helps with the transfer of carbon dioxide. Finally, biotin is helpful in maintaining a steady blood-sugar level.

Food sources of biotin are varied. Beans, peas, cauliflower, and avocados are good sources. So are bran cereals, bread, brown rice, oatmeal, and wheat germ. Mackerel, herring, and other fish are rich in biotin, as well as egg yolks, nuts, molasses, currants, and liver and kidney meats.

The RDA for biotin is 300 mcg (0.3 mg) per day for adults. The same dosage is recommended for pregnant and lactating women. (There is no recommended dose for children.) Although a shortage of biotin is very rare, it can happen and may result in dry and scaly skin, fatigue, loss of appetite, nausea and vomiting, mental depression, as well as tongue inflammation and high cholesterol. Researchers have found that biotin deficiency depletes the amino acid *glycine* from the process by which the cells' mitochondria are healthy and function properly.

Choline. Choline, considered one of the B-complex vitamins, functions with inositol, also considered a B-complex vitamin, as a basic constituent of *lecithin,* a lipid or fatty substance. Choline is present in the bodies of all living cells, and it is widely distributed in animal and plant tissues.

Choline appears to be associated primarily with the utilization of fats and cholesterol in the body. It prevents fats from accumulating in the liver and facilitates their movement into the cells. In the liver, choline combines with fatty acids and phosphoric acid to form lecithin. It is essential for the health of the liver and kidneys. Choline is also essential for the health of the myelin sheaths of the nerves. The myelin sheaths are the principal components of the nerve fibers. Choline plays an important role in the transmission of the nerve impulses. It also helps to regulate and improve liver and gallbladder function, and choline aids in the prevention of gallstones.

Lecithin is the richest source of choline, but other rich dietary sources are egg yolks, liver, brewer's yeast, and wheat germ. The daily requirements for choline are not known. The average American adult diet has been estimated to contain 500 to 900 mg of choline per day.

Folate. Folate (vitamin B_9) acid is part of the vitamin B complex and functions as a coenzyme, together with vitamins B_{12} and C, in the breakdown and utilization of proteins. Folate performs its basic role as a carbon carrier in the formation of *heme*—the iron-containing protein found in hemoglobin. It is also needed for the formation of nucleic acid, which is essential for the processes of growth and reproduction of all body cells. And folic acid is critical in the development of the fetus' spine and nervous system during pregnancy; a deficiency has been linked to spinal disorders.

Folic acid is a synthetic form of vitamin B_9.

Your body does not convert it into active vitamin B_9 very well, so unmetabolized folic acid may build up in your bloodstream. Researchers are concerned that high levels of unmetabolized folic acid may negatively affect health, but more studies are needed before any strong conclusions can be reached.

High-folate foods include asparagus, avocados, Brussels sprouts, and leafy greens like spinach and lettuce. However, for some people, such as pregnant women, supplements are an easy way to ensure adequate vitamin B_9 intake. The recommended allowance of folate is 400 mcg per day for adults, 800 mcg during pregnancy, and 600 mcg during lactation. There is no known toxicity associated with this vitamin. Many nutritional supplements use folic acid due to its lower cost.

Now you have a solid background on the B-complex vitamins. These vitamins are clearly very important to everything from basic metabolism of food to nerve function, mood, and eye health. Therefore, it is important to confirm with your doctor or nutritionist that you are getting adequate amounts.

Vitamin C

Vitamin C, also known as ascorbic acid, is a water-soluble nutrient. Although fairly stable in acid solutions, it is normally the least stable of the vitamins when exposed to air and is very sensitive to oxygen. Its potency can be lost through exposure to light, heat, or air, all of which stimulate the activity of the oxidative enzymes.

The primary function of vitamin C is to maintain the body's collagen, a protein necessary for the formation of the connective tissue in the skin, ligaments, bones, and, most importantly for this book's purposes, sclera of the eye. Vitamin C plays a role in the healing of wounds and burns because it facilitates the formation of connective tissue in scars. It also aids in the formation of red blood cells and the prevention of hemorrhaging. In addition, vitamin C prevents and cures some types of viral and bacterial infections and reduces the effects of some allergens. For these reasons, vitamin C is frequently used in the prevention and treatment of the common cold. And vitamin C promotes bone and tooth formation while protecting the dentine and pulp of teeth.

Vitamin C is present in most fresh fruits and vegetables. Natural vitamin C dietary supplements are prepared from rose hips, acerola cherries, green peppers, and citrus fruits. The level of ascorbic acid in the blood reaches a maximum about two or three hours after the ingestion of a moderate quantity of the nutrient, then decreases as the vitamin is eliminated in the urine and through perspiration. Most vitamin C is out of the body in three to four hours.

Because vitamin C is a "stress vitamin," it is used up even more rapidly under stressful conditions. Humans, apes, and guinea pigs are the only animals that must obtain vitamin C from their food because they are unable to meet the body's needs by synthesis alone. Ascorbic acid is readily absorbed from the gastrointestinal tract into the bloodstream. Two factors that influence its absorption are the manner in which the vitamin is administered and the presence of other substances in the intestinal tract. The normal human body, when fully saturated, contains about 5,000 mg

of vitamin C, of which 30 mg are found in the adrenal glands, 200 mg in the extracellular fluids, and the rest in varying concentrations throughout the cells of the entire body.

The RDA for vitamin C is 45 mg for adults. However, during his famous career, the researcher Dr. Linus Pauling suggested that the optimal daily intake of vitamin C for most human adults is from 2,300 to 9,000 mg. This wide range takes into account differences in weight, activity level, metabolism, ailments, and age.

One school of thought regarding the effects of vitamin C on the development of nearsightedness is that the vitamin fortifies the sclera of the eye, as the sclera is connective tissue. If there is a lack of vitamin C for an extended period of time, especially during the high growth years, the eye structure will weaken, allowing the pressure inside the eye (due to an increase in near-viewing tasks) to expand the length of the eye, which leads to nearsightedness. In addition, it is a fact that the fluid filling the anterior chamber of the eye—the space between the cornea and the lens—maintains a vitamin C level approximately twenty times higher than that of the blood plasma. This is considered significant in the nutrition of the lens, which has no blood supply and depends entirely on the aqueous fluid for its nourishment. It only stands to reason that the level of vitamin C should be upheld or increased as we age to maintain a clear and healthy lens within the eye.

Toxicity symptoms usually do not occur with high intakes of vitamin C because the body simply discharges whatever it cannot use. However, a daily intake of 5,000 to 15,000 mg may cause side effects in some people.

If present, toxicity symptoms of vitamin C include a slight burning sensation during urination, loose bowels, and skin rashes.

The body's ability to absorb vitamin C is reduced by smoking, stress, high fever, prolonged intake of antibiotics or cortisone, inhalation of petroleum fumes, and ingestion of aspirin or other painkillers. Baking soda destroys vitamin C, as does cooking with copper utensils. The signs of deficiency include shortness of breath, impaired digestion, poor lactation, bleeding gums, weakened tooth enamel or dentine, tendency toward bruising, swollen or painful joints, nosebleeds, anemia, lowered resistance to infections, and slow healing of wounds. Severe deficiency results in scurvy, which is a disease that causes a reduction of collagen creation in the body.

Vitamin D

Vitamin D is a fat-soluble vitamin that can be acquired both from food and through exposure to sunlight. It is known as the "sunshine vitamin" because the sun's UV rays activate a form of cholesterol present in the skin and convert the substance to vitamin D.

Vitamin D aids in the absorption of calcium from the intestinal tract, and in the breakdown and assimilation of phosphorus, which is required for bone formation. In the mucous membranes, vitamin D helps to synthesize enzymes that are involved in the active transport of available calcium. Vitamin D is necessary for normal growth in children, for without it, the bones and teeth do not calcify properly. But adults also certainly benefit from vitamin D. It is valuable for maintaining a stable nervous system, normal heart action,

increased imune support and normal blood clotting because all of these functions are related to the body's supply and utilization of calcium and phosphorus.

Most of the body's need for vitamin D can be met by sufficient exposure to sunlight and the ingestion of small amounts of fortified foods. In fact, fortified foods represent the major dietary sources of vitamin D, as very few foods naturally contain significant amounts of vitamin D. However, fish is an excellent source of this important vitamin.

The sun's action on the skin can be inhibited by such factors as air pollution, clouds, window glass, and clothing. The RDA for vitamin D is set at 400 IU per day, which should meet the requirements of most healthy individuals who are not regularly exposed to UV light. But because deficiencies have been found to be so common, experts expect the RDA to go as high as 2,000 IU. Vitamin D is best utilized by the body when taken with vitamin A. Fish-liver oils are the best natural sources of vitamins A and D.

Because vitamin D is fat-soluble, it can be stored in the body. Excessive blood levels of the vitamin often cause a rise in the blood levels of calcium and phosphorus, as well as excessive excretion of calcium in the urine. This leads to calcification and therefore loss of flexibility of the soft tissues and of the walls of the blood vessels and kidney tubules, a condition known as *hypercalcemia*. The symptoms of acute overdosage are increased frequency of urination, loss of appetite, nausea, vomiting, diarrhea, muscular weakness, dizziness, and calcification of the soft tissues of the heart, blood vessels, and lungs. These symptoms disappear soon after the discontinuation of overdosing.

A deficiency of vitamin D leads to inadequate absorption of calcium from the intestinal tract and inadequate retention of phosphorus in the kidneys. Without proper levels of calcium and phosphorus, the bones become soft and cannot withstand the stress of the body's weight, resulting in skeletal malformations. Proper absorption of vitamin D is associated with levels of Vitamin K_2; thus, both should be in any supplement. *Rickets,* a bone disorder in children which can lead to bowed legs, is a direct result of vitamin-D deficiency. Adult rickets, called *osteomalacia,* can also occur. As far as the eyes are concerned, one study showed that a vitamin-D deficiency might cause nearsightedness, although other studies do not support that conclusion. An imbalance of the vitamin with calcium is at the root of this disorder. Other possible effects are keratoconus (cone-shaped cornea), pinkeye, cataracts, and arteriosclerosis.

Vitamin E

Vitamin E, a fat-soluble vitamin, is composed of two groups of compounds called *tocopherols* and *tocotrienols*. Four forms of each—alpha, beta, gamma, and delta—exist in nature. Of these various forms, alpha tocopherol is the most common in nutritional supplements.

Vitamin E is an antioxidant, which means that it opposes the oxidation of substances in the body. (Antioxidants are specifically discussed on page 97.) It plays an essential role in the cellular respiration of the muscles, especially the cardiac and skeletal muscles. Moreover, it makes it possible for these muscles and their nerves to function with less oxygen, thereby increasing their endurance and stamina. Vitamin E also causes dilation of the blood vessels, permitting a fuller flow of blood to the heart, as well as to the other organs. As a diuretic, vitamin E helps to lower elevated blood pressure.

There are numerous skin and tissue benefits associated with vitamin E. It is effective against the formation of elevated scar tissue both on the surface of the body and within the body. In ointment form, it is used on burns to promote healing and to lessen the formation of scars in general. Similarly, it helps to remedy skin ulcers and abrasions. It is also helpful in counteracting premature aging of the skin. For maximum benefit, apply vitamin E to the skin in ointment form while also taking it orally, because it affects cell formation by replacing the cells on the outer layer of the skin.

Vitamin E also helps to counter the gradual decline in metabolic processes during aging. And it protects against the damaging effects of many environmental poisons in the air, water, and food. As if that weren't enough, it works to treat and prevent heart diseases, such as *coronary thrombosis,* which is a heart attack caused by vessels being blocked by blood clots. Vitamin E causes arterial blood clots to disintegrate. *Angina,* a condition in which chest pain results from an insufficient supply of blood to the heart tissues, is successfully treated with alpha tocopherol. And vitamin E is beneficial to people with *atherosclerosis*—a build-up of plaque in the vessels—if used as a therapy before irreparable damage occurs. It relieves pain in the extremities, speeds up blood flow, and reduces clotting tendencies. Vitamin E therapy has been suggested as beneficial in a number of other conditions, including bursitis (inflammation of a bursa resulting in joint pain), gout (defective uric-acid metabolism), arthritis, varicose veins, thrombosis (thickening of the blood resulting in blood clots), phlebitis (inflammation of the wall of a vein), nephritis (a problem of the kidneys), and even headaches.

The tocopherols occur in the highest concentrations in cold-pressed vegetable oils, whole raw seeds and nuts, and soybeans. Wheat germ oil is the source from which vitamin E was first obtained. The RDA for vitamin E is based upon *metabolic* body size—how fast of a metabolic rate the body has—and level of polyunsaturated fatty acids in the diet, rather than upon body weight or caloric intake. More specifically, the requirements increase along with any increases in the amount of polyunsaturated fatty acids consumed. The RDA is 4 to 5 IU daily for infants; 7 to 12 IU for children and adolescents; 15 IU for adult males; 12 IU for adult females; and 15 IU for pregnant and lactating females. However, many nutritionists consider these allowances exceedingly low and therefore recommend much higher doses for optimal benefits. Most sources suggest a daily dosage of 300 to 400 IU of vitamin E per day.

There are several substances that interfere with, or even cause a depletion of, vitamin E in the body. For example, when iron, especially the inorganic form, and vitamin E are administered together, the absorption of *both* is impaired. Chlorine in drinking water, ferric chloride, rancid oil or fat, and inorganic-iron compounds destroy vitamin E in the body. Mineral oil used as a laxative depletes vitamin E. As suggested above, large amounts of polyunsaturated fats or oils in the diet compromise vitamin E in the body; they increase the oxidation rate of vitamin E. In addition, the more unsaturated fats or oils that are consumed, the more vitamin E that is necessary.

The first sign of a vitamin E deficiency is the rupture of red blood cells, resulting from the cells' increased fragility. This can appear as fatigue, weakness, and paleness. A deficiency could result in a reduction of membrane stability and shrinkage of collagen. Also, a tendency toward muscular wasting or abnormal fat deposits in the muscles, and an increased demand for oxygen, can occur in a deficiency state. The essential fatty acids are altered so that blood cells break down and hemoglobin formation is impaired. In addition, the body's ability to utilize several amino acids is compromised, and the level of functioning of the pituitary and adrenal glands is reduced. Iron absorption and hemoglobin formation also are impaired. A severe deficiency can cause damage to the kidneys and liver. And a prolonged deficiency of vitamin E can cause faulty absorption of fat and the fat-soluble vitamins. Lastly, poor utilization of vitamin E or an increased demand for it can result in anemia.

There has been a concern in one research study about the over-dosage of vitamin E as a supplement to the diet. This isolated finding applied only to an older group of patients (over the age of seventy) with long histories of heart disease, stroke, or diabetes, who were also taking a combination of medications during the course of the study. In addition, a significant percentage of study participants were also cigarette smokers, further clouding the issue. Thus, the results of the study should be viewed in that light.

The Council for Responsible Nutrition continues to support the safe upper limits of vitamin E established by the Food and

Nutrition Board at the Institute of Medicine. The published safe daily upper limits (ULs) are 1,000 IUs of synthetic vitamin E and 1,500 IUs of natural vitamin E. However, under normal circumstances, a daily supplement of 200 IU is adequate.

Be aware of the type of vitamin E you take because, as just stated, there are natural and synthetic types. The *d-form* of vitamin E, derived from vegetable oils and other natural sources, is different from the *dl-form*, which is often called the synthetic form. The dl-tocopherols are actually a mixture containing the d-form and an l-form (usually a 1:1 mixture). The human body uses only the d-form. The dl-form, when present, does not confer any known health benefit and is normally excreted by the body. So, in essence, when consuming the dl-form of vitamin E, you obtain an *effective dose* of about half the vitamin E dosage reported on the label. But all in all, the prevention of vitamin E deficiency should not be a concern for most people in the United States, since the vitamin is found in a wide variety of foods.

Vitamin P (Bioflavonoids)

More commonly called the bioflavonoids, vitamin P is water-soluble and composed of a group of brightly colored substances that often appear in fruits and vegetables as companions to vitamin C. The members of the group are citrin, hesperidin, rutin, the flavones, and the flavonols. These micronutrients were first discovered as substances in the white part, not the juice, of citrus fruits. The solid part of citrus fruits contains ten times more bioflavonoids than the strained juice.

The bioflavonoids are essential for the proper absorption and use of vitamin C. They assist vitamin C in keeping the collagen in healthy condition. They also have the ability to increase the strength of the capillaries and to regulate the permeability of the capillaries. These actions help to prevent hemorrhages and ruptures in both the capillaries and the connective tissue, and to build a barrier that protects the body against infection. Importantly, the blood-vessel leakage that occurs within the retina of the eye—and is most often associated with diabetes, macular degeneration, and hypertension—may be reduced to some degree by the use of a combination of vitamin C and bioflavonoids.

The main sources of the bioflavonoids include lemons, grapes, plums, black currants, grapefruits, apricots, buckwheat, cherries, blackberries, and rose hips. The absorption and storage properties, daily requirements, deficiency symptoms, and body utilization of the bioflavonoids are all similar to those of vitamin C. So please see the section on vitamin C (page 80) for guidelines regarding supplementation.

Other Important Micronutrients

We've discussed a number of vitamins that are crucial to general health maintenance and, more specifically, to eye health. By now, it probably has become clear that a proper balance of these vitamins is as essential as the individual supplementation recommended for each. And the truth is, we're not done with our discussion of the micronutrients yet. There are additional natural substances to consider taking for optimal well-being and visual health.

Acetyl-L-Carnitine (ALC)

ALC is actually a delivery form for an amino acid called L-carnitine. It transports omega-3 long-chain fatty acids across the mitochondrial membranes into the mitochondria, which, remember, are the energy-producing parts of the cell. ALC also transports small-chain and medium-chain fatty acids out of the mitochondria in order to maintain normal coenzyme-A levels in these organelles within the cell. (Coenzyme A plays an important role in synthesizing and metabolizing fatty acids.) This is particularly important for maintenance of retina health, since the retinal cells have more mitochondria than any other cell in the body.

ALC levels may decrease with advancing age. However, because it is not an essential nutrient, true deficiency does not occur. There are natural dietary sources of ALC, the primary one being red meat. Vegetables and grains also contain a certain amount. Most research involving acetyl-L-carnitine supplementation has used 500 mg, three times per day, as the suggested optimal dose, though some research recommends double this amount.

Side effects from taking acetyl-L-carnitine are uncommon. However, skin rash, increased appetite, nausea, vomiting, agitation, and body odor have been reported in people taking it.

Coenzyme Q_{10} (CoQ_{10})

CoQ_{10} is a fat-soluble compound primarily synthesized by the body but also consumed in the diet. It is required for mitochondrial energy synthesis and functions as an antioxidant in cell membranes and lipoproteins. (As its name suggests, a lipoprotein is a structure of lipids—or fats—and protein that carries fats around inside the body.) But the primary function of CoQ_{10} is as a catalyst for metabolism—the complex chain of chemical reactions during which food is broken down into packets of energy that the body can use. Acting in conjunction with enzymes, this compound speeds up the vital metabolic process, providing the energy that the cells need to digest food, heal wounds, maintain healthy muscles, and perform countless other bodily functions.

Because of this nutrient's essential role in energy production, it's not surprising that it is found in every cell in the body. CoQ_{10} is especially abundant in the energy-intensive cells of the heart. In addition, CoQ_{10} acts as an antioxidant, much like vitamins C and E, helping to neutralize the cell-damaging free radicals.

CoQ_{10} may play a role in the prevention of cancer, heart attacks, and other diseases linked to free-radical damage. It's also used as a general energy enhancer and anti-aging supplement. CoQ_{10} does not directly affect the eye by itself. However, a study on age-related macular degeneration (AMD) showed that CoQ_{10} in combination with acetyl-L-carnitine and essential fatty acids can actually reverse the signs of macular degeneration!

Because levels of CoQ_{10} diminish with age (and with certain diseases), some doctors recommend daily supplementation beginning at approximately forty years of age. A standard daily dosage is about 30 mg per day. However, statin drugs, often prescribed for elevated cholesterol levels, deplete CoQ_{10} levels; therefore CoQ_{10} supplements (at least 100 mg daily) should be routinely taken with all statin drugs.

Lipoic Acid

Lipoic acid is both water- and fat-soluble and is a vital cofactor for the production of enzymes necessary for mitochondrial function. Also known as alpha-lipoic acid, it works together with other antioxidants such as vitamins C and E. Lipoic acid is important for growth, helps to prevent cell damage, and helps the body rid itself of harmful substances.

Lipoic acid therapy has also been used in the treatment of diabetes and its associated symptoms. Several studies suggest that supplementing with lipoic acid may help reduce *peripheral neuropathy*—pain, burning, itching, tingling, and numbness—in people who have nerve damage caused by diabetes. Lipoic acid has been used for years for this purpose in Europe. Other studies have shown that lipoic acid speeds the removal of glucose (sugar) from the blood of people with diabetes and that this antioxidant may prevent kidney damage associated with diabetes in animals.

The benefits of lipoic acid continue from there. It may prove useful in the treatment of chronic hepatitis, for lipoic acid has been found to relieve stress on the liver and help rid the body of toxins. There have been several case reports of use of alpha-lipoic acid in combination with silymarin (milk thistle) and selenium (a substance with liver-protecting and antioxidant properties) to help treat hepatitis C.

Because lipoic acid can pass easily into the brain, it has protective effects on brain and nerve tissue and shows promise as a treatment for stroke and other brain disorders involving free-radical damage. Animals treated with alpha-lipoic acid, for example, suffered less brain damage and

had a four-times-greater survival rate after a stroke than the animals who did not receive this supplement. While animal studies are encouraging, more research is needed to understand whether this benefit applies to people as well. Additional conditions for which alpha-lipoic acid may prove useful include heart failure, human immunodeficiency virus (HIV), cataracts, and glaucoma. More research is underway in these areas.

Good food sources of lipoic acid include spinach, broccoli, beef, yeast (particularly brewer's yeast), and certain organ meats (such as kidney and heart). While most of us get an adequate intake, a supplement of 150 mg per day is advised for general health maintenance.

Minerals

Minerals are nutrients that exist in the body and in food, in organic and inorganic combinations. In fact, all of the tissues and internal fluids of living things contain varying quantities of minerals. Approximately fifteen minerals are essential in human nutrition. There are two main divisions: macrominerals (which are needed in larger amounts) and microminerals (which are needed in smaller amounts). Although minerals make up only 4 or 5 percent of the human body's weight, they are vital to overall mental and physical well-being. Minerals are constituents of the bones, teeth, soft tissue, muscle, blood, and nerve cells. They are important in maintaining the physiological processes, strengthening the skeletal structure, and preserving the vigor of the heart, the brain, and all of the muscle and nerve systems.

Although we will discuss a number of minerals separately in the following pages, it is important to note that the actions of the minerals within the body are interrelated; no one mineral functions without affecting the others. Also, physical and emotional stress can cause a strain on the body's supply of minerals. A mineral deficiency often results in illness, which may be corrected by adding the missing mineral to the diet. Thus, maintaining adequate levels of minerals is a key to optimal health.

Calcium

Calcium is the most abundant mineral in the body. About 99 percent of the calcium in the body is deposited in the bones and teeth, with the remainder found in the soft tissues. To function properly, calcium must be accompanied by magnesium, phosphorus, and vitamins A, C, and especially D. Within cells, calcium is stored in the mitochondria.

Calcium's powerful effects are plentiful. This mineral is essential for healthy blood. It eases insomnia and helps to regulate the heartbeat. Calcium assists in the process of blood clotting and aids in preventing the accumulation of too much acid or alkali in the blood. It also plays a part in muscle growth, muscle contraction, and nerve transmission. Calcium assists in the body's utilization of iron, activation of several enzymes, and regulation of the passage of nutrients in and out of cell walls in a process called *cell signaling*. It also plays a role in the collagen build-up in the sclera of the eye.

Calcium absorption is very inefficient; usually only 20 to 30 percent of ingested calcium is absorbed. When it needs calcium, however, the body can absorb it more effectively. Therefore, the greater the need for calcium is and the smaller the dietary supply is, the more efficient the absorption is. Absorption is also increased during periods of rapid growth. Calcium absorption depends upon the presence of adequate amounts of vitamin D, which works with the parathyroid hormone to regulate the amount of calcium in the blood. Moreover, vitamins A and C, and small amounts of consumed fats, phosphorus, and protein all facilitate calcium absorption.

Excellent food sources of calcium include dairy products and dark green leafy vegetables such as spinach, collard greens, mustard greens, and turnip greens. The daily recommended dosage of calcium varies with age. It is suggested that infants intake about 200 mg of calcium per day. That dosage should then be increased by about 300 mg every few years. Adults require approximately 1,000 mg daily, while seniors need about 1,200 mg per day.

There is a possibility of "over-calcification" with the ingestion of excessive amounts of calcium over a long period of time. This condition can lead to kidney stones, mitral valve disease, and calcification of the small and large blood vessels, which includes the vessels of the eyes. If you wear gas permeable contact lenses (see page 341) and notice that they get deposits on them frequently, one possible cause may be an excess intake of calcium. Check with your contact lens professional.

It is important to understand that certain substances inhibit calcium absorption. When excessive amounts of fat combine with calcium, the result is an insoluble compound

DIABETES AND THE GLYCEMIC INDEX

Diabetes is a disease in which the body does not produce or properly use *insulin,* a hormone that is required to convert sugar, starches, and other food into energy needed for daily life. Insulin is secreted by the pancreas. The cause of diabetes continues to be a mystery, although both genetics and lifestyle factors such as obesity and lack of exercise appear to play roles. Some figures from 2018 report that about 34.2 million children and adults in the United States, or almost 10.5 percent of the population, have diabetes. Others state that 7.3 million people have the disease but are not aware of it, and perhaps 96 million more have pre-diabetes.

There are several types of diabetes. Type 1 diabetes results from the body's failure to produce the insulin that "unlocks" the cells of the body, allowing glucose to enter and fuel them. It is estimated that 5 to 10 percent of Americans who are diagnosed with diabetes have type 1 diabetes. At one time, this was called "juvenile" diabetes because it was most often found in children. However, with the increase in diabetes in children caused by obesity, more recently, this disorder simply has been called "type 1."

Type 2 diabetes is the most common form of diabetes. In type 2 diabetes, either the body does not produce enough insulin or the cells ignore the insulin. Sugar is the basic fuel for the cells in the body, and insulin normally takes the sugar from the blood into the cells. When glucose builds up in the blood instead of going into cells, it can cause two problems:

first, in the present, your cells may be starved for energy; second, over time, high blood-glucose levels may hurt your eyes, kidneys, nerves, and/or heart.

While diabetes occurs in people of all ages and races, some groups have a higher risk for developing type 2 diabetes than others. The disease is more common in African Americans, Latinos, Native Americans, and Asian Americans/Pacific Islanders, as well as the aged population.

Eye problems associated with diabetes will be covered in more detail in the section on diabetic retinopathy found in Part Two (see page 205). But let's cover a few facts here. People with diabetes are 40 percent more likely to suffer from glaucoma than people without diabetes. The longer someone has had diabetes, the more common glaucoma is. Also, while many people without diabetes get cataracts, people with diabetes are 60 percent more likely to develop this eye condition. And those who have diabetes also tend to get cataracts at a younger age and have them progress faster.

The glycemic index (GI) is a way of describing how a carbohydrate-containing food affects blood-glucose levels. Just like a car needs fuel, our body needs carbohydrates to run. When we eat carbohydrates, our body breaks them down to produce glucose. Our cells use this glucose as their main energy source. As described, for glucose to move from the blood into the body's cells, insulin is needed. Insulin is stimulated whenever there is glucose in the blood. However, if there is insufficient insulin, which occurs in individuals who have diabetes, glucose levels will rise. Insulin is not only involved in regulating blood-glucose levels, but also plays a key role in determining whether our bodies burn fat or carbohydrates for energy. High levels of insulin means the body is forced to burn carbohydrates rather than fat. Therefore, by controlling the rate of glucose being absorbed, we also control the amount of insulin secreted. This is where the glycemic index comes into play.

Foods and drinks that carry a high glycemic index trigger an undesirable insulin response. This reaction results in an excess of insulin in the bloodstream. Controlling the glycemic index of foods and drinks allows for control over food-driven insulin stimulation and then

reactive hypoglycemia (or low blood sugar). The GI of foods may have important implications for the prevention and treatment of the major causes of sickness and death in Western countries, including obesity, cardiovascular disease, and type 2 diabetes. Furthermore, considerable evidence exists sup- porting the value of a low-GI (below 55) diet for individuals with hyperlipidemia (high cholesterol) and for prolonging endurance during physical activity, improving insulin sensitivity, reducing food intake, and increasing colonic fermentation (important for those who are lactose intolerant). For more information on the glycemic index, see the inset on page 65 and visit websites such as www.glycemicindex.com, which provides the GI for many common foods.

that cannot be absorbed. Vitamin K_2 should be taken with calcium to assure that the mineral gets to the bones and not just lodged into the lining of the blood vessels. Calcium combined with oxalic acid, found in chocolate, spinach, and rhubarb, makes another insoluble compound that may form into stones in the kidneys or gallbladder. Other interfering factors are lack of exercise, excessive stress, and too rapid a flow of food through the intestinal tract.

One of the first signs of a calcium deficiency is a nervous affliction called *tetany*, which is characterized by muscle cramps, as well as numbness and tingling in the arms and hands. Some people may experience eyelid twitches as well. A calcium deficiency can result in bone

malformation, causing what is referred to as *rickets* in children and *osteomalacia* in adults. Another ailment that results from calcium deficiency is *osteoporosis*, in which the bones become porous and fragile because calcium is withdrawn from them, as well as from other body areas, faster than it is deposited. Moderate cases of calcium deficiency may lead to cramps, joint pains, heart palpitations, eyelid twitching, slow pulse rate, tooth decay, insomnia, impaired growth, and excessive irritability of the nerves and muscles.

Chromium

Chromium is an essential mineral found in concentrations of twenty parts of chromium to one billion parts of blood. It stimulates the activity of enzymes involved in the metabolism of glucose for energy and the synthesis of fatty acids and cholesterol. Chromium also appears to increase the effectiveness of insulin, thereby facilitating the transport of glucose into the cells. (For more on insulin and glucose uptake, see the inset on diabetes and the glycemic index, page 89.) In the blood, it competes with iron in the transport of protein. Chromium may also be involved in the synthesis of protein through its binding action with *ribonucleic acid (RNA) molecules*. RNA is the building block of protein that is formed from DNA in the nucleus of the cell.

The sources of chromium include corn oil, clams, whole-grain cereals, and meats. Fruits and vegetables contain trace amounts. Brewer's yeast provides a dependable supply without the problems of high carbohydrate intake and high cholesterol levels. But chromium is difficult to absorb. Only about 3 percent of dietary chromium is retained in the body, and the amount of chromium stored in the body decreases with age. The best form of supplemental chromium is called *polynicotinate,* and we need only about 200 micrograms (mcg) per day as a supplement.

A chromium deficiency may upset the function of insulin and result in depressed growth rates and severe glucose intolerance in diabetics. It is also believed that the interaction of chromium and insulin is not limited to glucose metabolism but also affects amino-acid metabolism. Chromium may inhibit the formation of aortic plaques, and a deficiency may contribute to atherosclerosis. Finally, chromium deficiency has also been shown to be found in cases of myopia.

Copper

Copper is a trace mineral in the body. This means that it is essential for good health, but that only a tiny amount is needed. When excess copper accumulates, it is stored in the eyes, brain, kidneys, and liver; damage usually occurs as a result. For example, excess copper that collects in the liver causes *cirrhosis* of the liver, which is a serious, life-threatening condition. While copper doesn't directly affect any eye condition, the blood vessels in the eye are comparable to the blood vessels in the kidney. In fact, in Chinese medicine, the same remedies are given for conditions that affect the kidneys and the eyes. So that is something to seriously consider when choosing a multiple vitamin supplement. Copper also facilitates zinc absorption, so there must be a balance of copper and zinc.

Copper is found in different amounts in a wide variety of foods. For example, most nuts (especially Brazil nuts and cashews) contain copper, as well as seeds (especially poppy and sunflower), chickpeas (garbanzo beans), liver, and oysters. The dietary supplement intake of copper should be less than 1 mg per day.

Wilson's disease is a hereditary disorder in which the body retains too much copper. However, Wilson's disease is treatable. Dietary restriction alone is usually not enough to control the disorder. Still, it is helpful to avoid copper-rich foods as much as possible if you suffer from Wilson's disease. In general, chronic copper poisoning is very rare, and usually involves patients with liver disease. The capacity for healthy human livers to excrete copper is considerable, and it is primarily for this reason that no cases of chronic copper poisoning in otherwise healthy individuals have been reported.

Iron

The mineral iron is part of *hemoglobin*, the oxygen-carrying component of the blood. In addition, although iron is part of the antioxidant enzyme *catalase,* iron is not generally considered an antioxidant because too much iron can cause oxidative damage. But on the other side of the spectrum, iron-deficient people tire easily because their bodies are starved for oxygen. Iron is also part of *myoglobin*, which helps muscle cells store oxygen. Without enough iron, *ATP*—the fuel the body runs on—cannot be properly synthesized. As a result, some iron-deficient people become fatigued even when their hemoglobin levels are normal.

Iron balance naturally declines with age. In fact, normal aging of the brain and neuro-degenerative (or brain-degenerative) changes share certain changes with the retina, including mitochondrial dysfunction, oxidative stress, and loss of iron balance. So signs of a declining iron level can be found in the eyes. Actually, it is becoming clear that many organs show various changes before hemoglobin levels change. *Heme*—a red pigment that is complex in nature and is composed of iron as well as other atoms that bind to oxygen—is synthesized in the mitochondria, and the decline in synthesis could explain the loss of iron in aging.

The most absorbable form of iron, called *heme iron,* is found in oysters, meat, poultry, and fish. *Non-heme iron* is also found in these foods, as well as in dried fruit, molasses, leafy green vegetables, wine, and most iron supplements. Acidic foods (such as tomato sauce) cooked in an iron pan can also be a source of dietary iron.

Vegetarians consume less iron than non-vegetarians, and the iron they ingest is somewhat less absorbable. As a result, vegetarians are more likely to have reduced iron stores. However, iron deficiency is not usually caused by a lack of iron in the diet alone; an underlying cause, such as iron loss due to the shedding of menstrual blood, often exists. Pregnant women, marathon runners, and people who take aspirin are likely to become iron deficient. So are those who have parasitic infections, hemorrhoids, ulcers, ulcerative colitis, Crohn's disease, gastrointestinal cancers, and other conditions that cause blood loss or mal-absorption of iron.

Yet individuals who fit into one of these groups—even pregnant women—shouldn't automatically take iron supplements. A nutritionally oriented doctor should assess the need for iron supplements, since taking iron when it isn't needed does no good and may do some harm. In fact, it is generally agreed these days that, unless you're a menstruating woman, you do not need any iron supplementation. But if a nutritionally oriented doctor diagnoses iron deficiency, iron supplementation is essential. A common adult dose is 100 mg per day. When iron deficiency is diagnosed, the doctor must also determine the cause. Usually, it's not serious; common causes include menstruation and the donation of blood. Many pre-menopausal women become marginally iron deficient unless they supplement with iron. In such cases, the 18 mg of iron present in most multivitamin/mineral supplements is often adequate. Occasionally, however, iron deficiency signals ulcers or even colon cancer.

Again, beware of assuming that an iron deficiency exists. Fatigue, the first symptom of iron deficiency, can be caused by many other things. As mentioned, too much iron is unhealthy. An increase in consumption of iron can increase the risk of cardiac disease, as well as problems with the blood vessels of the eyes. Excess iron has also been linked to advanced macular degeneration in one study, so caution should be used if it is decided that you should supplement with iron.

Magnesium

Magnesium is an essential mineral that accounts for about .05 percent of the body's total weight. Nearly 70 percent of the body's supply is located in the bones, together with calcium and phosphorus, while 30 percent is found in the soft tissues and body fluids. On the cellular level, most of the body's magnesium is found inside the mitochondria, where it activates enzymes necessary for the metabolism of carbohydrates and amino acids. More specifically, the mitochondria account for nearly one-third of total cellular magnesium. Magnesium is required for mitochondrial energy production.

As suggested above, magnesium is involved in many essential metabolic processes. It also helps to promote the absorption and metabolism of other minerals, as well as the utilization of the B vitamins and vitamins C and E. And it aids during bone growth and is necessary for the proper functioning of the nerves and muscles. By countering the stimulating effect of calcium, magnesium plays an important role in neuromuscular contraction. Finally, it helps to regulate the acid-alkaline balance in the body.

Magnesium is widely distributed in food sources, but it is found chiefly in fresh green vegetables, where it is an essential element of chlorophyll. Other excellent sources are unmilled raw wheat germ, soybeans, figs, corn, apples, and oil-rich seeds and nuts, especially almonds. Dolomite, a natural dietary supplement, is also rich in magnesium. However, magnesium oxide is preferred over dolomite. When dolomite is taken, additional supplementation with hydrochloric acid is needed to ensure that the dolomite is dissolved properly.

Despite magnesium's presence in numerous food sources, it is estimated that the typical American diet provides only about 120 mg per day. The RDA for magnesium is 350 mg for adult males and 300 mg for adult females. The amount for females increases to 450 mg during pregnancy and lactation. In general, because magnesium acts as an alkali, it should not be taken after meals.

Evidence suggests that the balance between calcium and magnesium is especially important. If calcium consumption is high, magnesium intake should be high. The magnesium requirement is further influenced by the amounts of protein, phosphorus, and vitamin D in the diet. For example, the need for magnesium increases when the consumption of protein is high. It also increases when the blood-cholesterol level is high.

Large amounts of magnesium can be toxic, especially if the calcium intake is low and the phosphorus intake is high. Excessive magnesium is usually excreted adequately, but in the event of kidney failure, there is a greater danger of toxicity because the rate of excretion is much lower. Yet while too much magnesium is not healthy, so is too little. Magnesium deficiency can occur in patients who have diabetes, pancreatitis, or kidney malfunction. It can also affect those who are alcoholic and those who consume a high-carbohydrate diet. Moreover, *moderate* magnesium deficiency is common, particularly among African Americans, and is associated with increased risk for hypertension and diabetes. Generally, a deficiency is related to coronary heart disease, since it results in the formation of clots in the heart and brain, and may contribute to calcium deposits. The symptoms of magnesium deficiency include apprehensiveness, muscle twitching, tremors, confusion, and disorientation.

Manganese

The mineral manganese is needed for healthy skin, bone, and cartilage formation, as well as glucose tolerance. And zinc and copper work together with manganese to activate *superoxide dismutase* (*SOD*), creating a very powerful antioxidant called SOD2. However, several minerals, such as calcium, iron, and zinc, reduce the absorption of manganese.

Manganese is found in nuts, wheat germ, wheat bran, leafy green vegetables, beet tops, pineapple, and seeds. While at least some of these foods are not uncommon in many diets, many people consume less than the *conservative* amount that is currently considered safe and adequate: 2.5 to 5 mg. It certainly is important to maintain a healthy level of manganese in your system, but whether most people would benefit from manganese supplementation remains unclear. The 5 to 20 mg dose often found in high-potency multivitamin/mineral supplements is generally considered to be a reasonable level for those wishing to supplement manganese.

Amounts of manganese found in supplements have not been linked with any toxicity. But excessive intake of manganese can lead to the rare side effects of dementia and psychiatric symptoms. Preliminary research suggests that individuals with cirrhosis may not be able to properly excrete manganese. Until more is known, these people should not supplement manganese.

Clear deficiencies of manganese are rare, but individuals with osteoporosis sometimes have low blood levels of manganese, which is suggestive of deficiency. We also know that inadequate manganese levels increase mitochondrial oxidation and subsequent mitochondrial decay, which can lead to premature aging and loss of energy. And low levels of manganese can be associated with impaired glucose tolerance, as well as altered carbohydrate and lipid metabolism, which are so important for diabetes control.

Selenium

Selenium is an essential mineral found in minute amounts in the body. It works closely with vitamin E in some of the latter's metabolic actions and in the promotion of normal body growth and fertility. Selenium is a natural antioxidant and appears to have the anti-aging effect of preserving the elasticity of tissue. It does this by delaying the oxidation of polyunsaturated fatty acids, which can cause solidification of tissue proteins.

In our bodies, the liver and kidneys contain four to five times as much selenium as do the muscles and other tissues. Excess selenium is normally excreted in the urine. Its presence in the feces is an indication of improper absorption.

Selenium is found in several common food sources: in the bran and germ of cereals; in vegetables such as broccoli, onions, and tomatoes; and in tuna. The RDA for selenium for adults is extremely minute. Consider that five to ten parts of selenium per 1 million parts of food or other minerals is considered toxic. This is due to the tendency of selenium to replace sulfur in biological compounds and to inhibit the action of some enzymes.

Another important fact is that selenium can be toxic in its pure form, so supplements should be taken with care. Reported instances of toxicity have occurred in areas where the selenium content of the soil is high. And while low doses of supplemental selenium are considered useful in preventing cataracts, higher doses have actually been found to induce cataracts. This emphasizes the importance of balance of nutrients in the diet.

Several reports have shown selenium deficiency causes defects in mitochondrial structure, integrity, and electron transport chain function. An increased risk of cancer and decreased immune system function has been associated with selenium deficiency. And a deficiency of this mineral may encourage premature aging. Again, this is because selenium preserves tissue elasticity. By the way, selenium's connection to tissue elasticity is of major significance for the lens within the eye, which becomes less flexible with age. (For a related discussion, see Part Two's section on "Presbyopia," page 308.)

Sodium

Sodium is an essential mineral found mostly in the extracellular (outside the cell) fluids such as the vascular fluids in the blood vessels and the interstitial fluids surrounding the cells. The body's remaining sodium is located within the bones. Sodium functions with potassium to equalize the blood's acid-alkaline (or pH) balance. Along with potassium, it helps to regulate the water balance within the body—that is, it helps to control the distribution of fluids on either side of the cell walls.

The role of sodium and its partner potassium is not limited to "pH" and fluid balance, however. Sodium and potassium are also involved in muscle contraction and expansion, as well as in nerve stimulation. An important function of sodium alone is keeping the other blood minerals soluble so that they will not build up into deposits in the bloodstream. Sodium helps to purge carbon dioxide from the body, aids digestion, and functions in the production of hydrochloric acid in the stomach. In addition, it acts with chlorine to improve blood and lymph health.

Sodium is found in virtually all foods, especially in sodium chloride (table salt). High concentrations are found in seafood, carrots, beets, poultry, and meat. Kelp is an excellent supplemental source of sodium.

There is no established dietary requirement for sodium, but it is generally observed that the usual intake far exceeds the need. The average American ingests 3 to 7 grams (g) of sodium and 6 to 18 g of sodium chloride each day. The NRC recommends a daily sodium-chloride intake of 1 g for every 1 kilogram (kg) of water consumed. A kilogram of water is 35 ounces (oz).

A daily intake of 14 to 28 g of sodium chloride is considered excessive. An excess of sodium in the diet may cause potassium to be lost in the urine. Abnormal fluid retention accompanied by dizziness and swelling of the legs or face can also occur. Diets containing excessive amounts of sodium contribute to an increase in blood pressure. The simplest way to reduce sodium intake is to eliminate table salt from the diet.

Fluid balance within the eye is crucial for patients who are at risk for glaucoma—that is, those with high eye pressure or a family history of glaucoma. Sodium balance can have a major impact on eye pressure. If you are in that category of high risk for glaucoma, be sure to monitor your sodium intake.

Zinc

Zinc is an essential trace mineral that occurs in the body in a larger amount than any other trace element except iron. (The human body contains approximately 1.8 g of zinc, compared to nearly 5.0 g of iron.) Zinc has a variety of functions. It is related to the normal absorption and action of the vitamins, especially vitamin A and the B complex. It is a constituent of at least twenty-five of the enzymes involved in digestion and metabolism. It is a component of insulin and a part of the enzyme that is needed to break down alcohol. It also functions in carbohydrate digestion and phosphorus metabolism. Lastly, it has an important role in general growth and development, the function of the prostate gland, the healing of wounds and burns, and the synthesis of deoxyribonucleic acid (DNA), which is discussed at length in the section titled "Nutrition and Your Genes" (page 104).

The best sources of zinc and of all of the trace elements in proper balance are natural unprocessed foods—especially those grown in organically enriched soil. Diets that are high in protein, whole-grain products, brewer's yeast, wheat bran, wheat germ, and pumpkin seeds are usually high in zinc. But as discussed below, many people do not obtain enough zinc from their daily diet. So supplementation is a good idea.

The RDA for zinc is 15 mg per day for adults. An additional 15 mg is recommended during pregnancy, and an additional 25 mg is recommended during lactation. Zinc is relatively nontoxic, although zinc poisoning can result from eating a food that has been stored in a galvanized container. High intakes of zinc interfere with copper utilization, causing incomplete iron metabolism. Importantly, when zinc is added to the diet, vitamin A is also needed in larger amounts.

Recent studies have used zinc as an eye-related supplement. In fact, a "gold standard" studies (called AREDS and AREDS2) that examined macular degeneration supplemented the participants with about 80 mg of zinc. However, this formula was produced in 1988, when the science behind macular degeneration was still new. We now know that 80 mg is extreme and, in fact, the hallmarks of macular degeneration include tissue deposits that contain excessive amounts of zinc. While zinc is important to use in conjunction with vitamin A, too much of this mineral is not a good thing.

The AREDS2 study (released in 2007) showed that there was no difference in the progression of AMD between one group that took 25 mg of zinc against another group that took 80 mg. It was interesting that the final conclusion was to continue with the higher dose (which is twice the maximum RDA recommendation) instead of going with the lesser dose. There were many questions and discussions about this recommendation, but the study's authors stuck with their conclusion.

On another front regarding the zinc recommendation, a group of researchers looks at the results of the original AREDS study and linked the genetic profiles of those who got better results compared with those whose AMD got worse. It is still a very controversial and complicated issue, but, in short, they found that certain genes preclude some AMD patients from taking ANY zinc in a supplement. Thus, we now have "non-zinc" formula vitamins for AMD patients. Some doctors disagree with the concept, stating that the data was skewed and the populations that they studied were different. The controversy still exists today, so you'll need to ask your doctor for advice on zinc supplementation for AMD. Many doctors can offer a genetic test in the office to see if your genes are set up to accept or reject zinc.

Many supplements incorporate the zinc oxide form of zinc into their formulas. However, that is the least biologically active form of zinc. Actually, it's the form used in the white sunscreen you put on your nose! Zinc oxide must be combined with the proper balance of copper to avoid severe reaction. Zinc monomethionine is the most bioavailable form of zinc and the only form that does not interfere with copper absorption. (A mineral that is bioavailable is more easily transported to the site at which it is needed.)

Low zinc intakes are common, as 10 percent of the American population ingests under 50 percent of the RDA. Zinc deficiency in human cells in culture has been found to cause significant oxidative damage to DNA. Zinc deficiency is also associated with cancer. Therefore, proper ingestion of zinc is very important to good health.

We have completed our discussion of the minerals that affect our general well-being and our eye health in particular. It has become clear that many of these minerals influence each other's productivity and also have specific relationships to certain vitamins. It is amazing to contemplate the complex work our bodies accomplish in order to allow for a vital, functional life.

We have also concluded our detailed section on the micronutrients. The important piece of information to remember is that they all work together in the body. Therefore, if you are considering supplementing with *any* nutrients, be aware that an excess in some nutrients can cause deficiencies in others. In nature, all the nutrients are mixed in the proper proportions in the foods we eat; the same should hold for any nutritional supplement pills you may take. Balance is the key to health!

THE POWER OF ANTIOXIDANTS

The term *antioxidant* has been repeated again and again over the course of this book thus far. It's finally time to explore it in greater detail. All of the vitamins and minerals that are antioxidants operate in a similar manner in the body. They play an important role in the body's basic defense system against disease, infection, premature aging, and possibly the adverse effects of strenuous athletic performance. Here is some background on how the antioxidants work.

Damage from Free Radicals

At the root of many diseases and the aging process is a group of highly reactive substances called *free radicals* or *reactive oxidant species* (*ROS*). These chemical compounds consist of two or more elements bound together by a chemical bond. Existing in that bond is an unpaired, or "extra," electron. The unpaired electron makes the free radical very reactive and unstable. To stabilize itself, a free radical seeks out and grabs an electron from a stable compound. This, in turn, creates a new free radical. A chain reaction begins, thus extending the damage of even a small number of these reactive compounds.

Free radicals attack cell components and cause damage to cells and tissues in the body. Common sites of attack are the polyunsaturated fatty acids in cell membranes. Free-radical-induced damage alters the structure and function of the cell membrane. The membrane is no longer able to transport nutrients, oxygen, or water into the cell, or to regulate the removal of waste products. Continued free-radical attack ruptures the cell membrane, causing the loss of the cellular components and rendering the cell useless. The intracellular chemicals leak into and damage the surrounding tissues. This process is associated with the initiation of numerous disorders from arthritis to cardiovascular disease. This scenario shows that the actual "brain" of the cell is not the nucleus but the membrane around the cell, where it interacts with the environment.

Free-radical damage to tissues in general, and molecules in specific, might be an initiating factor of atherosclerosis. The oxidative damage to the arteries attracts platelets (which are responsible for blood clotting) and inflammatory cells, while the damaged artery becomes a place for cholesterol to accumulate. Oxidized cholesterol particles—LDLs—might contribute to the process and increase adhesion at the site of the injury. So, contrary to the popular belief that a high LDL level is a direct cause of heart problems, it's more likely that it's the "oxidized" LDLs that become misshapen (actually developing a "spiked" texture) and cause small tears in the artery wall. This is where the inflammatory cells accumulate and attempt to heal the damage to the blood vessel—that is, form clots and the like.

We're not done with the frightening effects of free radicals yet. They also damage the cells' mitochondria, which we remember as the cells' energy factories. The damage results in limited or halted production of energy for all the cell processes. And free-radical damage to enzymes and other proteins limits the building of body tissues and causes the accumulation of protein fragments. Both of these conditions are noted in the premature aging of tissues. Finally, a cell cannot reproduce normally when its genetic code has been altered by free radicals. At best, the cell dies. At worst, the cell mutates into a cancerous cell. These are the devastating effects of free radicals. What can we do to avoid them?

Repair Throughout the Body

Unfortunately, free radicals are unavoidable. They are formed during the normal metabolic process. They also are obtained from some foods, inhaled with polluted air and tobacco smoke, and generated in the environment by smog, solar radiation, and herbicides.

Fortunately, the body has an anti-free-radical system that makes use of many helpful substances we call antioxidants: antioxidant enzymes such as superoxide dismutase (SOD) and glutathione peroxidase; vitamins such as C, E, and beta-carotene; minerals such as zinc and selenium; herbs such as bilberry and ginkgo; and other nutrients such as cysteine, pine bark extract, coenzyme Q_{10}, and the bioflavonoids. These antioxidants intercede, deactivating the free radicals and rendering them harmless before they can cause irreversible damage to the body's tissues. Antioxidants are currently being thoroughly investigated for their role in the prevention of many major diseases, including eye diseases such as cataracts and age-related macular degeneration.

Findings on Antioxidants and Eye Health

Two recently discovered powerful antioxidants are the carotenoids called *lutein* (LOO-teen) and *zeaxanthin* (zee-ah-ZAN-thin). Lutein and zea-xanthin are similar to beta-carotene in that they are found in spinach, kale, and other vegetables and fruits. However, they are not converted to vitamin A, but, again, they do serve as potent antioxidants, as well as high-energy blue light filters. More specifically, they make up the yellow pigment in the retina and appear to protect the macula in particular. In addition, research shows that higher dietary levels of lutein and zeaxanthin are associated with greater protection of the macula, which can help to prevent macular degeneration. Lutein

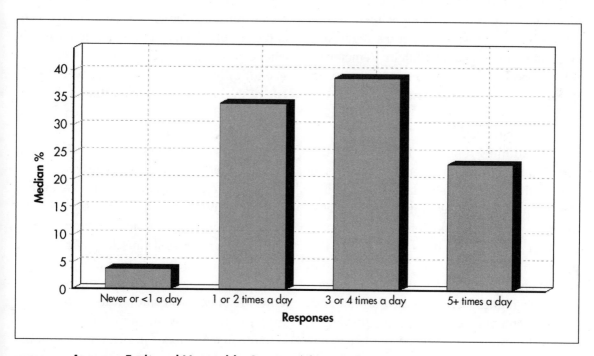

FIGURE 1.9 **Average Fruit and Vegetable Consumption per Day.**
Source: Centers for Disease Control.

and zeaxanthin have also been found in the lens of the eye and apparently lead to a lower level of cataract formation. The body is unable to manufacture lutein or zeaxanthin. But we can include these antioxidants in our diet and through supplementation. Let's discuss each one in greater detail.

Within the eye, lutein is highly concentrated in the macular region of the retina and is dispersed in lesser amounts throughout the entire retina, iris, ciliary body (the structure that produces the aqueous fluid inside the eye), and lens. There is currently no FDA-recommended daily intake level for lutein. However, research suggests that a minimum of 6 to 10 mg per day of lutein from dark green leafy vegetables or other sources is necessary to realize lutein's health benefits. Even if you eat a balanced diet, you would need a large bowl of fresh spinach to get about 6 mg of lutein. There are no reports of safety concerns regarding large amounts of intake of lutein. Remember, eating foods containing lutein or consuming dietary supplements that contain lutein are the only ways for your body to get it; your body cannot synthesize it.

Zeaxanthin's role is to help protect the eye from the harmful high-energy, blue-wave light in the same way sunglasses protect our eyes from sun glare. Zeaxanthin also protects the eye's vision cells and helps the eye repair itself. In fact, studies have shown that the portion of the macula with the highest concentration of zeaxanthin is the last to degenerate. The highest density of zeaxanthin is at the very center of the macula, thus affording it the greatest protection. Similar to lutein, there are no FDA-recommended daily intake levels for zeaxanthin. However, the recommended amount that most health authorities suggest is 4 mg daily for anyone diagnosed with macular degeneration and 2 mg for those taking it as a preventative measure. The best food sources of zeaxanthin are organic corn, egg yolks, goji berries, and green vegetables.

More recently, a new "player" in macular pigment has been discovered. Called meso-zeaxanthin, this carotenoid is created in the eye from a conversion from lutein. It is highly concentrated in the center of the macula and is very effective at protecting the retina from high-energy light. However, it is rare in the diet. Mostly found in shrimp shells, fish skin, and turtle fat, it is hardly a mainstay in the American diet. Some authorities believe it should be supplemented, but since it can be converted from lutein, other researchers just recommend adequate levels of lutein. Non-confirmed studies suggest that 20 percent of the population may not be able to make this conversion from lutein but that has not been scientifically verified. It was discovered than one of the enzymes in the "visual cycle" that converts light to nerve energy (to enable the visual process) is the same enzyme that converts lutein to meso-zeaxanthin. This is still a debated issue in the eyecare industry.

Another carotenoid, called astaxanthin has many studies that show it has the potential to increase muscle endurance and tone. Given that there are several muscle groups in the eye, and that eyestrain is typically associated with extensive use of the eyes looking at computer displays, astaxanthin does hold some promise for eye health and comfort. While it is found in many foods (it's responsible for the pink color in salmon and other food sources), the effective dosage would come more easily with supplementation. Only 6 mg of astaxanthin is needed to be effective and it is readily available in commercial over-the-counter supplements.

In addition, a carotenoid called capsanthin has recently gotten attention. This molecule is similar to other carotenoids, but has a unique structure that has been shown to not only reduce the effects of dry eyes but also lowers eye pressure. This would be a significant factor for those who have glaucoma or ocular hypertension. There have been few studies on the molecule, but it seems to have great potential.

It seems that as more research is conducted, the importance of antioxidants is only confirmed. Now you understand what antioxidants do in the body and, therefore, why they are so important to supply. Antioxidants scout out free radicals and disarm them, so to speak. They are crucial to maintaining health, including eye health. Luckily, we can bathe our bodies with antioxidants through both healthy foods and supplementation, the latter of which will be discussed in the following section.

THE NEED FOR SUPPLEMENTS

Today's food supply is stripped of a large amount of its nutritional value due to overworked soil, cold storage, food processing, and common cooking techniques. Therefore, the number of micronutrients provided even in the very best of daily diets cannot truly meet nutritional needs. So taking a full-spectrum supplement—one that contains all of the vitamins and minerals to maintain optimal health—in addition to eating clean, nutrient-dense food (meaning almost no junk food) and exercising

on a regular basis is the best investment you can make for both short- and long-term health.

A high-quality multivitamin should be the foundation for every supplement program. Despite all of the studies proving the efficacy of multivitamins in preventing disease and promoting optimal health, many physicians still don't take vitamin supplements seriously because they are too busy to read micronutrient studies published in nutrition and biochemistry journals. Additionally, many physicians recommend eating a balanced diet but don't suggest what that might look like. To some, a balanced diet might be fries with a burger!

A large amount of published scientific evidence suggests a full-spectrum multivitamin/mineral supplement is good insurance and markedly improves health. How? Well, research finds that such a supplement helps our bodies fight degenerative diseases of the eye, as well as heart disease, cancer, and poor immune function. This is particularly true for those who consume inadequate diets, which actually includes the majority of people in the United States. Figure 1.9 is based on data collected by the Centers for Disease Control (CDC) over the course of the "Healthy People 2000" research program. While it is now several years dated, it still speaks volumes about the need for daily supplementation.

But supplementation must be done carefully. Our bodies are made up of about 100 trillion cells. Each cell derives nutrients from foods and supplements, which are carried to them via the bloodstream. The semipermeable membrane that surrounds each cell allows only a select number of micronutrients to cross its barrier. Minerals are especially subject to this regulatory process, and they cross the cell's membrane based on the body's bioelectrical needs at any given time. Each nutrient we consume must compete for transport space, as well as for space within the cell. Therefore, long-term consumption of excessively high amounts of any single nutrient may cause a deficiency of another nutrient.

For the most part, our bodies are well equipped to handle nutrients in excess; the body simply excretes them as waste material. (I have alerted you, when necessary, about toxicity dangers due to overconsumption of the nutrients discussed in this book.) However, nutrient deficiencies caused by a poor diet or even excessive supplementation of other single nutrients cannot be compensated for. If there is not enough of a given nutrient crossing the cell membrane, the cell cannot make up for that deficiency by any other means. The concept of ratios tells us that all nutrients need to be present and available to our cells, and they need to be present in relative potencies. That can be quite complex. Remember, where supplements are concerned, more is not necessarily better!

The Design of a Supplement Plan

The Food and Nutrition Board at the National Academy of Science sets the recommended daily allowances (RDAs) or daily values at minimal levels needed to prevent diseases like scurvy and rickets. But research in the field of nutrition clearly indicates that the RDAs do not support *optimal* health. Higher doses of nutrients are needed to achieve the best nutrition we can get.

Unfortunately, most consumers notice very little difference in their health, their well-being, or their energy level when taking inexpensive, low-potency, one-pill-per-day formulations that include only the suggested RDA amounts of the most basic vitamins and minerals. And most of today's "baby boomers," and the aging population in general, are determined to maintain health and vitality through the aging process. That means that many people are currently custom-shaping supplement programs that address their own concerns and health goals. Are you?

Designing a supplement program is not as easy as one might think. There are literally dozens and dozens of nutrients to consider, and there are seemingly countless vitamin companies that make a multitude of supplements for various conditions. While the FDA prohibits vitamin companies from making claims that a nutrient will cure or address a particular disease, companies often "suggest" that a given product will help with a specific condition. However, as I discussed above, using a "single bullet" approach of one particular nutrient for a particular disorder is rarely effective and may actually be harmful.

If you wish to design a supplement plan, I suggest you work with a healthcare professional. There are many different professionals who are well-versed in nutrition, including but not limited to chiropractors, nutritionists, naturopaths, herbalists, and some medical practitioners (*if* they have special training in that area). Search for someone who has experience in nutrition and can review your specific diet. She should take detailed information on your eating habits and lifestyle, possibly using a "Food Frequency Intake" questionnaire. Also, she should be able to do some nutritional testing—for example, hair-mineral analysis, urine analysis, and/or blood testing—and make recommendations based on possible deficiencies. Ultimately, most of us need a full-spectrum supplement as a base and then additional nutrients as required by any deficiencies noted.

The Process of Choosing High-Quality Supplements

Once you have established your supplemental needs, you need to choose a high-quality product. Look for powdered multivitamin supplements presented in vegetable capsule form rather than hard-pressed pills. Why? Because the capsules are more readily absorbed and metabolized by the body. Also, always pay attention to the source or form of micronutrients in the "multiples." Current FDA label law requires that the source or form be identified for most micronutrients. A general rule of thumb is that absorption rate is associated with both the quality and cost of the raw-ingredient source. Hard-pressed, inexpensive "one-a-day" pills tend to have a lower absorption rate than higher-quality powdered formulations presented in vegetable capsules.

Look for supplements that include balanced amounts of the full-spectrum of both fat- and water-soluble vitamins, including the vitally important B complex. The first thing I look for is the form of vitamin A in a formula. It should be mostly (or all) retinal palmitate and little beta-carotene. Also, choose supplements that include a full spectrum of minerals, including the trace minerals. The enzymatic reaction created by balanced minerals becomes the catalyst for all energy production and proper metabolism of other micronutrients. Minerals

are vital for the production of biochemicals that send messages to our nervous system, thyroid, and adrenal glands. These messages are involved in the production of hormones as well as the efficient burning of calories. Amino acid agents support the absorption of minerals into cells to facilitate the energy cycle.

In addition, look for supplements with a large variety of plant-based antioxidants. As previously discussed, antioxidants help neutralize free-radical damage associated with chronic degenerative diseases, including cancer and diseases of the eye. The macula-specific *xanthophylls* (ZAN-tho-fills), which include lutein and zeaxanthin (discussed earlier), are antioxidants that are rarely included in "one-a-day" formulations. If they are included, it may be for marketing purposes and in amounts far less than those included in successful micronutrient studies. For example, one very popular product marketed to "silver" seniors claims to be formulated "with lutein." However, when you check the label, that product contains 250 mcg, which is about 100 times less than what would normally prove effective for an older adult. So be sure you're getting what you think you're getting; check the amounts of each nutrient, not just the number of nutrients, in any given supplement.

I recommend taking multiples twice per day, with meals. Our bodies use water-soluble micronutrients as they need them, and any extra is normally excreted within hours. Therefore, essential micronutrients should be replenished at least twice per day. One exception I make involves vitamin C, which I feel should be taken in 250 mg doses evenly throughout the day, four times per day. Quite differently, the fat-soluble vitamins—A, D, E and K—are stored in the liver and are slowly released as they are needed for metabolic function.

The bottom line on supplements is that, while they are crucial in assisting the maintenance of a good internal environment for growth and repair of the body, they cannot compete with double cheeseburgers and milk shakes. We crave food that tastes good and has appealing textures. And in truth, a good diet with the adequate number of fruits and vegetables is the proper starting point for healthful living. Supplementation is certainly important, but so is eating balanced, tasty meals.

NUTRITION AND YOUR GENES

When we think of the genes that make up our genetic code, we most often think of them as predictors of things to come. That is, if certain diseases "run in the family," then we believe we are doomed to have those diseases. And if our grandparents and parents were blessed with longevity, we assume we will enjoy it too. That is how science has viewed genes for the past fifty years. However, we now know that's not necessarily the case.

Our genes are formed from microscopic double strands of *deoxyribonucleic acid* (*DNA*). They are dependent on adequate nutrition for their structure and activity. We essentially all have the same genes, but they are all expressed differently based on several factors, including our environment, which means both our internal and external environments. By appropriately switching on and off, our genes direct the behavior of our body's 60 trillion cells. That switching on and off is called *transcription* in the "genome" research world. (See the discussion of the term "genome" on page 105.) Many genetic researchers consider our genes to be the Rosetta Stone of health and disease.

When we feed our genes with optimal amounts of the full spectrum of nutrients, they enable us to live a long life with a lower risk of disease. When we allow our genes to live in a nutritionally deficient environment, they send mixed up messages that accelerate our body's aging process and increase the risk and progression of degenerative diseases, including cancer, heart disease, Alzheimer's disease, Parkinson's disease, and many eye diseases. But how does this really happen?

The information in our genes is written in yet another language—one with which we need to become comfortable: the chemical language of DNA. The letters in the DNA alphabet are sequences of molecules called *nucleotides*. Each letter, or nucleotide, is constructed around one of four substances called *DNA nucleobases*: adenine (A), cytosine (C), guanine (G), and thymine (T). Different arrangements of these four bases spell different words in DNA language. For example, "TACGACCTGA" describes the genes that instruct our cells to make specific enzymes and proteins. The enzymes, in turn, catalyze a host of other biochemical reactions that eventually form proteins, and these proteins form the structure of hormones and tissue.

All of this amazing activity is dependent on nutrients. The DNA in the proteins we consume is broken down and reconstructed into our own distinctive DNA. Then, for example, vitamins B_3 and B_6 are needed for thymine synthesis; folic acid is necessary for guanine and adenine synthesis; and vitamin B_3 is required for cytosine synthesis. When we are deficient in any of these particular nutrients, DNA cannot be properly synthesized, and its instructions cannot be carried out.

Research suggests that breaks in a single strand of DNA can usually be repaired by specific nutrients if they are readily available. For example, as suggested by the information above, low intake of folic acid interferes with the production of thymine. When cells cannot make thymine, they replace it in our DNA with a substance called *uracil*. But when normal DNA-repair enzymes scan the DNA, they remove the uracil and that creates breaks in cellular DNA that could have been prevented by adequate amounts of folic acid. Unfortunately, a deficiency of folic acid is suggested to lead to large numbers of uracil deposits in DNA—so many deposits, in fact, that they dramatically increase the risk of double-strand DNA breaks. Double-strand breaks are not as easily repaired and are more likely to result in permanent damage to DNA and, ultimately, death of the cell.

The discovery of this exciting science led to a new area of research called *nutrigenomics*—the promising, cost-effective, nutritional approach to reducing the risk of diseases of aging associated with gene expression. This includes the study of the proteins that are inherited and linked to the inflammatory process now associated with degenerative disease, including degenerative diseases of the eye. Unfortunately, our DNA is easily damaged, and most of this damage is caused by free radicals. We have already discussed how free radicals are naturally formed as a byproduct of burning food for energy. Researchers also suggest that infections, ultraviolet sunlight, cigarette smoke, and internal and external pollutants also form free radicals. It is generally

agreed that free radicals delete sections of DNA, rearrange it, or cut it into pieces, and the end result is analogous to typographical errors that distort DNA's instructions and, no doubt, influence longevity. Large numbers of studies now suggest that supplemental antioxidants reduce the rate of DNA damage and slow age-related damage to the cells.

DNA damage also takes place during normal cell division. When a cell divides in a nutrient-deficient body, it replicates its DNA, but not perfectly. Cell division messages are sent by our individual DNA through *ribonucleic acid (RNA)*. RNA-message errors happen in nutrient-deficient environments during each cell division in the same way misspellings used to happen when we re-typed a written page. As the number of DNA errors increase, instructions for normal cell functions become more garbled. Fortunately for us, DNA that lives in a nutrient-rich environment has the remarkable ability to proofread itself and to send RNA messages to correct many errors before they become permanent.

The Human Genome Project (HGP) was a project to map and sequence the 3 billion nucleotides contained in the human genome and to identify all the genes present in it. The "genome"—the whole set of genes containing hereditary information and encoded in the DNA—of any given individual is unique (except for identical twins); mapping "the human genome" involves sequencing multiple variations of each gene. Of course, information is only as good as the ability to use it. Therefore, advanced methods for widely disseminating the information generated by the HGP to scientists, physicians, and others is necessary in order to ensure the most rapid application of research results for the benefit of humanity. Biomedical technology and research are particular beneficiaries of the HGP. In 2003, an accurate and complete human genome sequence was finished and made available to scientists and researchers two years ahead of the original Human Genome Project schedule. Today, this information is continuing to be developed and incorporated into our daily lives.

The bottom line in genomics is that we don't get sick because we "have a gene" for a specific disease, but there are genes that get expressed improperly due to our daily lifestyle and environment. So, it's up to each of us to maintain a proper working system within our bodies to continue to grow and age gracefully.

CONCLUSION

Nutrition is the relationship of foods to the health of the human body. Proper nutrition implies receiving adequate foods and supplements to convey the nutrients required for optimal health. Without proper nutrition, optimal health and well-being cannot be obtained. This statement is also true for the visual system. Our eyes are very complex organs and require an extremely high proportion of nutrients to maintain their proper function. With a little attention paid to general nutritional guidelines, you should be able to "feed your eyes" optimally and see well for years to come.

Herbal Therapies and Eye Health

Herbs, by definition, are plants that lack the woody characteristics of shrubs and trees. Over the years, many substances have been extracted from numerous herbs and used successfully to heal the human body. In fact, herbs are food for the body. They contain natural medicines, vitamins, and minerals, and they have remarkable histories of curative effects when used in the proper way. Not only have herbs been used medicinally for centuries, but also many of today's modern medicines have their foundations in herbal therapy.

The exact reasons for the positive effects that herbs exert on the human body are not always thoroughly understood. It is evident, however, that the nutrients stored within the plants' cellular structures are in forms that are easily metabolized by the body. And interestingly, it is an often-overlooked fact that the organic chemical structures of hemoglobin (the substance within red blood cells that carries oxygen and gives blood its red color) and chlorophyll (the substance within green plants that absorbs light and gives plants their green color) are very similar. The therapeutic actions of herbs come from *alkaloids,* which are organic compounds that cause certain chemical reactions within the body. Alkaloids also help the body to resist disease, strengthen tissues, and improve the nervous system. In addition, now that we know the genetic structure in humans, we can see that humans and plants have a majority of the same genes!

In this chapter, we will discuss herbs and herbal therapy. We will describe the nineteen most popular herbs used for the eyes, as well as the most common Western herbal combinations and the traditional Chinese herbal combinations used for eye problems. In addition, you'll find out what herbs to avoid so that your eyes can continue to work optimally.

BASIC BACKGROUND REGARDING HERBS

Before we enter into a very specific discussion on the herbs recommended for eye health, it is important to familiarize yourself with some basic definitions. First, we must clarify the difference between the terms "Western herbalism" and "Chinese herbalism." Then, we should review the various forms of herbs that are available to you, from liquids to compresses. So read on for a good background in the culture of herbal therapy.

Western Herbalism versus Chinese Herbalism

Western herbalism is a form of the healing arts that draws from the herbal traditions of Europe and the Americas. The term "Western," as used in the field of herbalism, really applies to the methods of using herbs rather than to the origins of herbs. That is why Western herb books often list substances from places such as Asia, Africa, South America, and Egypt.

In Western herbalism, individual herbs are used for their reputed health benefits. This form of herbalism emphasizes the study and use of herbs in the treatment and prevention of illness. Western herbalism is based on physicians' and herbalists' clinical experience and traditional knowledge of medicinal plant remedies preserved by oral tradition and in written records over thousands of years. Western herbalism, like the much older system of traditional Chinese medicine, relies on the synergistic and curative properties of the plant to treat symptoms and disease and to maintain good health.

Of course, herbs are grown all over the world, but some of the more popular herbs for therapy are referred to as "Chinese herbs." Throughout Chinese history, herbalists have sought out special *tonic herbs* that can be taken daily to improve the physical condition, enhance energy, increase resistance to disease, and prolong life. These particular herbs help to distinguish "Chinese herbalism" from other forms of the art, such as Western herbalism.

But Chinese herbalism, also known as "traditional Chinese medicine," involves more than herbal treatments for health maintenance. It arranges physical signs and symptoms into patterns of organ disharmony, which can then be treated with acupuncture (see page 332) and herbal combinations to restore harmony and balance in the human body. The treatment of disease by traditional Chinese medicine is generally a complicated procedure and should be performed only by an experienced practitioner. The herbal formulas are often adjusted as the symptoms change during recovery. Some of these formulas are meant for short-term therapy only.

Chinese tonic herbs are administered with very specific goals in mind—to improve and strengthen particular organs, systems, weaknesses, or the body as a whole. But compared to other herbs that are used for specific symptoms, most Chinese tonic herbs are nourishing and nutritive and can be taken regularly for long periods of time. Tonic herbs are *adaptogenic,* meaning that the body can regulate the beneficial herbal properties. The Chinese tonic herbs help us to adapt to whatever situations we are engaged in, whether they be physical, mental, or spiritual. Thus, Chinese tonic herbs are also used to increase the consciousness of energetic, psychological, and spiritual states in the individual.

Whether applied through the Western or Chinese herbal tradition, the benefits of botanical medicine may be subtle or dramatic, depending on the remedy used and the problem being addressed. Herbal remedies usually have a much slower effect than pharmaceutical drugs. But while many herbal remedies have a cumulative effect and work slowly over time to restore balance, others are indicated for short-term treatment of acute symptoms.

When compared to pharmaceutical drugs, herbal remedies prepared from the whole plant have relatively few side effects. This is due to the complex chemistry and synergistic action of the full range of phytochemicals present in the whole plant, and the relatively lower concentrations of chemicals that enter the body. Herbs are generally safe when used in properly designated therapeutic dosages, and less costly than the isolated chemicals or synthetic prescription drugs available from Western pharmaceutical corporations. There are several patented herbal medicines made in China and the United States that can be used to treat vision problems and benefit overall health. A qualified healthcare professional, however, should oversee their use.

Forms of Herbal Preparations

Whether referring to Western herbalism or Chinese herbalism, herbal preparations can be applied in many different forms. It is important to clearly define and understand these various forms so that you can properly follow directions whenever you use herbal therapies. The best forms are the tincture and the extract. And I refer to them as "the best forms" because they remain potent for longer periods than any other forms.

A *tincture* is an herb mixed in an alcohol solution. It is made by adding a powdered herb to alcohol, then adding enough water to make a 50-percent alcohol solution. If you prepare a tincture, you should let the mixture stand for two weeks, shaking the bottle once or twice each day, and then strain it before using it. It is important to emphasize that *a tincture should not be used in the eye.* No alcohol preparation should come into contact with the eye, as the eye is a delicate structure.

An *extract* is made by hydraulically pressing an herb, then soaking it in alcohol or water. The excess liquid is allowed to evaporate, and the result is a concentrated liquid. Before using an extract, dilute it in a small amount of water. Similar to the warning above, *never use an alcohol-based extract, no matter how diluted it is, directly in the eye.*

Then there are additional forms of herbal therapy. *Capsules* are a pleasant way to take herbs, especially when the herbs taste bitter or are mucus-forming. Capsules generally consist of a gelatin casing filled with powdered herb. If prepared capsules are purchased from a first-class herb company or health food store, the herbs generally are clean and combined in the correct proportions. To comfortably wash down and properly dissolve a capsule, take it with 8 ounces of pure water or herbal tea.

An *herbal compress* will achieve an effect similar to that of an ointment, but has the advantage of the therapeutic action of heat. To make a compress, bring 1 or 2 heaping tablespoons of the herb to a boil in 1 cup of water. Dip a cotton pad or piece of gauze in the strained liquid, allow the excess liquid to drain off, and then place the pad or gauze over the closed eyelid (or other affected area) while it is still warm but not too hot. Keep the compress in place until it has cooled off.

An *infusion* is made by pouring hot water over a dry or powdered herb, and then steeping the herb for several minutes to extract its active ingredients, as you do when steeping a tea bag. This method of preparation minimizes the loss of the herb's volatile elements. ("Volatile" simply means vulnerable to change under certain conditions.) The usual amounts are about $1/2$ to 1 ounce of herb to 1 pint of water. Use an enamel, stainless steel, porcelain, or glass pot with a tight-fitting lid to prevent evaporation and loss of the *essential oils*—the main medicinal part of some herbs. Steep the herb for about ten to twenty minutes. To drink an infusion, strain it into a cup, and drink it lukewarm or cool. For directions on how to prepare and use an infusion as an eyewash, see the inset titled "Herbal Eyewashes" found below.

A *decoction* is similar to an infusion. Instead of steeping the dry herb, however, simmer it

for about twenty to thirty minutes. Be careful not to boil the herb, as that would damage its potency.

A *poultice* is a warm, mashed, moist mass of fresh or ground herbs tied in a piece of muslin or other loosely woven cloth. It is applied directly to the skin to relieve inflammations, boils, and abscesses, and to promote proper cleansing and healing of the affected area. The skin should be oiled before applying a poultice. Because the skin around the eyes is very thin, make sure that the poultice is not too hot when

HERBAL EYEWASHES

Having herbal tea as a late-afternoon pick-me-up or just before bed to help release the tensions of the day has become as common in the United States today as tea time has been in England for centuries. But herbal tea can be used as more than a drink. Used as an eyewash, an herbal tea infusion or decoction can bring relief to a stressed eye through the direct application of the properties that make the herb so beneficial.

To prepare an herbal tea or other mixture for external application to the eye, use a piece of cheesecloth or filter paper, and strain the mixture repeatedly until it runs clear. This step is absolutely critical. In addition to being free of any debris that could scratch or irritate the eye, the mixture must be allowed to cool to room temperature before being used. Any leftover liquid can be stored in the refrigerator for future use. However, you should never use an herbal mixture that was prepared more than two weeks ago.

To apply an herbal mixture as an eyewash, use an eyedropper and simply put two drops of liquid in each eye. To do this, lean your head back, gently pull the lower lid down from the eye, and instill the drops in the pocket that is created. Another method is to instill the drops in the corner of the eye. Do not attempt to drop the liquid directly on the eye. The blink reflex is the quickest reflex in the body. Also, apply the eyewash to one eye at a time. Put the drops in the first eye, and then close the eye for about thirty seconds to keep the drops in contact with the eye tissue. Then repeat in the other eye.

You can use an eyecup instead of an eyedropper. Place a small amount of the herbal mixture in the cup, being careful to not overfill the cup, and place the cup up against your eye socket. Tilt your head back and look up, blinking a few times. Remove the cup, and keep the eye closed for another thirty seconds. Repeat with the other eye.

applying it to the eye area. A warm poultice is fine, but one that is too hot can easily cause a burn. Remember that the eyelid skin is some of the thinnest skin on the body. Once a poultice has cooled, discard it. A cooled poultice should never be reheated and reused.

Now you have enough background to enter into a discussion on specific herbal treatments. We have learned what the terms "Western" and "Chinese" mean in the world of herbalism. We have also defined the numerous ways in which herbs can be applied, from tinctures to teas. Now let's move on to a discussion about specific herbs that aid the function and health of the eyes.

HERBS TO USE FOR THE EYES

There are many herbs that are commonly used to treat eye conditions. In the following paragraphs, they are presented according to their most popular common names, with their Latin names following. Some of these herbs are meant to be used directly in or around the eyes, but many are taken orally to support eye function from the inside. Also included is general information on each herb, what each herb contains nutritionally, what conditions each herb is used to treat, and how the particular herb affects the eyes.

Alfalfa

Alfalfa (*Medicago sativa*) has been used by the Chinese since the sixth century to treat kidney stones and to relieve fluid retention and swelling. The leaves of this remarkable legume contain eight essential amino acids. Alfalfa has very rich supplies of vitamins A, D, and K. Its components are properly balanced to allow for complete absorption. Impressively, alfalfa is also the richest land source of trace minerals.

This perennial herb that grows throughout the world in a variety of climates helps the body to assimilate iron, phosphorus, potassium, protein, calcium, and other nutrients. In addition, it contains high levels of chlorophyll, and therefore it is a good body cleanser, infection fighter, and natural deodorizer. In fact, alfalfa alkalizes and detoxifies the body, especially the liver. It also breaks down poisonous carbon dioxide.

The beneficial effects of alfalfa don't stop there. Alfalfa is a good laxative and a natural diuretic. It is useful in the treatment of urinary tract infections and kidney, bladder, and prostate disorders. And it promotes pituitary gland function and contains an anti-fungus agent. Regarding the eyes, alfalfa's vitamin A content is particularly good for eye dryness and retinal function. Also, in traditional Chinese medicine, it is believed that anything that enhances the liver/kidneys also positively affects the eyes.

Bayberry

Bayberry (*Myrica cerifera*) can be useful in warding off colds at the first sign, especially when taken along with the herb capsicum (*Capsicum frutescens*). It is also helpful when used as a gargle for tonsillitis and sore throats. In addition to its anti-cold actions, there are many more health perks associated with bayberry. This herb has long been used as a tonic, stimulating the system to help raise vitality and resistance to disease. It has been touted as an aid to digestion and nutrition, and even to build the blood.

Bayberry is beneficial in the rejuvenation of the adrenal glands, cleansing of the bloodstream, and elimination of toxins. In India, the powdered root bark of bayberry is combined with ginger (*Zingiber officinale*) to successfully combat cholera. It kills germs and is stimulating to the mucous membranes, including those around the eye. Nutritionally, its healing benefits are rooted in its high amount of vitamin C. As we have learned in previous discussions, vitamin C is a powerful antioxidant. It is fuel for white blood cells, which then protect our bodies from infection and illness.

Bilberry

The bilberry plant is a small, shrubby perennial that grows in the woods and meadows of northern Europe. Bilberry (*Vaccinium myrtillus*) has been shown to be completely nontoxic, having no side effects and no contraindications. While this herb might sound mild, it has numerous health benefits. Bilberry's fruit contains flavonoids and anthocyanin, which serve to prevent capillary fragility, thin the blood, and stimulate the release of vasodilators. (*Anthocyanin* is a type of antioxidant that lowers blood pressure, reduces clotting, and improves blood supply to the nervous system.) The fruit of the bilberry also contains vitamins A and C, the bioflavonoids, and minerals. And bilberry contains *glucoquinine*, which has the ability to lower blood sugar.

This herb acts as a potent antioxidant, improves blood circulation, and has anti-inflammatory properties. In addition to these wonderful perks, bilberry has specific eye-health benefits. It enhances the regeneration of rhodopsin (visual purple) in the retina.

Moreover, bilberry has long been a remedy for poor vision. Some of bilberry's benefits include improving night vision and preventing and treating cataracts, diabetic retinopathy, eyestrain, macular degeneration, and glaucoma. Clinical tests confirm that, given orally, this very powerful antioxidant improves contrast sensitivity (that is, reduces glare) in healthy eyes, and it can help those with eye diseases such as glaucoma (see page 233).

Borage Oil

Borage (*Borago officinalis*) is especially soothing in cases of bronchitis and digestive upset. But it also promotes the activity of the kidneys and adrenal glands. Borage oil contains *gamma-linolenic acid* (*GLA*), a fatty acid that the body converts to a hormone-like substance called *prostaglandin E1* (*PGE1*). PGE1 has anti-inflammatory properties and may also act as a blood thinner and blood vessel dilator. But borage oil does need a balance of omega-3 fatty acids to work effectively.

What about borage oil's effects on the eyes? When combined with omega-3 essential fatty acids, it is directly responsible for an anti-inflammatory effect that increases tear production. This is especially beneficial to those who suffer from dry eyes. Borage oil also contains calcium and potassium, making it soothing to the mucous membranes, especially those in the covering of the eye.

Comfrey

Comfrey (*Symphytum officinale*) is one of the most valuable herbs known to botanical medicine. Comfrey is rich in vitamins A and C. It is high in protein, calcium, phosphorus, and potassium. This herb also contains copper, iron, magnesium, sulfur, and zinc, as well as eighteen amino acids. Clearly, it packs a nutritional punch.

Comfrey has been used successfully for centuries as a wound healer and bone knitter. It helps to maintain the calcium-phosphorus balance, promoting strong bones and healthy skin. In addition, comfrey encourages the secretion of the digestive enzyme pepsin and is a general aid to digestion. Actually, comfrey has a beneficial effect on all the parts of the body and is therefore used as an overall tonic. It feeds the pituitary with a natural hormone, and it helps to strengthen the body skeleton.

Topically, comfrey traditionally has been used to treat minor skin irritations and inflammation. It has also been used as a wash or topical application for eye irritations and for treating conjunctivitis. But internal use of the herb is a little more complicated. Comfrey can contain toxins called *pyrrolizidine alkaloids.* Due to variations in pyrrolizidine alkaloid content, root preparations are unsafe for internal use unless they are guaranteed to be pyrrolizidine-free. Although comfrey root tea has been used traditionally, the danger of its pyrrolizidine alkaloids is significant. Therefore, comfrey root and young leaf preparations should not be taken internally.

Eyebright

Eyebright (*Euphrasia officinalis*) was and continues to be used by herbalists primarily as a poultice for the topical treatment of eye inflammations, including blepharitis, pinkeye, and styes, all of which are discussed in Part Two. It is also credited with helping to stimulate the liver to cleanse the blood and relieve the conditions that affect the clarity of vision. Therefore, eyebright has traditionally been used as a remedy for eye problems such as failing vision, pinkeye, ulcers, and even eyestrain and eye fatigue. In addition, herbalists have recommended eyebright for problems of the respiratory tract, including sinus infections, coughs, and sore throat.

This herb is useful against inflammations because of its cooling and detoxifying properties. Plus, it has antiseptic properties that fight infections of the eyes. Traditionally, a compress made from a decoction of eyebright is used to give relief from redness, swelling, and visual disturbances due to eye infections. A tea is sometimes given internally along with the topical treatment.

Eyebright is so health-enhancing because it is extremely rich in vitamins A and C. And it contains the vitamin B complex, vitamin D, and some vitamin E. Adding to its nutritional value, this herb also has copper, iron, silicon, zinc, and a trace of iodine. But there is a lack of research that proves the efficacy of eyebright beyond its nutritional contents. While there are many chemicals that may be active in eyebright, none of them has been *proven* to have any effect on eye inflammation or irritation. Some herbal texts suggest that the astringent actions of eyebright may reduce eye irritation, while others suggest that eyebright may also have antibacterial actions when administered topically. To date, and despite its name, there are no clinical studies to support or refute these proposed actions. In fact, none of the traditional uses of eyebright have been studied in clinical research.

Ginkgo Biloba

Medicinal use of ginkgo (*Ginkgo biloba*), one of the most popular herbs to be used in the United States, can be traced back almost 5,000 years in Chinese herbal medicine. The nuts of the ginkgo tree were most commonly recommended and used to treat respiratory tract ailments. The use of the leaves is a modern development originating in Europe. Ginkgo is well known for its positive effect on memory and thinking (cognitive function). It may enhance cognitive performance in healthy older adults, in people with age-related cognitive decline, and in people with Alzheimer's disease. Thus, its benefits seem to be varied and powerful.

In general, ginkgo biloba extract (GBE) regulates the tone and elasticity of blood vessels, making circulation more efficient. The medical benefits of GBE are attributed primarily to two groups of active constituents: the *ginkgo flavone glycosides* and the *terpene lactones*. Ginkgo flavone glycosides, which typically make up approximately 24 percent of the extract, are primarily responsible for GBE's antioxidant activity and may mildly inhibit platelet aggregation (stickiness of the blood). These two actions may ultimately help GBE prevent circulatory diseases, such as atherosclerosis, and support the brain and central nervous system. In addition, GBE's antioxidant action may also extend to the brain and retina of the eye. Preliminary trials have suggested that people with macular degeneration and diabetic retinopathy can potentially benefit from ingesting the extract, but only in the early stages of the diseases.

As for GBE's terpene lactones, known as *ginkgolides* and *bilobalide*, they typically make up approximately 6 percent of the extract. They are associated with increasing circulation to the brain and other parts of the body, and thus also can contribute to eye health. And the terpene lactones may exert a protective action on nerve cells.

Goldenseal

Goldenseal (*Hydrastis canadensis*) has been used to boost a sluggish glandular system and to promote youthful hormone harmony. The active ingredient of the herb goes directly into the bloodstream and helps to regulate liver function. And goldenseal has a natural antibiotic ability to stop infection and to kill poisons in the body. It is valuable against all of the mucus-forming conditions that occur in the nasal, bronchial, throat, intestinal, stomach, and bladder areas. In fact, goldenseal has the ability to heal mucous membranes anywhere in the body, including the external eye tissue.

Goldenseal contains vitamins A and C. It also has the B-complex vitamins and vitamin E; the minerals calcium, copper, iron, manganese, phosphorus, potassium, sodium, and zinc; and unsaturated fatty acids. When taken along with other herbs, its tonic properties are increased for whatever ailment is being treated. However, there may be some negative interactions when taking doxycycline or tetracycline antibiotics, so be sure to consult your physician or herbalist before using goldenseal if you are taking antibiotics. Finally, be aware that due to overharvesting, goldenseal is now considered an endangered species. Therefore, it is used very rarely by responsible herbalists. As you can imagine, due to its rarity, goldenseal is very expensive.

Hawthorn

Hawthorn (*Crataegus oxycantha*) is a vasodilator that opens the blood vessels of the heart and also lowers the cholesterol level. It is found across the globe, in North America, Europe, northern Africa, and western Asia. Its healthful contents are as varied as its locations; hawthorn contains vitamins B_1, B_2, B_3, B_6, B_{12}, and C, as well as citric acid, choline, the flavonoids, folic acid, PABA, and selenium. It increases the intracellular vitamin C level, and it is useful against anemia, cardiovascular and circulatory disorders, high cholesterol, and lowered immunity.

As for the eyes, hawthorn's enhancement of immunity allows it to help prevent eye infections. The vasodilator effects can increase blood flow to the retina, as well. Hawthorn does have a contraindication, however; it should not be taken with Digoxin, which is also a vasodilator that, therefore, increases circulation to the eye.

Marigold

Marigold (*Calendula officinalis*) has been harvested in gardens and pots since the Middle Ages, due to its beautiful blossoms. And marigold—also commonly called calendula—grows equally as well in the wild. Its various types are all high in phosphorus and contain vitamins A and C. Flavonoids, also found in high amounts in marigold, are thought to account for much of its anti-inflammatory activity. Other potentially important constituents include the *triterpene saponins*—the main constituents of the essential oils of many types of plants and flowers—and the carotenoids.

Marigold is very useful as a first-aid

remedy. It has been used as a tea for acute ailments, especially fevers, and is effective as a tincture when applied to bruises, sprains, muscle spasms, and ulcers. This herb relieves earache, boosts the heart and circulation, and cleanses the lymphatic system. And when it comes to the eyes, there are more benefits associated with this herb. Traditionally, a sterile tea was topically applied in cases of pinkeye, also commonly known as conjunctivitis. It is now common knowledge that the petals of the marigold flower have a significant amount of lutein, the yellow pigment found in the retina that can protect the retina against damage from high-energy blue light.

Passionflower

In actuality, the name of this herb is related to the "passion of Christ." Various marks on and parts of the flower are given symbolic meaning linked with the crucifixion of Jesus. Native to Texas, Mexico, and Central America, passionflower has a centuries-long history of healing. But what constituent of this herb is responsible for its effects? Passionflower contains the flavonoids, which are actually a subgroup of the bioflavonoids.

Despite its name, passionflower (*Passiflora incarnata*) is used to treat insomnia and hysteria, as well as hyperactivity and convulsions in children. It is an herb that is quieting and soothing to the nervous system. It should be recommended to patients who wish to wean themselves from synthetic sleeping pills or tranquilizers. Passionflower also helps to reduce high blood pressure and tachycardia (racing of the heart), and it is an effective anti-spasmotic. As for eye treatments, when taken orally, passionflower is good for inflamed eyes and eyestrain.

Red Clover

Once you realize how many nutrients red clover (*Trifolium pratense*) contains, it is easy to understand why it has become a versatile natural remedy. Red clover is a good source of vitamin A. It is high in iron, and contains the B-complex vitamins, vitamin C, the bioflavonoids, and unsaturated fatty acids. It is valued for its high mineral content. For example, it is rich in calcium, copper, and magnesium, and contains some cobalt, manganese, nickel, selenium, sodium, and tin. However, it should not be taken while pregnant or breast-feeding.

Red clover has a multitude of applications. It is useful as a tonic for the nerves and as a sedative for nervous exhaustion. Yet this herb also has been credited with resolving a lack of vitality. And it is effective against coughs, a weak chest, wheezing, and bronchitis. When mixed with honey and water, it is useful as a cough syrup. It is good as an aid for strengthening the respiratory systems of delicate children. In addition, Native Americans used the plant as a tea for sore eyes and as a salve for burns. It has even been included in some well-known cancer mixtures.

Rose Hips

Rose hips (*Rosa canina*) are actually the fruit of a rose that develops after the petals have fallen. In fact, rose hips contain a natural fruit sugar. They have been a staple food item for Native American tribes; rose hips are not only used for tea, but in soups, stews, and as even

as a side dish because they are so health-enhancing. When compared with other herbs, rose hips have the highest vitamin C content. Actually, they have more vitamin C than an orange! They are also extremely rich in vitamins A and E, and very high in the vitamin B complex. Moreover, rose hips contain vitamin D and the bioflavonoids, a lot of calcium and iron, and some potassium, silica, sodium, and sulfur.

This herb plays an important role in treatments where vitamins A, C, and E are needed. It helps to prevent infections, and also aids in treatment when an infection has already developed. And rose hips are very nourishing to the skin and all epithelial-type cells, including those on the surface of the eye.

Rosemary

Rosemary (*Rosmarinus officinalis*) is often used in cuisine, due to its woodsy flavor. In legends from the past, it had been linked with extending memory, so rosemary became a tradition at key ceremonies, including weddings and funerals. But it contains a lot more than a delicious flavor and sentimental value. Vitamins A and C are present in rosemary. In addition, rosemary is high in calcium and contains iron, magnesium, phosphorus, potassium, sodium, and zinc.

This herb is a stimulant, especially of the circulatory system and pelvic region. It is considered a proven heart tonic and a treatment for high blood pressure, which provides a link to the eyes. Any herb that helps keep blood pressure at a healthy level also contributes to eye health, as high blood pressure is damaging to the eyes. In cases of colds or flu, rosemary can be taken in the early stages as a warm infusion, and it may be used as a cooling tea when the symptoms include restlessness, nervousness, and insomnia. Rosemary has been credited with being one of the most powerful remedies to strengthen the nervous system. It is a good tonic for the reproductive organs and has also been effective against diarrhea, especially in children. Externally, rosemary is used on bites and stings.

Rue

Rue (*Ruta graveolens*) has the ability to expel poisons from the system, and therefore it has been used for snake, scorpion, spider, and jellyfish bites. Old lore held rue as a powerful protector against evil. Thus, it has had its place in a variety of traditions over the centuries. And its reputation as a trigger for creativity has caused many great artists to add a little to their meals. Importantly, rue must be used in small doses only, as it is actually poisonous in larger amounts.

When properly administered, rue is very health-enhancing. It contains a large amount of *rutin*. Rutin is a bioflavonoid that is known for its ability to strengthen the capillaries and veins—especially those in the eyes. It is also commonly used in a homeopathic preparation (see the next section of Part One for more information on homeopathy). Rue also helps to remove deposits that tend to form in the tendons and joints, especially in the wrist joints, with age. It has even been found to be effective at treating high blood pressure, and helps to harden the bones and teeth. As for eye health, in addition to the blood pressure benefits, rue has been rumored to be very effective at preserving sight by strengthening the eye

muscles. However, there has been no clinical confirmation of this effect.

Sarsaparilla

Sarsaparilla (*Smilax officinalis*) grows in the moist rain forests of Central and South America, as well as in Jamaica and the Caribbean. It has been part of the healing arts in those locations for centuries. Yet sarsaparilla is also found in temperate zones across the globe, in places such as Australia and parts of southeast Asia. It not only has many native locations, but also many healthful contents. Sarsaparilla contains vitamins A, C, and D, as well as the B complex, and it has copper, iodine, iron, manganese, silicon, sodium, sulfur, and zinc.

This is a valuable herb used in glandular-balancing formulas. Its stimulating properties are noted for increasing the metabolic rate. Sarsaparilla also contains precursors of both the male and female hormones. But in regard to the eyes, it has been used internally to relieve sore eyes. The relief of soreness is due to its anti-inflammatory properties and its ability to deliver some amount of pain relief.

Siberian Ginseng

Siberian ginseng (*Eleutherococcus senticosus*) is very effective at increasing circulation, especially around the heart, normalizing blood pressure, and combating stress and fatigue. This thorny shrub has been very well studied, especially in Russia where it has been valued for its ability to aid the body under stressful circumstances. It increases brain and physical efficiency, improves concentration span, and increases speed and accuracy in work. This popular herb also strengthens the adrenal and reproductive glands. It stimulates the production of T-cells, which support the immune system, and it improves blood-lipid levels. Lastly, Siberian ginseng is a powerful antioxidant. The antioxidant effect can reduce the potential development of eye conditions, such as macular degeneration and cataracts.

There are several ginsengs available, but the plants are distinct. Many consumers do not realize that Siberian ginseng possesses different properties than American and Asian ginsengs. Siberian ginseng contains the B-complex vitamins, vitamin E, and *eleutherosides*, which are a type of complex sugar molecule with beneficial effects.

Taheebo

Taheebo (*Tabebuia impetiginosa*) also goes by several other names: pau d'arco, lapacho, and ipe roxo. It is found in South America, and it is a very powerful antibiotic with virus-killing properties. There is actually a taheebo tree, and the medicinal part of the herb discussed here is found in the bark. The Aztec and Incan tribes are historically some of the earliest tribes to recognize the herb for its healing effects. Taheebo contains a high amount of iron, which aids in the proper assimilation of nutrients and the elimination of wastes. Finally, it contains flavonoids.

Taheebo is said to contain compounds that seem to attack the causes of diseases. One of its main actions purportedly is to put the body into a defensive posture, to give it the energy needed for defense against and resistance to disease. It's a general "tonic" for building the immune system—which is always good for the eyes as well.

Wild Cherry

It's actually the bark of the wild cherry (*Prunus serotina*) tree that is credited with being an antioxidant and a remedy for a number of ailments. Native Americans traditionally made a tea with this bark and used it as a medicine for problems as varied as cold symptoms, diarrhea, and even labor pains. Wild cherry was considered a sedative.

Today, this herb continues to be considered very useful, especially as an expectorant. It is a valuable remedy for all mucus-forming conditions, and it is beneficial against bronchial disorders caused by hardened accumulations of mucus. Wild cherry contains a volatile oil that acts as a local stimulant in the alimentary canal and aids digestion. In general, it is a useful tonic for persons convalescing from diseases. It can also balance the tear film in any inflammatory eye condition.

After reading highlights on the previous herbs that, among other benefits, contribute to eye health, you have a solid foundation for further investigation into herbal therapies. Of course, there are many, many additional herbs that generally contribute to health. A huge amount of information on herbs is available, whether you are on the Internet or in a health food store. Just be sure to rely on reputable sources and practitioners if you decide to pursue herbal therapies. When buying an herb, make sure that you have selected the correct variety, since quite a few herbs are known by more than one name. If you are unsure of the specific herb that should be purchased, or if you have questions about the action of an herb, you should certainly consult an herbalist.

Most herbs can be purchased in bulk from health food stores or by mail order. For reliable mail-order companies, see Recommended Suppliers on page 409. Store bulk herbs in airtight containers in a dark, cool place.

HERBS TO AVOID

As much as we can reap positive effects from herbal remedies, we also need to take some precautions in their use. We must realize that the potency of herbs works both ways—they can be very effective treatments, but they can also be irritants and cause unwanted reactions. This holds true in a discussion about the eyes as much as it does for the rest of the body and its systems. So below you will find warnings about certain herbs that will result in undesirable effects on the eyes.

Herbs That Have Steroid-Like Effects

Steroids can be prescribed for many inflammatory conditions, but they are not without serious side effects. They are therefore used sparingly. The following herbs have the same anti-inflammatory effects as steroids *and* can cause the same ocular problems. These include but are not limited to cataracts, glaucoma, herpes simplex keratitis (corneal inflammation), light sensitivity, and retinal-blood-vessel problems.

- bethroot
- blue cohosh
- damiana
- false unicorn root
- fenugreek
- figwort
- ginseng
- goldenrod
- licorice
- red sage
- saw palmetto
- wild yam

Herbs That Have Aspirin-Like Effects

Aspirin is used for everything from relieving headaches to thinning blood. Some herbs have the same effects as aspirin (salicylates), as well as the same ocular effects of blurred vision, disturbed accommodation, optic atrophy, retinal edema (that is, retinal swelling), and visual-field constriction. These herbs are listed below:

- birch
- black cohosh
- black willow
- blue flag
- chickweed
- crampbark
- meadowsweet
- pansy
- sweet violet
- wintergreen

Diuretic Herbs

Diuretics are substances that affect the fluid and electrolyte balances in the body. They can cause blurred vision, disturbed accommodation, dry eyes, light sensitivity, xanthopsia (that is, yellow vision), and nearsightedness. The following herbs act as diuretics:

- bearberry
- birch
- blue flag
- boldo
- broom tops
- buchu
- bugleweed
- carline thistle
- cleavers
- hydrangea
- juniper
- licorice
- night-blooming cereus
- pansy
- parsley
- saw palmetto
- sea holly
- shepherd's purse

- corn silk
- couch grass
- dandelion
- fumitory
- gravelroot
- stone root
- sweet violet
- wild carrot
- yarrow

- bistort
- coltsfoot
- cudweed
- daisy
- eyebright
- golden root
- goldenseal
- ground ivy
- mouse ear
- myrrh
- pokeroot
- Scots pine

Herbs With Potent Oils

Some herbs contain volatile or aromatic oils that can cause ocular effects. Such effects include excessive tearing, irritation, contamination of contact lenses, and disorders of the central nervous system. These herbs are listed below:

- cinnamon
- clove
- cudweed
- echinacea
- fennel
- garlic
- ginger
- pennyroyal
- peppermint
- prickly ash
- queen's delight
- red sage
- rosemary
- selfheal
- skunk cabbage
- tansy
- thyme
- southernwood
- valerian
- wild carrot
- willow
- wintergreen

Herbs That Cause Dryness

Certain herbs have a drying effect on the eye tissue. This can, in some cases, be detrimental, especially if you have a dry eye condition or are wearing contact lenses. The following list identifies some of the drying herbs:

Other Herbs With Possible Side Effects

There is an assortment of additional herbs that possibly can affect the eyes in adverse ways. The list below associates specific symptoms with various herbs. Of course, different people will have different degrees of reactions, and some will not react at all to the herbs below. However, it is very important to consider the possibilities.

Herbs can certainly have medicinal-type actions on our bodies and I don't want to diminish the fact that we can use herbs to treat disease while avoiding many of the negative side effects of medications. But, as the above information indicates, like medications, herbs can also be harmful if taken inappropriately. Therefore, you should be prudent when choosing an herbal therapy. I strongly recommend consulting a qualified herbalist to discuss your options before taking any herb for any reason. And that certainly also applies to combinations of herbal therapies, which are discussed below.

WESTERN HERBAL COMBINATIONS FOR EYE PROBLEMS

While some herbs should be taken alone, many can be combined to make effective remedies.

ADDITIONAL HERBS AND THEIR POSSIBLE SIDE EFFECTS

HERB	ASSOCIATED SYMPTOMS
Arnica	Eye irritation.
Bittersweet	Blurred vision, dilated pupils, loss of accommodation, glaucoma, light sensitivity.
Bladderwrack	Metabolic changes due to altered thyroid activity, which includes bulging eyes associated with Graves' disease.
California poppy	Constricted pupils.
Canthaxanthine	Abnormalities in visual field, retina function, and dark adaptation.
Chamomile	Severe pinkeye/conjunctivitis.
Datura	Dilated pupils.
Echinacea	Eye irritation, pinkeye/conjunctivitis.
Ephedra	Dilated pupils, dry eyes, increased eye pressure.
Figwort	Lazy eye, blurred vision, central blind spot, double vision, disturbed color vision, disturbed accommodation, light sensitivity.
Hawthorn	Lazy eye, blurred vision, central blind spot, double vision, disturbed color vision, disturbed accommodation, light sensitivity.
Ginkgo biloba	Retinal hemorrhage, internal eye bleeding.
Kava	Blurred vision, red eyes, and dilated pupils.
Licorice	Transient visual loss.
Lily of the valley	Lazy eye, blurred vision, central blind spot, double vision, disturbed color vision, disturbed accommodation, light sensitivity.
Night-blooming cereus	Lazy eye, blurred vision, central blind spot, double vision, disturbed color vision, disturbed accommodation, light sensitivity.
Shepherd's purse	Blurred vision, red eyes, constricted pupils.
Squill	Lazy eye, blurred vision, central blind spot, double vision, disturbed color vision, disturbed accommodation, light sensitivity.

Herbal combinations have more than one benefit in the fight against eye problems, since they consist of several substances that each has its own benefits, and those substances then work together in natural harmony. When taken over a period of time, an herbal combination will condition the body to react in a way that is comparable to the effects produced by certain medications, but in a less drastic manner and without the unwanted side effects. Below you will find two herbal combinations from the Western tradition. They are suited to enhancing eye health.

When using an herbal combination, follow

the same precautions outlined for single herbs earlier in this chapter. A number of pre-mixed herbal combinations are available from health food stores and by mail order, but you can also mix a combination yourself if you are careful to keep your ingredients, tools, and work area clean. The usual recipe calls for approximately equal amounts of the different herbs. To prepare a tea, infusion, or other desired mixture, follow the procedures described for single herbs in "Forms of Herbal Preparations" on page 109.

Combination Number One

The first herbal combination consists of three herbs: bayberry, eyebright, and goldenseal. Bayberry is high in vitamin C; it kills germs and stimulates the mucous membranes so that irritants can be trapped in mucus and removed from the body. Eyebright boosts the body's immunity to eye problems. Lastly, goldenseal acts as a natural antibiotic against eye infections.

Bayberry, eyebright, and goldenseal are three of the more common herbs used for external eye conditions. Although each one used separately is effective, the combination benefits several types of eye problems, which make this combination a good choice if you are not sure of exactly what is wrong with your eyes. Specifically, this combination has been shown to be good for cataracts, iritis, pinkeye, and weak eyes.

Combination Number Two

The second herbal combination consists of the three herbs from the combination discussed above—bayberry, eyebright, and goldenseal—plus raspberry and capsicum. Raspberry is effective against styes, and its astringent action helps to stop discharge. Capsicum acts as both a stimulant (to increase blood flow) and a relaxant (it relieves pain). In addition, it is high in vitamin A and a number of minerals.

Use caution with this herbal combination. Capsicum is a very powerful herb and can cause severe damage to delicate tissues if not used properly. If the eye is very inflamed and has a discharge, use a very small amount of capsicum in the mixture. This combination will help to increase the eye area's circulation and thus rid the tissue of toxins. Consult an herbalist if you have any concerns or questions about the proper combination of herbs to use.

Herbal combinations work because the herbs trigger neurochemical reflexes in the body that, over time, become automatic and continue even after the person stops taking the herbs. One advantage of using an herbal combination instead of a medication is that the herbs help the body to bring about its own recovery and make the body unlikely to be susceptible to the same complaint during or after convalescence. Unlike medications, which treat symptoms, herbal combinations go right to the root of the disorder and treat its cause.

TRADITIONAL CHINESE HERBAL COMBINATIONS

As touched upon earlier, Chinese medicine is a science and art form that is well over 5,000 years old. The procedures and symptomology of Chinese medicine differ significantly from those of Western medicine. For example, a

Chinese medical practitioner generally asks different types of questions and performs different diagnostic tests than does a Western medical practitioner. The emotional aspects of illness are often of more concern to Chinese practitioners than to Western practitioners, and Chinese and Western practitioners often find different patterns in the health of the patient to be of interest. Oftentimes, there is no correlation between our Western medical terminology and diagnoses and those of traditional Chinese medicine.

It is rare for Chinese practitioners to use one herb alone. Some of the traditional Chinese herbal combinations contain only herbs, which are chosen because of the way they interact

TRADITIONAL CHINESE HERBAL COMBINATIONS AND THEIR USES

HERBAL COMBINATION	APPLICATIONS
An mian pian	Cools liver "heat"; helps to relieve anxiety, red eyes, and eye irritation.
Er ming zuo ci wan	Treats liver deficiency that is causing symptoms such as headaches, high blood pressure, pressure behind the eyes, insomnia, thirst, and eye irritation.
Long dan xie gan wan	Purges liver and gallbladder "heat"; relieves headaches, red and burning eyes, ringing in the ears, sore throat, fever blisters on the mouth, scanty urination, and constipation.
Ming mu di huang wan	Replenishes the energy in the liver and kidneys; relieves dry eyes, red and itchy eyes, poor eyesight, light sensitivity, excessive tearing, and eye diseases such as glaucoma and cataracts.
Ming mu shang qing pian	Dispels "heat"; clears the vision; sedates the liver; reduces liver "heat" that is affecting the eyes, causing redness, itching, tearing, and swelling (including pinkeye).
Nei zhang ming yan wan	Benefits the clarity of vision; nourishes the liver and kidneys; reduces "heat"; helps circulation; improves impaired vision due to a liver deficiency; aids recovery from eye surgery; helps treat cataracts, glaucoma, disturbed day or night vision, and itchy, painful eyes.
Niu huang shang qing wan	Relieves systemic "heat" rising from the liver that causes headaches, eye pain or eye redness, sore throat, toothache, or a fever with thirst.
Qi ju di huang wan	Nourishes the kidneys, boosting their energy; helps remedy blurred vision, dry and painful eyes, pressure behind the eyes, and disturbed night vision; aids in treating dizziness, headaches, pain behind the eyes, and restlessness.
Shi hu ye guang wan	Improves vision, especially eyesight that is beginning to become blurry or is affected by dizziness; serves as a valuable treatment in the early stages of cataract formation; relieves tearing eyes, red or itchy eyes, dry eyes, or hypertensive (high blood pressure) changes within the eyes.
Xiao yao wan	Remedies stagnation of the liver due to a blood deficiency; relieves diverse symptoms, including digestive dysfunction, menstrual and premenstrual disorders, vertigo, headaches, fatigue, blurred vision, and red, painful eyes; treats food allergies, chronic hay fever, and hypoglycemia.
Zhong guo shou wu zhi	Acts as an excellent tonic for the blood, nourishing the liver and kidneys and benefitting the eyes and tendons.

with one another. In fact, certain combinations include as many as twenty-five different herbs. A number of combinations also include non-herbal ingredients, such as minerals, plants, and animal organs. Many of the combinations listed in the table on page 123 are not used strictly for eye conditions. Since Chinese medicine strives to treat the whole person—the body, mind, and spirit—the treatment oftentimes is also directed toward a whole other set of symptoms, which may or may not be apparent.

The Chinese use terminology from their observations of nature to describe the workings of the inner body. For example, if a practitioner talks about "heat from the liver," he may be describing a series of conditions caused by an emotional constraint or blockage of energy in the liver. This "heat from the liver" may manifest as an inflammation (a Western medical term) in the head area—for example, a sore throat, earache, red eyes, or irritability. A person's condition is a very individualized expression of a disorder, and different people may display completely different combinations of symptoms. The different combinations of symptoms that are possible are what have given rise to the various herbal combinations used in traditional Chinese medicine. Some of the more common traditional Chinese herbal combinations that may have beneficial effects on eye conditions are discussed in the table on the previous page.

Since these and any other herbal preparations are not "pure" substances, you need to use caution when taking them. A problem to consider is that different parts of the herbs—the roots, leaves, pods, bark, seeds, flowers—are often used, giving different batches varying degrees of potency, or strength. In some cases, the potency of the active ingredient in an herb matches or exceeds that of the medication that is manufactured using that ingredient. Furthermore, some companies package and market their products in a way that fosters misuse of natural products by consumers who believe that "natural" means "weak" and "safe." And, of course, some products do have undesirable side effects, which can lead to dire consequences. Therefore, I highly recommend consultation with an experienced herbalist before taking any herb or herbal combination.

CONCLUSION

The use of and search for drugs and dietary supplements derived from plants have accelerated in recent years. Pharmacologists, microbiologists, botanists, and natural-products chemists are combing the earth for phytochemicals that could provide treatment for various diseases. In fact, according to the World Health Organization, approximately 25 percent of modern drugs used in the United States have been derived from plants. Most herbalists concede that pharmaceuticals are more effective in emergency situations, when time is of the essence. But many people prefer the "natural" approach of herbs that have been shown, over the centuries, to truly help heal the human body.

Homeopathic Remedies and Eye Health

Homeopathy (ho-me-OP-a-thee) is a system of medicine whose principles are even older than Hippocrates. Homeopathic medicines are prescribed according to an age-old standard that recognizes the body's ability to heal itself. This system seeks to cure in accordance with the natural laws of healing, and it uses medicines made from natural animal, vegetable, and mineral substances. The remedies are prepared in such a way that they are nontoxic and do not cause side effects.

This approach was discovered in the early 1800s by a German physician named Samuel Hahnemann. It was extremely popular in the United States in the nineteenth century, but its popularity then declined because of the new drugs and other political and economic changes in the practice of medicine. The holistic movement that surfaced in the early 1970s has been advocating a return to the natural laws of healing and has sparked a revival of interest in this scientific system of medicine.

Because you may not be familiar with the process used to produce homeopathic remedies and the system of diagnosis and treatment, we will review the laws of homeopathy in this chapter. We will also discuss the specific remedies that can be used to help the eyes and the

visual system. Toward the end of the chapter, I will offer a few comments on the relationship between homeopathy and herbalism, the latter of which you studied in the previous section. I hope these thoughts will be useful if you are considering either of these options.

THE LAWS OF HOMEOPATHY

Like any science, the system of homeopathy is governed by certain "laws" that dictate how the process works—laws which have not been changed or improved upon for over 200 years. These laws must be followed in order for the process to be considered homeopathic. There are three laws of this system: the Law of Similars; the Law of Proving; and the Law of Potentization.

The Law of Similars

The term "homeopathy" comes from the Greek *homoios*, meaning "similar," and *pathos*, translated as "suffering" or "sickness." The fundamental law upon which homeopathy is based is called the Law of Similars, which states that "like is cured by like." According to the Law of Similars, a remedy can cure a disease if it produces, in a healthy person, symptoms that are similar to those of the illness.

The basic concept of the Law of Similars is attributed to Hindu sages from the tenth century BCE. Those sages explained, "Through the like, disease is produced, and through the application of the like, it is cured." The following is an example of how the law works. Let's imagine that a person develops a fever, along with a flushed face, dilated pupils, a rapid heartbeat, and a feeling of restlessness. The homeopathic physician studies all of these symptoms, then searches for a remedy that, under scientifically controlled conditions, has produced all of these symptoms in a healthy person. The remedy is administered and, within a short time after taking the remedy, the patient's fever drops and she begins to feel well again. In other words, using the Law of Similars, a classic homeopathic physician selects the one necessary medicine by matching the symptoms of the patient's disorder to the symptoms the remedy is known to induce.

The Law of Proving

The second law of homeopathy, the Law of Proving, refers to the method used to test a substance to determine its medicinal effect. To "prove" a remedy, half of a group of healthy people is given a dose of the test substance, and the remaining half is given a placebo (an inactive substance). Conforming to the standard double-blind method used in pharmacological experiments, neither the subjects nor the researchers know which substance a particular person is taking. Every day, all of the subjects carefully record the symptoms they experience.

When the experiment is complete, it is determined who took what substance. All of the symptoms experienced by the persons taking the substance are listed as a characteristic remedy picture in the reference book. To treat a patient, a homeopathic physician looks up the remedy picture in the reference book and, when the symptoms fit, applies the Law of Similars.

The Law of Potentization

The third law of homeopathy, the Law of Potentization, refers to the method of preparation of a homeopathic remedy. All homeopathic remedies are prepared using a controlled process consisting of dilution followed by succussion (shaking), which may be repeated until the resulting medicine contains few or no molecules of the original substance. The original tincture is an alcohol-based extract of the substance as it comes directly from the plant, animal, or mineral. The dilutions are called *potencies.* Lesser dilutions are known as low potencies, and greater dilutions are known as high potencies. As strange as it may seem, the more a remedy is diluted, the greater is its potency.

The potencies are designated by a number followed by an "x" or "c." The "x" represents 10, and it signifies that the original tincture has been diluted to 1 part in 10. The "c" represents 100, and it signifies that the original tincture has been diluted to 1 part in 100. The number preceding the "x" or "c" indicates the number of times the remedy has been diluted. Thus, a 3x-potency remedy has been diluted three times, and a 6x-potency remedy has been diluted six times. For purposes of consistency, the recommended homeopathic remedies in this book are all 6x and should be used three to four times daily.

When the currently-used process of potentization was devised roughly 200 years ago, the idea that medicine containing an infinitesimal amount of matter could be curative was inconceivable. In this nuclear age, however, the power of minute quantities is all too well established. The dose of vitamin B_{12} that is used to treat certain anemias contains one-millionth of a gram of cobalt. Trace elements, essential for physical development and functioning, are present in the body in barely measurable amounts. The human body manufactures only fifty- to one-hundred-millionth of a gram of thyroid hormone each day, yet a small deviation in the amount can seriously affect the health of an individual.

The power of the infinitesimal dose is not clearly understood, but neither are the actions of many modern medications. The process of potentization makes it possible to use as medicines substances such as certain metals, charcoal, and sand, which are inert in their natural states. Potentized remedies do not contain sufficient matter to act directly on the tissues, which means that homeopathic medicines are nontoxic and cannot cause side effects.

The background you have read on homeopathy will help you better understand and use the remaining information in this section. It is important to be familiar with the philosophies or concepts behind the system in order to appreciate its approach. But before we get to the remedies, we should consider how homeopathy applies to the eyes in particular. Read on.

SINGLE REMEDIES AND HOW TO ADMINISTER THEM

Although we have been emphasizing that the eyes are an integral part of the body and that, like the body, they respond to nutritional influences and environmental factors, there are not very many homeopathic remedies specifically for the disorders that afflict the eyes. Many of the homeopathic recommendations you will see listed for various disorders in Part Two may be considered general—that is, prescribed for general symptoms. The remedy may not be directed at the specific eye disorder or even at the chief complaint, but at the person's well-being as a whole. That being said, the correct homeopathic remedy may act instantaneously, like an electric spark, upon the defense mechanism or vital force, and the effects of one dose may last for a month.

Homeopathic remedies come in liquids, creams, pellets, and tablets. The liquid form is an alcohol-based extract of a specific remedy and therefore should not be used directly on the eye. It generally is placed under the tongue with an eyedropper, which usually comes with the bottle. Because the oral liquid remedies contain alcohol, they should be given to children only in small doses. The liquid can also be used to make a cream, ointment, or salve, which is done by mixing the liquid with a cream or gel base. Creams, ointments, and salves are almost never used on the eye tissue itself.

Tablets and pellets, which are made with a base of lactose (sweet milk sugar), are dissolved in the mouth, usually under the tongue, without chewing. They are excellent for use with children. However, they should not be

COMMON HOMEOPATHIC REMEDIES FOR EYE PROBLEMS

REMEDY	INDICATIONS
Aconite	Any kind of pain or injury, conjunctivitis, conditions that appear rapidly, red eyes.
Agaricus	Dimmed vision.
Allium cepa	Eye allergies; headaches, mostly in the forehead area.
Anacardium	Swollen eyes.
Antimonium crudum	Eyelid inflammation.
Apis mellifica	Bee stings, eye allergies, puffy swelling around the eyes, red eyes.
Argentum nitricum	Pinkeye (conjunctivitis), sticky eyelids.
Arnica montana	Any kind of bruising, eye injuries, black eyes.
Arsenicum album	Dry eyes, foggy vision, late stages of head colds, red eyes.
Aurum	Any kind of pain, double vision.
Belladonna	Dilated pupils, light sensitivity, red eyes.
Bryonia	Dry, hard coughs; headaches.
Calcarea fluorica	Appearance of flickering lights.
Calcarea sulfuric	Discharge from any kind of infection.
Calendula officinalis	Corneal abrasions and erosions, general dryness associated with irritants.
Carboneum sulfuratum	Any kind of swelling.
Causticum	Impurities in any kind of tissue.
Chamomilla	Irritations in any kind of tissue.
Cinchona officinalis	Dilated pupils.
Cineraria maritima	Cataracts; red, irritated eyes.
Cocculuc	Floaters.

REMEDY	INDICATIONS
Conium	Heavy-eye feeling.
Cyclamen	Tense eye muscles.
Euphrasia officinalis	Any kind of burning and irritation.
Ferrum phosphoricum	Early stage of any kind of inflammation, red eyes.
Gelsemium sempervirens	Aching all over the body, tired eyes.
Glonoinum	Red eyes.
Graphites	Light sensitivity.
Hyoscyamus	Double vision.
Hypericum perforatum	Any kind of shooting pain, eye injuries.
Ignatia amara	Emotional stress, severe headaches.
Kali muriaticum	"Gritty" feeling in eyes.
Kali sulfuricum	Red eyes.
Lac caninum	Blurred vision.
Lachesis	Dull vision.
Ledum palustre	Eye pain, if Arnica montana fails to relieve it.
Lycopodium	Eye pain, tearing.
Magnesia carbonica	Red, inflamed, burning eyes.
Magnesia phosphoric	Double vision, general feeling of tiredness.
Mercurius corrosives	Eye discharge.
Mercurius vivus	Red eyes with no discharge, swollen glands.
Natrum muriaticum	Difficulty reading/poor accommodation, eye pain.
Natrum sulfuricum	Light sensitivity.
Nitricum acidum	Tearing.
Nux vomica	Dry eye, headaches, light sensitivity.

REMEDY	INDICATIONS
Petroleum	Eyelid inflammation.
Physostigma	Tense eye muscles
Pulsatilla	Dry eye related to hormone fluctuation, sticky eyelids, yellowish eye discharge.
Rheum	Any kind of muscle twitching.
Rhus toxicodendron	Light sensitivity and tearing.
Ruta graveolens	Eyestrain followed by headache, red eyes.
Sanguinaria	Eye pain.
Senecio	Any kind of muscle weakness.

REMEDY	INDICATIONS
Sepia	Dry eye related to hormone fluctuation, excessive tearing.
Silicea	Eye pain accompanied by light sensitivity.
Spigelia	Eye pain.
Staphysagria	Any kind of infection.
Stramonium	Dilated pupils.
Sulphur	Allergies, dry eyes, red eyelids.
Symphytum	Injuries to the eyeball, pain from a blow to the eye.
Veratrum album	Cold sweats, dry eyes.
Zincum metallicum	General dryness, foggy vision.

touched, as this may decrease their effectiveness. For infants, dissolve a pellet or tablet in water and administer it using an eyedropper.

The best time to take a homeopathic treatment is at least thirty minutes before or after eating. Also, strong "flavors" are believed to decrease the effectiveness of homeopathic remedies. Examples of such flavors include mint or camphor, odors from perfumes and paints, and caffeine.

Homeopathy requires personal observation to determine the length of treatment. If no change occurs in a chronic ailment after a week, switch to another remedy. If improvement is noted, continue with the remedy until all the symptoms disappear. Please note that an initial worsening of symptoms can occur. This is known as a "healing aggravation" and is seen as a good sign by the homeopathic doctor, for it signifies that the correct remedy was chosen and that healing will follow.

It is very important to be continually aware of the symptoms because the remedy should be changed as the symptoms change. For example, a sore throat may turn into a headache, which may turn into sneezing or coughing, which may lead to a runny nose. Each of these symptoms has a separate remedy that is specific for that symptom. For a list of common homeopathic remedies and the symptoms for which they can be used, see pages 128 to 129.

As is evident in the table, there can be many different remedies for the same symptoms. That is why a series of questions must be answered to determine which specific remedy is most appropriate for your condition. This type of approach takes extensive training and should be applied only by a homeopathic physician or a specialist.

COMBINATION REMEDIES AND WHY THEY DEVELOPED

Contrary to the current medical practice of prescribing two or more medicines for use at the same time, the majority of homeopaths recommend only one remedy at a time. The single-remedy approach is called "classic homeopathy." But because the effective practice of homeopathy takes a lot of training, plus a fair amount of time to accurately determine the one correct remedy, homeopaths and pharmacists began combining several remedies indicated for particular conditions. It was found that these combination remedies were effective in a large percentage of cases. Thus, the resurgence of homeopathy today is largely a result of the popularity of combination remedies, and they can be found in virtually every pharmacy, grocery, and health food store in the United States. Classic homeopaths caution that remedies in combination have not been proven. But most homeopaths agree that they are often effective, cause no harm, and are a better choice than pharmaceutical drugs, which often cause adverse side effects.

Combination therapies are categorized or labeled according to the symptoms they are designed to treat. For example, you can find homeopathic remedies for "Colds," "Flu," and "Teething." These combination remedies may be as effective as single remedies, but in most cases, they are not. They are simply more marketable and easier for the consumer to get than single remedies that are prescribed by a classic homeopath.

HOMEOPATHY VERSUS HERBALISM

Many people are confused about the differences between homeopathy and herbalism because both systems use herbs as medicines. There are, however, significant differences between the two. Let's review them.

First, the targeted therapeutic mode of action of the two systems is completely opposite. Herbs provide a natural pharmacologic and/or nutritional effect. Homeopathic medicines attempt to trigger the body's self-regulating mechanisms to respond with its own capabilities to heal itself or regain balance. Second, the methods of preparing the remedies are very different. Herbalists utilize the actual plant in material doses. Homeopaths utilize micro-dilutions.

The methods of preparing the remedies are also very different. An herbalist may use an age-old formula for making an herb tea or a poultice, but she can also improvise like a cook, personalizing the recipe. In addition, using intuition and experience, herbalists often combine a number of herbs to increase the desired effect. (Remember, in prescribing the remedies, herbalists draw on thousands of years of experience, pharmacologic data, and/or established formulas to achieve the desired effect.) Homeopathy is somewhat more scientific; its remedies are prepared, tested, and prescribed in accordance with specific laws and procedures.

Some herbs, by themselves, are toxic, particularly when they are ingested in large amounts. Herbalists should not use these herbs in large doses. In contrast, although many homeopathic remedies are made from poisonous herbs or plants, the potentized remedies contain only minute amounts of the original substances and are nontoxic. Yet it cannot be overemphasized that caution should be taken with any self-remedy. And although a homeopathic remedy may be harmless because of its low potency, it can also be ineffective at treating a disorder. This is why it is important to work in conjunction with a trained homeopathic physician.

CONCLUSION

Homeopathic treatment is different from traditional Western medicine in many ways. Homeopathic remedies treat each symptom distinctly, without necessarily assigning a "syndrome" name to the condition. Part Two will continue to identify certain homeopathic approaches for various symptoms/disorders. You might be tempted to try to treat your own symptoms based on the conditions listed in this book and the remedies given for each. However, a homeopathic practitioner may see a whole other set of symptoms, based on further questioning, that might indicate the need for a different remedy. She will take your overall physical condition, personality, and emotional state into consideration. So, it is best to consult a trained homeopathic practitioner before attempting any treatment on your own. It can save you some time, perhaps some money, and possibly even your eyesight!

PART TWO

Disorders of the Eye

You have learned a lot about how the eyes work, when certain ocular (or eye-related) abilities develop, and what types of natural, noninvasive approaches can enhance eye health. So far, we've discussed the healthy eye and then a few basic problems, such as refractive errors, that can degrade your vision. But what about specific eye injuries, disorders, and diseases?

We will begin Part Two of this book with information that surely warrants being kept in a handy place. A quick-reference Troubleshooting Guide lists common eye symptoms and possible causes. Next, there's basic first aid for common eye problems such as burns and abrasions, as well as common contact lens problems such as adherent lenses and severe eye redness. The step-by-step instructions are invaluable to have at your fingertips. Please be sure to read the first-aid guide carefully and follow the steps as closely as possible if you have an eye emergency.

It is also very important to talk about how various medications can affect your eyes. There are many ocular side effects caused by systemic medications, but the average consumer does not necessarily associate those side effects and the related medicine in a timely manner. When it comes to the eyes, timing can be everything. So, check the table on ocular side effects of particular medications any time that you begin taking one of the listed treatments.

Finally, Part Two serves as an A-to-Z guide to eye disorders. Numerous maladies of the eyes are discussed in detail, from simple styes to the complex eye-related symptoms of diabetes, just to name two topics. In fact, there are over fifty disorders discussed. Each disorder is described in layman's terms. Solid and practical treatment advice is given, and easy-to-read tables provide information on everything from nutritional supplementation to homeopathic remedies. Special recommendations are offered in bulleted lists, so that you can access extra tips quickly.

Please be aware that Part Two is offered solely to aid you in deciding what you can do to help yourself and assist your doctor in solving your problem. Be careful when attempting to diagnose your own condition. Remember that a missed diagnosis can cost valuable time and, possibly, valuable eyesight.

Troubleshooting Guide

Most likely, you will never simply notice an eye problem, walk into your eye doctor's office, and offer a complete and accurate diagnosis of your own condition. However, if you do have an eye problem, it would be helpful to enter the office with a general idea of what your symptoms are, what conditions they might indicate, and what requires immediate attention. The following table lists some of the visual symptoms that most commonly occur and mentions conditions that can be the root cause of each problem.

EYE SYMPTOMS AND THEIR POSSIBLE CAUSES

SYMPTOM	POSSIBLE CONDITION
Blind spots	Glaucoma, lazy eye (from tobacco or alcohol), migraine headaches, optic atrophy, retinitis pigmentosa.
Blinking, frequent	Accommodative insufficiency, anxiety, contact lens irritation, dry eye disease, farsightedness, foreign body in eye, Parkinson's disease, stroke.
Blurred distance vision	Albinism, astigmatism, cataracts, central serous retinopathy, corneal ulcer, dry eyes, keratoconus, lazy eye, macular degeneration, nearsightedness, optic atrophy.
Blurred near vision	Accommodative insufficiency, astigmatism, computer vision syndrome, convergence insufficiency, dry eyes, keratoconus, lazy eye, presbyopia.
Blurred vision	Astigmatism, central serous retinopathy, keratoconus, computer vision syndrome, myopia.
Burning	Chemical burn, computer vision syndrome, dry eye disease, eyestrain, pinkeye.
Color vision, disturbed	Acute optic neuritis, cataract, medication allergy, primary optic atrophy.
Discharge, sticky	Dry eye disease, pinkeye (bacterial).

Symptom	Possible Condition
Discharge, watery	Allergy, blocked tear duct, foreign body in eye, pinkeye (viral).
Double vision	Binocular vision disorder, convergence insufficiency, diabetes, Graves' disease (hyperthyroidism), high astigmatism, lazy eye, optic nerve defect, orbital (eye socket) fracture, strabismus.
Drooping eyelid	Aging, botulism, diabetes, eyelid or head injury, hypothyroidism, muscle weakness, optic nerve defect.
Eye dryness	Computer vision syndrome, drug reaction, hormone imbalance, keratocon–junctivitis sicca (inflammation of cornea and conjunctiva), Sjögren's syndrome (salivary gland disorder), Stevens-Johnson syndrome (hive-like rash on mucous membranes), xerophthalmia (dry, thickened, wrinkled cornea and conjunctiva).
Eye movements, involuntary	Acute optic neuritis, albinism, alcohol intoxication, lupus erythematosus.
Eyelid, swelling around	Blunt trauma, excessive salt consumption, pinkeye (allergic), smoking, swollen tear duct.
Eyelid, swelling of	Chalazion, stye.
Flashing lights	Blunt trauma, migraine headache, retinal detachment, vitreous detachment.
Headaches	Astigmatism, computer vision syndrome, convergence insufficiency, farsightedness, migraine.
Itching	Dry eye disease, pinkeye (allergic), trichiasis (irritation of eyeball by eyelashes).
Light sensitivity	Computer vision syndrome, eyestrain, farsightedness, iritis (inflammation of the iris), pinkeye.
Night blindness	Nearsightedness, retinitis pigmentosa, vitamin-A deficiency.
Pain, sharp	Corneal abrasion, corneal ulcer, foreign body in eye, torn or broken contact lens.
Protruding eyes	Graves' disease (thyroid eye disease), intraorbital tumor.
Pupils, different-sized	Glaucoma, intracranial tumor, iritis, meningitis, nearsightedness, nerve defect.
Redness	Computer vision syndrome, corneal abrasion, dry eye, iritis, pinkeye, subconjunctival hemorrhage.
Tearing	Acute optic neuritis, blocked tear duct, corneal abrasion, dry eye disease, foreign body, iritis, pinkeye.
Tired eyes	Accommodative insufficiency, computer vision syndrome, convergence insufficiency, farsightedness, presbyopia.
Yellow eyes	Jaundice.
Yellow spot in eye	Pinguecula (yellow patch on sclera).

First Aid for Common Eye Problems

Things happen, and things happen to the eyes. However, not everything that happens to the eyes is an emergency. Therefore, it is important to know which conditions are true emergencies, requiring prompt or immediate attention, and whether you should see an optometrist, ophthalmologist, or emergency-room physician.

Of course, the best way to handle an eye emergency is to prevent it from happening in the first place through the use of appropriate safety procedures and protective eyewear. This is especially important to consider when working on home improvements, playing sports, using high heat such as when cooking, and roughhousing with children. But accidents happen, and you should know how to recognize the kinds of problems they can cause.

The first part of this section covers potentially serious eye injuries, while the second offers guidance on treating eye ailments that are *usually* manageable at home but certainly require that you treat them to some degree. I also have dedicated a segment to potential problems arising through the use of contact lenses. Because so many of us rely on contact lenses on a daily basis to correct our vision, it is important to highlight some of the hazards

that can result from their use. All in all, by the end of this section, you will feel confident that you are prepared to intelligently handle most common worries concerning injury and irritation to the eye.

EYE EMERGENCIES

If you know you have a serious injury—one involving obvious major eye damage, loss of vision, or extensive bleeding—go to your nearest hospital emergency room immediately. A chemical burn is really the only type of serious injury you should try to treat before going to the emergency room by rinsing the eye for fifteen minutes. (See "Burn," page 138.) For less pressing but serious concerns, call your optometrist or ophthalmologist and ask for an appointment as soon as possible. If you clearly state the problem and don't diminish the facts, a good practitioner will see you promptly or, if unable, will refer you to someone who can.

Both optometrists and ophthalmologists can handle minor eye injuries, such as a foreign body superficially imbedded in the eye. Like ophthalmologists, optometrists also can prescribe certain medications, such as topical antibiotics, to treat minor eye injuries. If the situation arises that requires a surgical intervention, an optometrist will send the patient to an ophthalmologist in whom he is confident. So, if you think you have a serious injury, but don't know an ophthalmologist, contact your optometrist for a referral. Most optometrists have working relationships with ophthalmologists.

The following discussion covers eye injuries that have the potential to be very serious. If you experience any of these, assess the situation calmly and seek appropriate medical attention. These problems are further discussed later in Part Two, so be sure to check for treatment information in the specific sections on these emergencies as well.

Burn

Since the blink reflex is one of the fastest reflexes we have, the eye is rarely burned by fire. Most eye burns are caused by chemicals or radiation. Chemical burns fall into two categories: acid burns and alkali burns. Acid substances that burn the eyes include battery acid, such as car-battery acid; industrial chemicals; and liquid bleach. Alkali burns are most often caused by lye-based drain cleaners. Both acid and alkali substances can splash into unprotected eyes and do a great deal of damage in a short time. Alkali burns, however, are a lot worse than acid burns. Acids penetrate the eye more slowly than alkali chemicals and can more often be washed out before doing any major damage.

Speed is crucial with a chemical burn. Immediately begin flushing the eye with water. Rinse the eye, continually and gently, for *at least fifteen minutes.* If possible, hold the eye open under slowly running water. If you do not have water available, use anything, even milk, tea, or soda pop. Do not make calling for assistance or leaving for the emergency room your first priority. Again, your initial action should be to flush your eye for fifteen minutes. If you take the time to call for help before washing out the eye, significant damage can occur to the eye. In addition, do not use an eyecup for flushing. An eyecup will allow the chemical to remain in contact with the eye, therefore reversing any of the positive effects of the flushing. For the same reason, do not bandage the eye. Leave the eye uncovered, since a bandage will also keep the chemical in contact with the eye.

When you have finished flushing the eye, get to an emergency room. The doctor will probably complete irrigating the eye, as well as apply an antibiotic ointment, and give you medications to reduce the inflammation and pain. Your eye will be closed and patched under pressure to help relieve the pain and to allow healing to take place.

The other type of burn that affects the eyes is a radiation burn. This type of burn can come from too much exposure to radiation such as UV, infrared, nuclear, and X-ray radiation. As is true regarding other injuries, prevention is the best medicine. Never stare directly at the sun, especially during an eclipse or as reflected off glass or water. You can permanently damage your retinas and cause complete loss of your central vision this way. When I was a Navy optometrist, one young sailor thought he could get an easy discharge by causing himself some "minor" eye damage by staring at the sun. He ended up nearly blind, although he did get his discharge—a psychiatric one!

Rather, make sure you always protect your eyes. Wear appropriate eyewear if you work around excessive UV, infrared, or other radiation. If you indulge in sunbathing, whether in natural sunlight or in a tanning booth, be sure to wear opaque goggles.

Radiation burns leave the eyes feeling gritty and tearing excessively for several hours after exposure to the source of the radiation. You may also experience spasm of the eyelid muscles that makes it difficult to open your eyes. Your eyes will be sensitive to light. If you experience these symptoms, contact your optometrist or ophthalmologist as soon as possible and explain what is happening. The standard medical treatment consists of pain medication, bed rest, cold compresses, and topical antibiotics.

Corneal Abrasion

A *corneal abrasion* is a scrape on the cornea, most often caused by a foreign body such as a grain of sand, piece of dirt, ill-fitting contact lens, baby's fingernail, twig, or mascara wand. A person with a scraped cornea will often tell his eye doctor that he feels something under the upper eyelid. Usually, the foreign body is no longer present, but the patient feels discomfort whenever the upper eyelid passes over the damaged part of the cornea.

If you have a corneal abrasion, you will probably feel a great deal of pain. Generally, when the injury first occurs, your eye will tear profusely, in an attempt to wash out the foreign body that caused the abrasion. However, the offending object might have become trapped in your eye. You can try washing out your eye further with purified water or commercial eyewash. Do not use commercial eye-whitening drops—they have a cosmetic, not a healing, purpose. If you or someone else can see the cause of the problem, such as a speck of dirt, you can try to remove it with a clean handkerchief, a damp cotton swab, or a tissue.

Scratches on the cornea usually cannot be seen with the naked eye. Your eye doctor will examine the injury under magnification and may also use a fluorescein (FLOOR-ess-seen) stain to make the abrasion visible. You may be given a topical antibiotic, in the form of an ointment or drops, to help prevent infection. I tell my patients to get plenty of rest and to take an over-the-counter pain medication for any discomfort.

Doctors used to routinely patch an eye that suffered a corneal abrasion, but many now feel that the eye is better off healing without a patch. One reason is that a patch keeps the eye warm, which increases the chance of an infection developing. Also, it is easier to monitor progress and apply medication if the eye is not covered. On the other hand, patching makes the eye more comfortable.

Most corneal abrasions heal within a few days, although those from a plant material such as wood or from a very dirty substance may take longer. Even if you remove any foreign body from an eye, it's always safer to consult your eyecare professional to confirm that there is no residual damage. Better safe than sorry, as they say!

Corneal Ulcer

A *corneal ulcer* is an open sore on the cornea and involves a deeper invasion of the corneal tissue than an abrasion. (See "Corneal Abrasion," previous page.) It may start with a corneal abrasion that becomes infected, or with a bacterial or viral infection that was not preceded by an injury.

Actually, corneal ulcers can result from a number of different situations. Complications from contact lenses are a frequent cause of corneal ulcers today. Wearing lenses that were improperly disinfected or improperly fitted, or leaving daily-wear lenses in while sleeping, can cause corneal ulcers. But any eye injury, such as one from a twig or fingernail, can result in a corneal ulcer. Also, one very serious type of corneal ulcer results from the herpes simplex virus, which is the virus that causes cold sores and genital ulcers. You can transmit a herpes infection to the eye if you touch a herpes sore and then touch your eye.

Most corneal ulcers are painful, and some can be seen with the naked eye as a round depression or white spot. Corneal ulcers resulting from the herpes virus actually cause the cornea to *lose* sensitivity in the area of the ulcer, so you may not have pain as a clue that something is seriously wrong. However, your eye will be red and sensitive to light. Your vision in the affected eye also will be blurred, but this is hard to notice unless the unaffected eye is temporarily covered for some reason. Under magnification, an ulcer from a herpes virus has a distinctive branching pattern, but this cannot be seen without special instruments and sometimes even a fluorescein stain.

Corneal ulcers must be treated immediately, or else scarring or loss of vision can result. Generally, the treatment includes an antibiotic or antiviral medication. If the cornea is irreparably damaged, a corneal transplant may need to be performed. (The cornea is the only part of the eye that is donated to eye banks.) In a corneal transplant, the central eight to ten millimeters of the cornea are cut out. The new cornea is then cut into the same diameter and sewn onto the eye. The thread used for this procedure is extremely thin and strong. Rejection is possible, though not as common as in other kinds of transplants. Most corneal transplants are successful, and vision can go from extremely poor to extremely good. See "Corneal Transplant" on page 353 for more information.

Cuts In and Around the Eye

Most of us have experienced abrasions around and on the superficial surface of the eye, perhaps from a baby's fingernail or something similarly sharp. Cuts around the outside of the eye bleed a lot and look very frightening, but they heal well, as do cuts in the conjunctiva. Even though such abrasions are common, you really should see your eye doctor to assess the seriousness of an eye-area injury.

If you experience a large cut on or even near the eye, you should confirm with your doctor that you have no hidden damage to your eye, and do so within a short amount of time. For general lacerations immediately around the eye, bandage the cut lightly and seek a doctor at once. Do not wash the eye out with water. Any penetration into the eyeball opens the eye to infection, and tap water contains bacteria. Moreover, if you do get a large object stuck in your eyeball itself, it is important that you do not attempt to remove the penetrating object from the laceration if that object is still there. If the object penetrates the eyeball (into the interior), then the fluids inside the eye might leak out and cause a dangerous drop in the pressure inside the eye. This can cause all kinds of additional problems, including a detached retina or other major visual loss. Let the doctor remove the object because he has the proper equipment to handle the situation.

Hyphema

A *hyphema* (high-FEE-mah) is a condition in which blood leaks into the anterior chamber of the eye, in front of the iris. The iris, or colored part of the eye, may just look "dark," but this is caused by the accumulating blood. It almost always is a result of being struck in the eye with a blunt object, such as a racquetball or soccer ball. You don't feel the hyphema itself. Rather, you feel the pain from the injury that caused it.

A hyphema is a true eye emergency, requiring medication, immediate patching of the eye, and bed rest for up to a week. These measures are intended to minimize your eye movements, promote the absorption of blood, and prevent further bleeding. Without treatment, your eye may be stained with blood, resulting in permanent loss of vision. Glaucoma and/or a serious inflammation of the iris can also result from an unsuccessfully resolved hyphema. If you suspect you have a hyphema, or if you have sustained any kind of blunt injury to your eye, see an eyecare professional or emergency room physician right away. Have someone drive you to the doctor, and avoid any excessive head or eye movements en route. It's also extremely important to follow the doctor's recommendations after the visit.

Retinal Detachment

Retinal detachment is the peeling away of the retina from the back of the eye, the way wallpaper might peel away from a curved surface. The retina detaches when it has a hole or tear that allows fluid to collect between it and the back of the eye. The separation that results is similar to what happens when water gets behind wallpaper.

Retinal detachment can occur for many reasons, not all of them injuries, although a blunt or penetrating injury to the eye is a common cause. Extremely nearsighted eyes and prominent eyes are more prone to retinal detachment, probably because their retinas are more tautly stretched. Recent cataract surgery is another risk factor.

The retina can be reattached by a surgeon if the detachment is caught in time, and that critical amount of time depends on the extent of the detachment. If there is only a small hole in the retina, a laser can be used to seal it. If there is a large tear and the retina is actually peeling away from the eye, a freezing probe will be used to make the retina adhere to the eye again.

It is vital to know the symptoms of retinal detachment because failure to seek treatment immediately can result in blindness in the affected eye. A developing retinal detachment is heralded by flashes of light that look like sparks or flickers, a large number of floaters in the field of vision, and a shadow or curtain that spreads from the edge of the visual field to the central vision. A shimmering effect, similar to what you would see if you looked through gelatin, may also be noticed in the visual field. No pain will arise from the retina itself because the retina does not contain pain receptors. (You may, of course, feel pain from elsewhere in the eye if the detachment was caused by an injury.) If you experience this eye emergency, it is important to lie very still, preferably face up, with as little movement as possible.

The conditions and situations discussed above are true ocular emergencies and warrant medical attention. Do not hesitate to call an eye-care professional. Too many people assume their symptoms will go away if they simply rest their eyes for a few hours. But these eye emergencies are exactly that—emergencies—because serious and permanent damage is very likely if a timely and effective eyecare protocol is not followed.

EYE INJURIES

There are some common eye problems that are often, but not always, manageable at home. It all depends on how severe the injuries are. Many of us have experienced a black eye at some point in our lives, whether from a careless friend's elbow or a tumbling box of food we were sneaking from a high shelf in the cabinet. Maybe you've even broken a few tiny capillaries in an eye while you were suffering with a severe cold. The next few paragraphs review these very injuries and offer guidance on what to do if the situation is not too serious. Of course, *if you even suspect that the injury should be assessed by a professional because you are in pain, you are unsure of how deep the problem goes, or you are having vision problems, seek medical attention right away.*

Black Eye

For a bruising injury from a blunt object—commonly referred to as a black eye—apply an ice bag or cold compress during the first twenty-four to forty-eight hours following the injury. This will help to constrict the damaged blood vessels in and around the eye, and to reduce further bleeding and swelling. That is why applying a steak to an injured eye has been used time and again in movies, family stories, and the like—a frozen or refrigerated steak is nice and cold. Actually, a bag of frozen peas works very well too!

Once the swelling has largely subsided, which usually takes a few days, apply heat to the eye. Heat will cause the blood vessels to dilate (open) and to absorb the fluid that is causing the remaining swelling. The dilated blood vessels will also bring in infection-fighting cells from elsewhere in the body. One way to make a hot compress is to wet a clean washcloth and microwave it for thirty to forty-five seconds. Gently apply to the closed eye with light pressure and hold securely, preferably by lying down.

While you might resolve the condition with these suggestions, it's still important to make sure no collateral damage was done. Thus, a check-up with your eye doctor is highly recommended.

Subconjunctival Hemorrhage

A *subconjunctival* (SUB-con-junk-TIE-val) *hemorrhage* is actually bleeding from small broken blood vessels under the conjunctiva of the eye, between the conjunctiva and the sclera. This is a case where the problem looks much more serious than it is. Subconjunctival hemorrhages can occur from a jarring injury, such as a blow to the head, or from anything that increases the pressure in the delicate blood vessels of the conjunctiva, such as intense coughing, sneezing, vomiting, or labor contractions.

The area where the bleeding occurs appears as a bright red patch on the white sclera. There is no pain, and vision is not affected. To hasten the resolution, use a cold compress for the first day or so. Apply heat on and off when you reach the fourth day, or even later. Depending on the amount of blood that leaked out, the blood will be absorbed, and the eye will return to normal within one to three weeks. Of course, if you have any symptoms that concern you, such as pain or visual disturbances, see your eye doctor.

It should be clear from the brevity of this particular section that not many eye injuries are harmless enough *not* to warrant quick medical attention. However, there are a few that can generally be self-treated at home. And if truth be told, many of us try to manage mild injuries on our own anyway. This advice is conservative wisdom on how to do so. But it can never hurt to check with your eyecare professional, even if you are confident that you can assess and care for the injury at home. If you are self-treating, be sure to give yourself the rest needed to recover; pamper your eyes for a little while.

CONTACT LENS CONCERNS

Today, millions of people wear corrective contact lenses on a daily basis. With proper hygiene and regular eye care, contact lenses are really very safe and effective. However, there are certain problems that can occur, whether due to carelessness, injury, or simply bad luck. And problems with contact lenses can be a special type of concern because of the close proximity of the lenses to the eye tissue. Although many of the following problems can arise even if you don't wear contacts, they require special attention if you do.

Adherent Lenses and Dry Eyes

Contact lenses must remain wet, especially when riding on the tear film of your eyes. If allowed to dry out, they will adhere, or stick, to the eyes themselves. If your lenses are soft lenses, they can dry out due to a number of environmental factors. These include high heat, infrared radiation, wind, and a low-humidity and/or air-conditioned environment. A dry eye condition, such as dry eye disease, can also cause dryness in the eyes and, ultimately, dry lenses.

What should you do if your contacts dry out and stick to your eyes? Do not attempt to remove them before they are re-hydrated. Use a lubricant specifically designed for your type of lenses or an artificial tear solution. If possible, increase the humidity in the room—turning on the shower in the bathroom often works well. Gas permeable lenses can also dry out, but they don't adhere to the eye quite as easily. Wet these types of lenses with the appropriate eye drops. Ask your eye doctor to recommend the best type of eye drops to use.

Blurred Vision

Contact lenses are designed to enhance your vision, making clarity possible. They should not make your vision blurry or distorted. If your vision becomes worse when you wear your contacts, the first thing you should do is remove and clean them. If you reinsert the lenses and your vision is still blurred or distorted, check to make sure the lenses are sitting correctly on your eyes and are not inside out (this applies to soft lenses only). Heavy deposits on your lenses can blur your vision, as can creams and oils from soap or perfumes. If the lenses are clean and positioned correctly on your eyes and you still cannot see properly, contact your eye doctor. Obviously, there is another reason for the problem, and that reason must be identified in a timely manner.

Broken Lens

Any trauma to the eye can be significant and cause severe damage. In one sense, having a contact lens on the eye affords a certain level of protection from external blows. However, if the lens is a rigid lens and it is broken while in the eye, the eye can be cut. Soft lenses are less likely to break, but they also offer less protection to the eye.

No matter what type of lens you wear, if you suffer a blunt trauma that results in a broken lens, see your eye doctor. It's okay to attempt to flush out the eye in order to remove the torn or broken lens, but do *not* put any pressure on the eye—that is, no rubbing! Swelling or lacerations may make removal of the lens or lens pieces difficult.

Chemical Splash

All contact lenses are permeable to gases and also absorb all types of liquids. If a chemical splashes into your eye while you are wearing your contacts, remove the affected lens immediately. If you don't, the lens will hold the chemical in contact with your eye tissue for an extended period of time, making the problem worse.

After removing the lens, hold the lids apart and irrigate the eye continuously with clean water for at least fifteen minutes. If you are alone, irrigate your eye before calling for help because rinsing the chemical from your eye is more important than rushing to get medical assistance. For more information on how to handle a chemical splash, see the previous section entitled "Burn" on page 138.

Dust Irritation

Dust particles are notorious for becoming trapped underneath contact lenses, especially the smaller gas permeable lenses. This can happen if there is a lot of debris in the air, but also just from normal environmental particles that get trapped as you are inserting your contact. Dust can be very uncomfortable, feeling larger and sharper than you would usually imagine and quite often causing blurriness of vision.

If your eyes become red or uncomfortable, remove your lenses and irrigate your eyes. If your eyes clear up, clean the lenses and reinsert them. If your eyes remain red or uncomfortable, be sure to consult your eye doctor before reinserting the lenses.

Exposure High Heat and UV Light

Many tales have been passed down about contact lenses becoming "fused" to the eyes of welders because they work with such high and concentrated heat. These stories are not true; this has never happened. However, welding *arcs* can cause several other types of damage. Arc welding uses a welding power supply to create an electric arc between an electrode and the base material in order to melt the metals at the welding point.

I'm not sure where the stories of contact lenses and arc welding started, but it's likely due to the inflammation that can happen with over-exposure to ultraviolet (UV) light. The brightness of the weld area leads to a condition called *arc eye*, in which ultraviolet light causes inflammation of the cornea and can burn the retinas of the eyes. Goggles and helmets with dark face plates are worn to prevent this exposure. In recent years, new helmet models have been produced that feature a face plate that self-darkens immediately upon exposure to high amounts of UV light.

If you are exposed to an arc of any kind and do not have protective filters in place, remove your lenses before your eyes begin to become inflamed. Inflammation is usually a delayed reaction. If no symptoms develop within twenty-four hours, you can reinsert your lenses. If symptoms do develop, consult your eye doctor first.

Lost Lens

If you fear that you may have lost a contact lens, first check the eye itself. The lens may be displaced on the conjunctiva or caught under the upper lid. If it is, carefully re-center the lens. It is very unlikely that the lens will go "behind" your eye (unless you have been hit with a baseball bat). The conjunctiva forms a continuous loop between the surface of the eye and the inside of your eyelids, so there is a "sac" under your eyelids to trap anything from going behind the eyeball. Why would the lens get displaced in the first place? Your eye might be dry. In such a case, you should lubricate your eye with the appropriate drops first so that you are able to easily slip the lens back to the desired location.

If the lens is not displaced, check your clothing and the surrounding floor. If you find the lens, clean it and evaluate it for damage. Soft lenses that are not cracked can be re-hydrated and successfully worn again. Just soak the lens for at least four hours before attempting to reinsert it. If the lens feels uncomfortable in your eye, remove it immediately and call your doctor. It very well might be damaged and have to be replaced.

Red, Sore Eyes

Redness and soreness in the eyes while wearing contact lenses are indications of some type of eye problem. If your eyes become red or sore and the problem persists, remove your lenses. Once the condition clears, if it does, try to reinsert the lenses, being attentive to any discomfort. If the discomfort returns, remove the lenses and contact your eye doctor. Never wear lenses when your eyes are red or sore.

After reading about the possible problems involving contact lens wear, it might seem that wearing glasses is the safer and better option. But actually, the science of contact lenses has become highly sophisticated and most people do not run into serious problems with their lenses. It is simply important to maintain the lenses well and be proactive about preventing eye damage if the lenses are compromised. If you or your children wear contact lenses, hopefully the above information will convince you to be extra vigilant concerning them. You can read more about contact lenses, including the types of contacts that are available, on page 338 of Part Three.

CONCLUSION

Eye emergencies are serious; it is not unlikely for them to result in some degree of damage. Fortunately, nature has provided us with a sure-fire alarm system for most eye emergencies—pain! If you feel any pain around your eyes, it is best to play it safe and have an eye doctor check it out. And even a mild eye injury can be problematic if you do not take proper care to rest and relieve the eye. No matter what the injury or resulting level of pain, it is best to err on the side of caution and see an eyecare professional if you so much as suspect that the situation might be more damaging than it appears.

How Medications Can Affect Your Eyes

It should be obvious by now that the eyes are an integral part of the human body. Whatever we eat or ingest in any way affects all the parts of our body, including our eyes. This is especially true of medications. Many of us are on prescription and over-the-counter medications for symptoms and disorders not even closely related to the eyes. Yet those seemingly harmless treatments might be compromising your eye health on a daily basis.

The following table lists some of the more common medications taken today for a number of different physical conditions. Included in the table are the brand name and generic name of each medication, as well as what it is used for and how it affects the eyes. Some of these medications may have variations and updated formulas on the market. Therefore, please check with your physician before taking any medication or changing any medications so that you are aware of any possible visual effects. Contact your physician immediately if you notice any new visual sensations when taking any of the medications.

COMMON MEDICATIONS AND THEIR OCULAR SIDE EFFECTS

BRAND NAME	GENERIC NAME	INDICATIONS	OCULAR SIDE EFFECTS
Accutane	Isotretinoin	Difficult cases of cystic acne; keratinization disorders; folliculitis; psoriasis.	Redness, dry eyes, corneal opacities, tearing, optic neuritis, light sensitivity, floaters, contact lens intolerance, night blindness.
Achromycin	Tetracycline	Acne; chlamydia.	Retinal hemorrhage, decreased vision, headaches, light sensitivity, nearsightedness, enlarged blind spot.
Actifed	Pseudoephedrine	Allergic rhinitis; allergic conjunctivitis and skin manifestations; motion sickness.	Hallucinations, decreased eye pressure, dilated pupils, dry eyes.

Brand Name	Generic Name	Indications	Ocular Side Effects
Adipex	Phentermine	Obesity/extra weight.	Decreased vision, headache, cataracts, hallucinations, double vision, disturbed accommodation.
Aricept	Donepezil	Alzheimer's disease.	Cataracts, glaucoma, retinal hemorrhages, conjunctival hemorrhages, eye irritation, blepharitis, dry eyes, floaters.
Arimidex	Anastrozole	Breast cancer.	Cataracts.
Atrovent	Ipratropium bromide	Rhinitis.	Worsened narrow-angle glaucoma, pinkeye, dry eyes, blurred vision, eye pain.
Benadryl	Diphenhydramine	Allergic rhinitis; allergic conjunctivitis and skin manifestations; motion sickness.	Visual-field constriction, hallucinations, retinal hemorrhage.
Betoptic	Betaxolol	Open-angle glaucoma.	Hallucinations, decreased tear flow (dry eyes), redness, double vision, drooping eyelids.
Cafergot	Ergotamine	Migraines.	Spasm and constriction of blood vessels in all parts of the eye.
Cardizem	Diltiazem	Angina due to coronary-artery spasm; mild to moderate hypertension.	Eye pain, redness, dizziness, hallucinations, tearing, irritation.
Catapres	Clonidine	Hypertension.	Eye irritation, dry eyes, hallucinations, dilated pupils.
Celebrex	Celecoxib	Inflammation.	Visual field defects, blurred vision.
Coumadin	Warfarin sodium	Venous thrombosis; atrial fibrillation with embolization; pulmonary emboli; coronary occlusion.	Tearing, cataracts, hemorrhage, decreased vision, yellowing of eyes.
Desyrel	Trazodone	Depression.	Optic neuritis, lazy eye, retinal or subconjunctival hemorrhage, light sensitivity, dry eyes, decreased vision.
Detrol	Tolterodine tartrate	Lack of bladder control.	Headaches, dry eyes, hallucinations, blurred near vision, glaucoma.
Diabinese	Chlorpropamide	Diabetes.	Optic neuritis, yellowing of eyes, disturbed color vision, retinal hemorrhage, light sensitivity, double vision.
Dilantin	Phenytoin	Epilepsy.	Retinal hemorrhage, nystagmus, yellowing of eyes, double vision, poor accommodation, flashing lights, glare sensitivity, poor color vision.

BRAND NAME	GENERIC NAME	INDICATIONS	OCULAR SIDE EFFECTS
Dimetapp	Brompheniramine	Coughs and upper respiratory symptoms, including nasal congestion, associated with an allergy or common cold.	Different-sized pupils, visual-field constriction, hallucinations, dry eyes, double vision.
Diuril	Chlorothiazide	Hypertension; edema associated with congestive heart failure, cirrhosis, or corticosteroid or estrogen therapy.	Ocular edema, retinal hemorrhage, disturbed accommodation, nearsightedness, yellow vision.
Donnatal	Phenobarbital	Epilepsy; anxiety.	Blind spots, hallucinations, lazy eye, optic neuritis, involuntary eye movements, blurred vision, dilated pupils.
Elavil	Amitriptyline	Depression.	Hallucinations, retinal hemorrhage, lazy eye, optic neuritis, dry eyes, yellowing of eyes, increased eye pressure.
Enduron	Methyclothiazide	Hypertension; edema associated with congestive heart failure, cirrhosis, premenstrual tension, or corticosteroid or estrogen therapy.	Ocular edema, retinal hemorrhage, decreased vision, disturbed accommodation, redness, light sensitivity.
Fosamax	Alendronate sodium	Osteoporosis.	Inflammation of the sclera, uveitis.
Humulin	Insulin	Diabetes.	Decreased pupil reaction, double vision, involuntary eye movements, blurred vision.
Imitrex	Sumatriptan	Migraines.	Eye muscle weakness, accommodative disorder, dilated pupils, ocular hemorrhage, eye pain, conjunctivitis, ocular edema, corneal opacities.
Inderal	Propranolol	Hypertension.	Drooping eyelids, double vision, decreased vision, hallucinations, dry eyes, headache.
Ismelin	Guanethidine	Hypertension.	Light sensitivity, burning, double vision, accommodative spasm, flashing lights.
Lamictal	Lomtrigine	Seizures.	Dizziness, ataxia, sedation, involuntary eye movements, blurred vision, double vision.
Lanoxin	Digoxin	Congestive heart failure; atrial fibrillation or flutter; atrial tachycardia.	Optic neuritis, disturbed color vision, blurred vision, headache, yellow vision, hallucinations, glare sensitivity, halos around lights, double vision.
Lasix	Furosemide	Hypertension; water retention.	Blurred vision, dizziness, headache.
Librium	Chlordiazepoxide	Anxiety.	Disturbed depth perception, retinal hemorrhage, disturbed accommodation, yellowing of eyes.

BRAND NAME	GENERIC NAME	INDICATIONS	OCULAR SIDE EFFECTS
Lipitor	Atorvastatin	Elevated cholesterol.	Swelling around eyelids, red eyes, itching, myasthenia gravis, headaches, light sensitivity.
Lithobid	Lithium	Manic phase of bipolar disorder.	Blind spots, retinal or subconjunctival hemorrhage, hallucinations, light sensitivity, involuntary eye movements, dry eyes.
Mellaril	Thioridazine	Psychosis.	Night blindness, blind spots, cataracts, blurred vision, hallucinations, lazy eye, crossed eyes, light sensitivity, yellowing of eyes, optic atrophy, discolored eyes.
Mevacor	Lovastatin	Elevated cholesterol.	Cataracts, blurred vision, headache.
Motrin	Ibuprofen	Osteoarthritis; pain; fever.	Blind spots, visual field constriction, lazy eye, retinal hemorrhage, optic neuritis, dry eyes.
Niaspan	Niacin	Elevated cholesterol.	Blurred vision, toxic lazy eye, central blind spot, glaucoma, protruding eyes.
Norpramin	Desipramine	Depression.	Hallucinations, lazy eye, optic neuritis, dryness, blurred vision, headache, light sensitivity, yellowing of eyes, disturbed accommodation.
Norvasc	Amlodipine	Hypertension; angina.	Blurred vision, headache, vertigo, visual distortion, yellowing of eyes.
Ortho-Novum	Norethindrone	Birth control.	Optic neuritis, blind spots, halos around lights, cataracts, headache, yellowing of eyes.
Orudis	Ketoprofen	Rheumatoid arthritis.	Decreased vision, eye hemorrhage, eye pain, hallucinations, visual-field constriction, pinkeye.
Paxil	Paroxetine hydrochloride	Depression.	Dry eyes, abnormal vision, blurred vision, headache, dizziness.
Pepcid	Famotidine	Duodenal ulcer; benign gastric ulcer.	Decreased vision, hallucinations, retinal or subconjunctival hemorrhage, light sensitivity, yellowing of eyes.
Plaquenil	Hydroxychloroquine	Malaria; rheumatoid arthritis; lupus erythematosus.	Cataracts, eye pigmentation, focusing difficulty, eye blisters, eye muscle paralysis, accommodative difficulty, halos around lights, hallucinations, night blindness, flashing lights.
Pravachol	Pravastatin sodium	Elevated cholesterol.	Headache, muscle weakness, dizziness.
Premarin	Estrogen	Menopause; osteoporosis; female hypogonadism; atrophic vaginitis; breast cancer; prostate cancer.	Optic neuritis, blind spots, disturbed color vision, yellowing of eyes, nearsightedness, dry eyes, fluctuations in vision, contact lens intolerance.

Brand Name	Generic Name	Indications	Ocular Side Effects
Prozac	Fluoxetine	Depression.	Eye pain, light sensitivity, dry eyes, iritis, cataracts, double vision, drooping eyelids.
Restoril	Temazepam	Insomnia; anxiety, tension, agitation; skeletal-muscle spasms.	Eye pain, disturbed accommodation, yellowing of eyes, hallucinations, tearing, burning, light sensitivity, nystagmus.
Retin-A	Tretinoin	Acne.	Skin dryness, light sensitivity, red eyes, red eyelids.
Ritalin	Methylphenidate	Attention deficit/hyperactive disorder.	Retinal or subconjunctival hemorrhage, dilated pupils, hallucinations, blurred vision, redness.
Rogaine	Minoxidil	Hair loss.	Increased eye pressure, decreased vision, optic neuritis, blurred vision.
Synthroid	Levothyroxine	Hypothyroidism.	Decreased vision, double vision, drooping eyelids, yellowing of eyes, dry eyes.
Tagamet	Cimetidine	Ulcers.	Hallucinations, light sensitivity, blurred vision, redness, irritation, dry eyes.
Tavist	Clemastine	Mild allergy symptoms.	Decreased vision, dry eyes, light sensitivity, eyelid swelling, hallucinations, different-sized pupils.
Tenormin	Atenolol	Hypertension (beta-blocker).	Decreased vision, hallucinations, dry eyes, burning, redness, yellow eyes.
Timoptic	Timolol maleate	Glaucoma.	Dryness, burning, blurred vision, pupil size variations, droopy eyelids, nearsightedness, hallucinations.
Topamax	Topiramate	Seizures.	Glaucoma, increase tearing, double vision, myopia.
Tylenol	Acetaminophen	Fever; mild pain.	Hallucinations, disturbed color vision, double vision, redness.
Viagra	Sildenafil	Erectile dysfunction.	Blurred vision, yellow vision, sensitivity to light, blue vision, double vision, hemorrhages, burning eyes.
Voltaren	Diclofenac	Rheumatoid arthritis; osteoarthritis; post-eye surgery symptoms.	Blurred vision, night blindness, lazy eye, blind spots, bleeding in the eye, itching, tearing, light sensitivity.
Xanax	Alprazolam	Anxiety; depression.	Disturbed color vision, disturbed accommodation, eye pain, hallucinations, uncontrolled eye movements, yellow eyes.
Zantac	Ranitidine	Gastric ulcers.	Disturbed color vision, hallucinations, blurred vision, eyelid swelling, yellowing of eyes, redness.

Brand Name	Generic Name	Indications	Ocular Side Effects
Zestril	ACE Inhibitor	Hypertension.	Yellow eyes, dizziness, headache.
Zocor	Simvastatin	Elevated cholesterol.	Blurred vision, worsened cataracts, eye muscle weakness.
Zoloft	Sertaline	Depression.	Eye pain, blind spots, dry eyes, light sensitivity, double vision, increased tearing.
Zyrtec	Cetirizine	Allergies.	Ocular melanoma, glaucoma, ocular hemorrhage, loss of accommodation, dry eyes, headache, loss of visual field.

Your A-to-Z Guide to Common Eye Disorders

The following A-to-Z guide was designed to familiarize you with over fifty common disorders of the eye; their conventional treatments, such as prescription eyeglasses, medication, and surgery; and any alternative means of self-treatment that are available, including nutritional supplements, herbs and herbal supplements, homeopathic remedies, and other potentially effective modes of therapy. Also included are recommendations for simple lifestyle changes, such as dietary modifications, that can make a significant impact not only on your eye health, but also on your overall well-being. While not every condition is amenable to self-treatment or nutritional remediation, the best available support is listed. Whether you are looking for information on a specific problem or are simply leafing through the different discussions, it is important to remember that this material was provided to help you better understand your eye condition and assist you in working with your doctor towards a successful outcome. It was not meant to replace diagnosis and treatment by a qualified eyecare professional.

ACCOMMODATIVE INSUFFICIENCY

One of the most fascinating aspects of the eye is its ability to change focal power. This changing of focal power enables us to see things clearly at a distance (20 feet or more away) and also at a near point (16 inches or even closer). This change of power is called *accommodation*.

The eye's ability to accommodate usually follows a normal pattern of degeneration with age, being at its maximum when we are young and gradually decreasing as we get older. If you are over forty years old and your eyes are beginning to lose their ability to accommodate, you have presbyopia, a different condition than what is discussed here. (For a discussion of presbyopia, see page 308.) Occasionally, the focal power of the eyes is not up to par for our age. This is most commonly seen in school-aged children who

Accommodation is the ability of the eyes to change focal power between distance and near point. When relatively young people have difficulty changing focal power—when they can't clearly see the print in a book, for instance—the condition is called *accommodative insufficiency*.

153

have difficulty focusing on their reading materials. In this case, the condition is called accommodative insufficiency.

There can be many causes for this condition, and while most of them are not medically related, a full eye exam is certainly warranted. Most often there is a spasm of the focusing muscles, thus leaving less muscle power available to focus clearly. This can happen when children read for extended periods of time without taking breaks to allow their focusing muscles to relax.

CONVENTIONAL TREATMENT

Either prescription eyeglasses or vision therapy can be used to treat accommodative insufficiency. In some cases, a doctor may prescribe both forms of treatment.

There are two procedures that should be considered for treating accommodative insufficiency. The first is the conventional prescribing of reading glasses. The lenses in reading glasses are designed to mimic the shape of the lenses inside the eyes. In this way, the glasses take over much of the work of near-point vision, allowing the lenses in the eyes to relax and making near-point work easier to do.

The theory behind reading glasses sounds fine, but glasses really accomplish little in the way of helping people to overcome accommodative insufficiency. The eyes and their lenses should be worked, but not overworked when viewing at a close distance. Glasses, especially if they are too strong, may simply allow the eyes to relax too much, making them more dependent on glasses for clear near-point viewing. This should not be misconstrued as a statement against reading glasses. In many cases, glasses are prescribed to assist the eyes in reading with greater ease, and are used alongside the second treatment, which is discussed below.

The second treatment method is vision therapy. (For a complete discussion of vision therapy, see page 385.) Although vision therapy is considered to be much more than simply eye exercises, in this case techniques are used to work the lenses together with their associated muscles in an effort to achieve their full potential. Vision therapy can help you learn how to better control your eyes so that you can use them more efficiently.

As mentioned above, and depending on the severity of the problem, a doctor may prescribe glasses *and* vision therapy. This combination treatment may be the ideal remedy if the accommodative system is so weak that the vision therapy program must be prolonged. The reading glasses will help you with normal near-point viewing, and the vision therapy will teach you how to better control your eyes. If this combination treatment is successful, eventually you will not need the glasses.

SELF-TREATMENT

The core of the vision therapy program for accommodative insufficiency is a technique called the accommodative rock. This technique helps to improve the eyes' ability to change focus and to see clearly at close points and at a distance. For complete instructions for doing the accommodative rock, see page 389.

NUTRITIONAL SUPPLEMENTS

SUPPLEMENT	DIRECTIONS FOR USE	COMMENTS
Vitamin B_2	Take 75 mg daily.	Good for the nerves, muscles, and fatigue.
Vitamin C	Take 250 mg, 4 times daily.	Nourishes the lens within the eye.
Vitamin E	Take 300 IU daily.	An antioxidant.
Lutein	Take at least 10 mg daily.	An antioxidant that is found in the lens.
Astaxanthin	Take 6 mg daily.	Supports muscle strength and function.

HOMEOPATHIC REMEDIES

REMEDY	DIRECTIONS FOR USE	COMMENTS
Cocculuc 6c	Place 3–4 pellets under the tongue, 3–4 times daily.	Good for accommodative insufficiency associated with nausea.
Gelsemium sempervirens 6c	Place 3–4 pellets under the tongue, 3–4 times daily.	Good for accommodative insufficiency associated with headache.
Natrum muriaticum 6c	Place 3–4 pellets under the tongue, 3–4 times daily.	Good for accommodative insufficiency associated with anger or irritability.

RECOMMENDATIONS

• Get a thorough eye examination that includes near-vision testing.

• Don't confuse accommodative insufficiency with presbyopia. If you are near or past your fortieth birthday and are having difficulty focusing at the near point, your condition is probably presbyopia.

• If your child is having difficulty with school due to accommodative insufficiency, don't hesitate to get glasses and vision therapy for the child. If the child won't cooperate with the vision therapy, then he can use just the glasses to at least make reading easier. When the child matures somewhat, the vision therapy can still be useful as a long-term treatment.

AGE-RELATED FARSIGHTEDNESS

See Presbyopia, page 308.

AGE-RELATED MACULAR DEGENERATION

See Macular Degeneration, page 273.

ALBINISM

The word albinism (also called oculocutaneous albinism) refers to a group of conditions resulting from the presence of little or no pigment in the eyes, skin, and hair. In some cases, only the eyes are affected. People with albinism have inherited genes from their parents that do not work correctly. These genes do not allow their bodies to make the usual amounts of melanin. Melanin is a dark-brown to black pigment.

Worldwide, 1 in 17,000 people have some type of albinism. About 18,000 people in the United States are affected. Albinism can be found in every race. The majority of those afflicted were born to parents with normal hair and eye colors.

When most of us think about albinism, we think about how vulnerable the skin is in those who have the condition. People with albinism sunburn easily, since the skin needs pigment for protection against sun damage. In tropical areas, many people with albinism who do not protect their skin get skin cancer. What many don't realize is that the eyes are also considerably affected. The eyes need pigment to develop normal vision. It is the melanin in the retina that facilitates the conversion of light energy to a nerve impulse that begins the visual process.

Common eye problems associated with albinism include:

- Extreme far- or nearsightedness

- Astigmatism

- Nystagmus (involuntary back-and-forth eye movements)

- Strabismus (inability of the eyes to fix on and track an object)

- Light sensitivity

People with albinism have impaired vision because their eyes do not have the normal amount of pigment. In fact, they often have several eye-related problems. First, they are generally very far- or nearsighted, or have astigmatism. Their visual acuity ranges from 20/30 (nearly normal) to 20/400 (legally blind). This latter state is considered having "low vision" (see page 271) and requires special accommodation. Second, they often have nystagmus (nis-TAG-mus), which is an involuntary back-and-forth movement of the eyes. (For a complete discussion of nystagmus, see page 292.) They can also have strabismus (strah-BIZZ-muss), which is an inability of the eyes to fix on an object and track together. Despite having this condition, people with albinism have some depth perception, although at close distances it is not as sharp as when the eyes work together. (For a complete discussion of strabismus, see page 320.) Last, they are light sensitive. Their irises allow "stray" light to enter the eyes and cause sensitivity. Contrary to popular belief, light sensitivity does not prevent people with albinism from going out in the sunlight but the exposure time must be limited. (For a complete discussion of light sensitivity, see page 268.)

It is a common notion that people with albinism have red eyes. In reality, the color of their irises varies from dull gray to blue to brown. (Brown irises are common in races with darker pigmentation.) In some types of albinism and under certain lighting conditions, a reddish or violet hue may be reflected through the iris. The reddish reflection comes from light bouncing off the retina, which lines the inner surface of the eye. It is similar to what occurs when a flash photograph is taken of a person looking directly at the camera—the "red eye." In such cases of albinism, the red color can reflect back through the iris as well as through the pupil.

The key problems of the eye in albinism involve a lack of development of the macula and a change in the development of the nerves that connect the eye to the brain. It is not fully clear why the macula does not develop in people with albinism. What we do know is that the developing eye needs melanin to organize the macula, as well as to route the nerves from the retina to the areas of the brain where vision is processed. Studies have shown that the nerve impulses of people with albinism follow an unusual route from the eye. The nerve connections from the eye to the vision areas of the brain are disorganized. This unusual route probably prevents the eyes from working well together, which can cause strabismus.

In most cases, ocular albinism is X-linked, which means the gene for it is on the X chromosome. "X-linked ocular albinism" occurs almost exclusively in males. It is passed to sons from mothers who carry the gene. Each time a mother who carries the gene for ocular albinism gives birth to a son, there is a one-in-two chance that the son will have ocular albinism.

> Because albinism is linked to the X chromosome, it occurs almost exclusively in males.

CONVENTIONAL TREATMENT

Optometrists and ophthalmologists can help you compensate for eye problems related to albinism, but they cannot cure the problems. To help with visual acuity, eye doctors experienced with treating low vision can prescribe a variety of devices. No one device serves the needs of every patient, since different occupations and hobbies require the use of vision in different ways. The choice of optical aids for a child or adult is an individual one.

Many adults with albinism use ordinary glasses or bifocals with a strong reading correction. Some children may do well with ordinary glasses as well. For older children and adults, glasses with small telescopes mounted on the lenses may help with both close and distant vision. Such lenses are referred to as *bioptics*. They can be adapted for near-point work as well as for distance vision. Contact lenses sometimes provide additional correction that glasses cannot.

For nystagmus, research has not yet found an effective treatment. Attempted treatments to control nystagmus have included biofeedback, rigid contact lenses, and surgery. However, research has not proven any specific treatment to be effective for all people.

For light sensitivity, eye doctors can prescribe dark glasses, which shield the eyes from bright light. They can also prescribe photochromic lenses, which darken as the light becomes brighter. There is no proof that dark glasses improve vision, even when used at a very early age. Still, they can improve comfort. (It is important to note that many children with albinism do not like tinted glasses.) Specially tinted contact lenses can also be designed to mask the iris and create a more normal appearance. While this will likely reduce uncomfortable glare it will not likely improve visual acuity.

Also important in the treatment of ocular albinism is attention to emotional and social adjustment. Often those who have albinism, and the parents of children with albinism, feel anger and shame about the condition and try to deny it or pretend it does not exist. For those with albinism, this denial can result in low self-esteem, difficulties in relationships with others, and low functioning in school and work. Thankfully, there are many support groups and helpful organizations that exist. See page 416 of the Resource Organizations section for more information.

Because albinism is linked to the X chromosome, it occurs almost exclusively in males.

If you are a parent of a child with albinism, definitely look into all available options at your child's school regarding visual aids and support. Most children with albinism can function in a mainstream-classroom environment, provided the school addresses their special visual needs. The majority of them do not require Braille. Rather, children with albinism often prefer to read with the head tilted and the page held close to their eyes. Sometimes it is difficult to get them to use their glasses, so alternatives are important to offer. Honest, open conversation about their eye problems should certainly be encouraged. The following recommendations are for parents of children with ocular albinism who suffer from low vision.

RECOMMENDATIONS

• Ask your child's teacher to use high-contrast written materials. Children with low vision often have a hard time reading low-contrast materials. Black on white is best, and photocopying with high quality copies often makes reading easier.

• Ask your child's school to order large-print textbooks. Schools can obtain large-print editions of most of their regular textbooks directly from the publishers. Because children with albinism often have difficulty keeping track of their place on the page when shifting back and forth between a textbook and a worksheet, request permission for your child to write in her textbooks.

• Ask the teacher to provide your child with a paper copy of all the board notes. Your child can then read the notes up close while the rest of the class reads from the board.

• Request that the school purchase optic devices to make reading assignments easier for your child. Hand-held monoculars, telescopic lenses mounted on eyeglasses, video-enlargement machines, and other types of magnifiers often help children with low vision. The prescription of appropriate classroom visual aids requires teamwork among the student, parents, classroom teacher, vision-resources teacher, and an optometrist or ophthalmologist experienced in working with children with low vision. The American Foundation for the Blind maintains a directory of low-vision clinics in the United States.

• Children with albinism should begin keyboarding skills early, since computers with software for large character screen display can help greatly with writing projects.

If your child has albinism, speak to the school about providing necessary visual aids and support. Reading and schoolwork can be difficult for children with albinism.

AMBLYOPIA

See Lazy Eye, page 264.

ANISOCORIA

Anisocoria (an-is-oh-KOR-ee-ah) is a condition in which the pupils of the two eyes are unequal in size. This has potentially dangerous implications because nerves in the brain control the size of the pupils. In a healthy person, both pupils are equal in size and response. That is, when a light is shined into just one eye, both pupils should react equally.

When light is shined into one eye, the pupils of both eyes should react equally. If they don't, a professional evaluation is warranted.

It is possible to have a slight difference in the sizes of the two pupils and still be perfectly healthy. Therefore, if you notice a slight difference, don't be alarmed. However, unequal size warrants a thorough evaluation, so be sure to get a professional opinion as soon as possible. Pupil size can be affected by a number of physical, psychological, environmental, and emotional conditions. Some drugs can also affect pupil size. Anisocoria is actually just a sign that there may be a disorder affecting the nerves within a certain part of the brain. In the treatment sections below, there is also information on how anisocoria is diagnosed.

CONVENTIONAL TREATMENT

Testing pupil response is part of all routine eye examinations. There is always a comparison between the pupils to see if there is an extreme difference in size or reaction to light. The doctor simply shines a light into one eye and checks the reaction of the pupil, and then does the same with the other eye. Pupil response is a good indicator of how well the central nervous system is functioning. If there is any question regarding the size or reaction of the pupils, the doctor will probably order a visual field test, just to rule out other potential issues.

The retinal nerve fibers, some of which branch off to the control centers for pupil response, can be evaluated by testing the visual field of each eye. This is similar to the peripheral vision test that we discussed in Part One but more scientific and detailed. A visual field test is something like a mapping of the side vision to determine if all of the nerves are functioning properly. It can be a somewhat tedious test, but it is well worth the trouble, since good results indicate that there is no problem with nerve or brain function.

If the doctor finds that your pupils are significantly different in size but there are no other abnormalities, there is really no problem—unless you notice excessive glare on the side of the larger pupil. In extreme cases, a contact lens with an "artificial" pupil can be worn to cut out too much glare.

SELF-TREATMENT

While there is no self-treatment for anisocoria, you can test yourself for the condition. Stand in front of a mirror and flash a small light into one of your eyes. Look at the pupil of that eye to see if it constricts (closes) when the light enters it. Shine the light into that same eye again, but this time look at the other eye. The pupil of the other eye should also constrict.

Next, shine the light into both eyes, one at a time, alternating between the two eyes and using a steady back-and-forth motion of the flashlight. Both pupils should remain constricted. If there is a problem with the transfer of information along one of the optic nerves, one pupil may actually dilate (open) when the light is shined into it. If one of your pupils dilates while doing this, immediately phone your eye doctor for an appointment, just to make sure there is nothing unusual going on.

HOMEOPATHIC REMEDIES

REMEDY	DIRECTIONS FOR USE	COMMENTS
Argentum nitricum 6c	Place 3–4 pellets under the tongue, 3–4 times daily.	Good for dilated pupils.
Belladonna 6c	Place 3–4 pellets under the tongue, 3–4 times daily.	Good for dilated pupils.
Calcarea fluorica 6c	Place 3–4 pellets under the tongue, 3–4 times daily.	Good for dilated pupils.
Cinchona officinalis 6c	Place 3–4 pellets under the tongue, 3–4 times daily.	Good for dilated pupils.
Gelsemium sempervirens 6c	Place 3–4 pellets under the tongue, 3–4 times daily.	Good for dilated pupils.
Stramonium 6c	Place 3–4 pellets under the tongue, 3–4 times daily.	Good for dilated pupils.

RECOMMENDATIONS

- Periodically check your pupil reaction with a flashlight to make sure your pupils constrict properly.

- If you notice signs of anisocoria during self-tests, do not delay in calling your eye doctor for an appointment. Explain that this is a priority situation and that you need to see the doctor promptly. On the chance that you have a serious health concern, time is essential.

Periodically check your pupil response to make sure that your eyes are reacting to light in a healthy way. If they are not, be sure to visit your eye doctor for an examination.

ANISOMETROPIA

Anisometropia (an-is-oh-met-ROH-pee-ah) is a visual condition in which the refractive error of each eye is different. Most people's eyes have slightly different refractions, but in anisometropia, the difference is great. For example, one eye might be farsighted and the other eye nearsighted. Or both may be farsighted or nearsighted, but of considerably unequal amounts. Additionally, one eye may have some astigmatism while the other doesn't, or both may have astigmatism but of differing amounts. Anisometropia has many variations.

Because the eyes send their images to the brain independently of each other and the brain must fuse the two images together so that only one picture is seen, it is important for both images to be approximately equal in size and clarity. If there is a significant difference between the two images, the brain cannot put them together properly and will either suppress one or cause double vision. (For complete discussions of suppression and double vision, see pages 328 and 209, respectively.) While suppression results in seeing just one picture again, it is not a desirable state for proper visual function. The ideal situation is to have both eyes seeing clearly and both images fusing into one picture.

CONVENTIONAL TREATMENT

Contacts are a more viable solution to anisometropia than eyeglasses. When someone with this condition wears eyeglasses, it may be difficult for the brain to fuse the two images taken in by the eyes into a single image.

In treating anisometropia, many doctors simply prescribe glasses with the correct prescription for each eye. However, as the refractive error of an eye becomes greater, the thickness of the eyeglass lens increases. When two lenses are of significantly different thicknesses, the result is images of two different sizes, even if both eyes are corrected to 20/20. The brain may then have difficulty fusing the two images into a single picture. So, for significant anisometropia, glasses are not an ideal solution.

Contact lenses have shown to be a much more viable solution to anisometropia. Because contact lenses are much thinner than the lenses in eyeglasses, and because contact lenses rest directly on the eyeball, the images seen by the eyes are almost identical. These identically sized images are easier for the brain to fuse, therefore facilitating more comfortable binocular vision.

SELF-TREATMENT

The type of treatment you should self-administer depends on what type of anisometropia you have. In most cases, you might consider contact lenses to compensate for the size difference described above.

RECOMMENDATIONS

- If your child is school-aged, make sure that she does not tilt the head significantly while reading or writing. Also, check if the child holds a hand over one eye while doing near-point tasks. If so, an eye examination including an evaluation of binocular-vision skills, is in order. This condition happens when children have difficulty coordinating their eyes, so she'll likely need a course in vision therapy to train her eyes to work together efficiently.

ARCUS SENILIS

The condition of arcus senilis (ARK-us see-NIL-us) most often develops during the later years of life, but it is not uncommon in middle age or even younger. In arcus senilis, an opaque white ring encircles the periphery of the cornea. It usually happens in both eyes but often is more advanced in one eye. If you look closely at a case of arcus senilis, you can see a clear section of cornea between the edge of the ring and the white sclera. This is due either to the deposition of fat granules in the cornea or to hyaline degeneration, the latter of which is a type of tissue degeneration that results in rounded masses or broad bands of translucent tissue (like the cornea).

Arcus senilis—a whitish ring around the cornea—generally occurs in the elderly. When seen in younger people, it may be a sign of elevated cholesterol.

Arcus senilis generally is not considered to be dangerous. However, from a biochemical viewpoint, it represents a specific metabolic disturbance and is a valuable indication of fat and cholesterol metabolism. The general consensus among eye doctors is that arcus senilis is normal in older adults, but it can be a sign of elevated cholesterol in middle-aged or younger (pre-fifty) individuals.

CONVENTIONAL TREATMENT

Arcus senilis is cosmetically unappealing but not threatening to the sight. Therefore, it is most often noted but not treated by eye doctors. There is no cosmetic surgical option.

NUTRITIONAL SUPPLEMENTS

SUPPLEMENT	DIRECTIONS FOR USE	COMMENTS
Chromium	Take 400–600 mcg daily.	Lowers the cholesterol level and improves picolinatethe HDL-LDL ratio.

L-carnitine	Take 1,000 mg, 3 times daily, with meals.	Supports cholesterol metabolism, transports essential fatty acids, and aids liver and gallbladder function.
Lecithin	Take 1,200 mg, 3 times daily, before meals.	Emulsifies fat in the body.
Niacin	Take 1,000 mg before bed.	Raises good cholesterol. Confirm with your doctor.
Phosphatide	Take 1,500 mg daily.	Emulsifies fat in the body.

HERBS AND HERBAL SUPPLEMENTS

HERB	DIRECTIONS FOR USE	COMMENTS
Garlic	Take as directed on the label.	Reduces the cholesterol level.
Ginger	Take as directed on the label.	Reduces the cholesterol level.

RECOMMENDATIONS

• Keep your cholesterol levels checked and in check.

• Always use good quality sunglasses when outdoors—and especially around water.

• Keep the cornea moist at all times, even if it means using lubricating eye drops (not eye whiteners).

AMD

See Macular Degeneration, page 273.

ASTHENOPIA

See Eyestrain, page 222.

ASTIGMATISM

Astigmatism (ah-STIG-mah-tis-em) is a refractive error of the eye; the image that is focused on the retina is distorted. In Latin, *a stigma* means "without point." The distortion of astigmatism comes most often from the cornea being shaped more like a barrel than a ball. The light rays in the vertical orientation focus on one spot, while the light rays in the horizontal orientation focus on a different spot. There is a blur between the two points, and the resulting picture is distorted.

It has been reported that up to 80 percent of the American population has some degree of astigmatism. However, not all of these cases are severe enough to require an optical correction. Slight astigmatism is often of no consequence and just an example of the imperfections in nature. Yet, for many people, the degree of astigmatism can be severe enough to cause headaches and other symptoms.

The unique aspect of this problem is that a person may have significant astigmatism and not be aware of it. This is due to the fact that the optical disparity manifests as a distortion rather than a blur. Because of the distortion, the brain, when it receives the image, makes a perceptual adjustment, so the person thinks that everything is clear and properly oriented. This is part of the brain's attempt to make the visual world comfortable. I have seen cases in which young people thought that their vision was "pretty good," when in fact it tested at 20/60!

Although up to 80 percent of Americans have some degree of astigmatism, for many people, the astigmatism is so light that it does not require optical correction. Other people with this condition can benefit from the use of eyeglasses, contact lenses, surgery, or vision therapy.

CONVENTIONAL TREATMENT

The most conventional way to treat astigmatism is with eyeglasses. The curvatures of the eyeglass lenses roughly correspond to the curvatures of the eyes, and the optical distortion is resolved back into a "point" image. This can be very effective, allowing clear vision. However, if you have new glasses for astigmatism, there are a few things that you need to understand about your vision.

First, since your brain has already adjusted to compensate for the distortion in your uncorrected vision, new glasses may make things seem rather strange. This is because the visual images are now being realigned by the glasses, and your brain must readjust its perception to allow the glasses to do their job. It may take some time, and until the readjustment is complete, your vision through the glasses will be disorienting. You may notice the floor sloping up, and straight lines may appear curved. These distortions will disappear with time, usually in a week or so, depending on the degree of astigmatism. To make the readjustment easier, simply wear your new glasses as much as is comfortable initially, and gradually increase your wearing time as you adapt.

Second, the correction for astigmatism is in the central portion of the eyeglass lens—that is, the part through which you look when focusing straight ahead. However, when you look off to the side, up, or down, the thicker portions of the lens will create different types of astigmatism and may cause additional distortion. You may feel as if your whole world is moving when you move your head around. This situation will also disappear as you adapt to the lens prescription.

Another treatment for astigmatism is contact lenses. Contact lenses have a few advantages over eyeglasses—for astigmatism and most other problems that require optical correction. Because the contact lenses sit directly on the eyes, you're always looking through the optical center of the lens. This makes the image on your retina more like "real life" and avoids extra distortions. The different types of contacts and the different problems for which they are effective are discussed in detail in "Contact Lenses" on page 338. In recent years, advances in contact lenses have made the use of both the gas permeable (rigid) and soft varieties routine treatments for astigmatism.

There is also a surgical option for the treatment of astigmatism. LASIK and other refractive surgeries designed to reduce nearsightedness can be modified to treat astigmatism. These procedures are discussed in detail in "Refractive Surgery" on page 371.

SELF-TREATMENT

Since most types of astigmatism are related to the curvature of the cornea, conventional wisdom holds that nothing short of surgery can effectively correct the condition. Glasses and contact lenses can compensate for the visual problems while they are being worn or used, but they will not reverse the actual condition. Though this may be true in some cases, sometimes astigmatism can be dealt with successfully using a program of vision therapy. For complete details of how astigmatism can be addressed using such a program, see "Vision Therapy" on page 385.

Orthokeratology, a corrective program utilizing a series of contact lenses to reshape the eye, can also have an effect on the curvature of the cornea. Thus it aims to actually reduce the degree of astigmatism in the eye. This program is covered in detail in "Orthokeratology" on page 370.

RECOMMENDATIONS

● Have a complete eye examination to determine if you have astigmatism and, if you do, ask if it's enough to warrant correction.

- Discuss all of the treatment options—including eyeglasses, contact lenses, vision therapy, surgery, and orthokeratology—with your eye doctor.

BLEPHARITIS

The word blepharitis (blef-are-EYE-tis) comes from *blepharon*, the Greek word for "eyelid," and *itis*, a suffix that means "inflammation." In blepharitis, the tiny glands and hair follicles that open onto the surface of the eyelids are inflamed. The eyelids are red, sore, and sticky. There may be little ulcers on the eyelids, and some eyelashes may fall out. Styes, chalazia, and dandruff of the scalp often occur along with blepharitis. (For complete discussions of chalazia and styes, see pages 185 and 324, respectively.) Figure 2.1 offers a simple illustration of an eye with blepharitis.

Blepharitis has two primary causes. When the blepharitis is accompanied by ulceration (open sores) of the eyelid skin, the cause is usually a bacterial infection. The other primary cause of blepharitis is a waxy, greasy form of dandruff that affects the scalp and can also involve the eyelids, eyebrows, external ears, and the area around the nose and lips. There are additional causes of blepharitis as well. It can be an allergic reaction caused by exposure to dust, smoke, irritating chemicals, or other allergens.

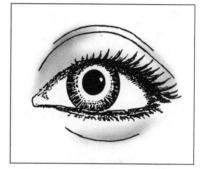

FIGURE 2.1
An Eye Affected by Blepharitis.

CONVENTIONAL TREATMENT

When the cause of blepharitis is a bacterial infection, prompt treatment with a topical antibiotic is necessary. You might also be advised to apply warm compresses on the eye or to scrub your eyelids with a special solution.

If the cause of your blepharitis is the dandruff condition described above, you may be instructed to scrub your eyelids frequently using a washcloth or cotton-tipped applicator dipped in a solution of warm water and baby shampoo. This treatment will remove the crusty material and mucus from the eyelids. An anti-dandruff shampoo is usually recommended to bring the scalp condition under control. There are now specific eyelid "scrubs" that are recommended to treat this form of blepharitis. However, "scrubbing" the lids is often misinterpreted as hard rubbing, when a gentle massaging technique is more appropriate. A newer treatment is to use a diluted solution of tea tree oil. CAUTION: DO NOT USE FULL STRENGTH TEA TREE OIL

NEAR THE EYES. Only a pre-made diluted solution should be used, and only on the lids, not the eye itself.

SELF-TREATMENT

If your blepharitis is caused by environmental irritants such as dust, smoke, irritating chemicals, or allergens, antibiotics won't help. But you can remove yourself from the irritating environment, plus use warm compresses—just warm water on a washcloth. If these self-treatments bring no improvement, ask your doctor about anti-inflammatory medications.

NUTRITIONAL SUPPLEMENTS

SUPPLEMENT	DIRECTIONS FOR USE	COMMENTS
Linoleic acid	Take 500 mg of black currant seed oil.	Supports skin tissue.
Vitamin A	Take 2,500 IU daily.	Good for dry skin.
Vitamin-B complex	Take 75 mg daily.	Promotes healthy skin and proper circulation. Aids in cellular reproduction.
Vitamin C with bioflavonoids	Take 3,000 mg daily, in divided doses.	An antioxidant. Protects the eyes and reduces inflammation. Note: Use powdered buffered ascorbic acid.
Zinc (monomethionine) and copper	Take 20 mg of zinc and 2 mg of copper daily.	Enhances immune function. Note: The copper supplementation is needed to balance the zinc supplementation. Caution: Do not take more than 40 mg of zinc daily.

HERBS AND HERBAL SUPPLEMENTS

HERB	DIRECTIONS FOR USE	COMMENTS
Dulse	Apply as a compress.	High in iodine.
Goldenseal	Apply as a compress.	Soothes the tissues. Caution: Do not take internally for more than 1 week. Do not use during pregnancy.
Horsetail	Apply as a compress.	Tones the skin.
Rosemary	Apply as a compress.	Stimulates the skin.
Sage	Apply as a compress.	An astringent.

HOMEOPATHIC REMEDIES

REMEDY	DIRECTIONS FOR USE	COMMENTS
Antimonium crudum 6c	Place 3–4 pellets under the tongue, 3–4 times daily.	Good for all skin conditions.
Apis mellifica 6c	Place 3–4 pellets under the tongue, 3–4 times daily.	Good for all skin conditions.
Argentum nitricum 6c	Place 3–4 pellets under the tongue, 3–4 times daily.	Good for all skin conditions.
Arsenicum album 6c	Place 3–4 pellets under the tongue, 3–4 times daily.	Good for blepharitis associated with anxiety or burning.
Calcarea sulfurica 6c	Place 3–4 pellets under the tongue, 3–4 times daily.	Good for all skin conditions.
Carboneum sulfuratum 6c	Place 3–4 pellets under the tongue, 3–4 times daily.	Good for all skin conditions.
Euphrasia officinalis 6c	Place 3–4 pellets under the tongue, 3–4 times daily.	Good for blepharitis associated with soreness.
Graphites 6c	Place 3–4 pellets under the tongue, 3–4 times daily.	Good for all skin conditions.
Hepar sulphuris 6c	Place 3–4 pellets under the tongue, 3–4 times daily.	Good for all skin conditions.
Lycopodium 6c	Place 3–4 pellets under the tongue, 3–4 times daily.	Good for all skin conditions.
Petroleum 6	Place 3–4 pellets under the tongue, 3–4 times daily.	Good for all skin conditions.
Rhus toxicodendron 6c	Place 3–4 pellets under the tongue, 3–4 times daily.	Good for all skin conditions.
Sulphur 6c	Place 3–4 pellets under the tongue, 3–4 times daily.	Good for all skin conditions.

RECOMMENDATIONS

• Try to avoid rubbing your eyes, even if they feel itchy. (Itching might be a sign of an allergy, so use a cold compress to relieve the itchy feeling.)

• Apply a warm compress to your eyes a few times a day, for at least ten minutes each time. To enhance the effect, make a tea of your chosen herb, soak a clean cloth in the tea, and apply the cloth as the compress. When finished, gently wipe your eyelids with the compress to remove any excess debris. Never re-use a compress.

- Stay away from irritants such as smoke, wind, excessive sunlight, and bright lights.

- Eat a well-balanced diet that emphasizes fresh raw vegetables, plus whole grains, legumes, and fresh fruits.

- Get sufficient sleep, and avoid eyestrain.

BLEPHAROSPASM

Blepharospasm (BLEF-ah-ro-spaz-em) is a condition involving the uncontrollable closing of the eyelids. It is a dystonia (dis-TONE-ee-ah)—that is, a positional disorder caused by abnormal, involuntary, sustained muscle contractions and spasms, also known as "tics." Moreover, this disorder is both cranial, because it involves the head, and focal, because it is confined to one specific part of the head. *Blepharo* comes from the Greek word for eyelid. Patients with blepharospasm have normal, healthy eyes. The visual disturbance is solely the repeated forced closure of the eyelids. It usually affects both eyelids but can affect just one eyelid in some conditions.

Blepharospasm usually begins gradually with excessive blinking and/ or eye irritation. In the early stages, it may occur only in the presence of specific stressful conditions, such as bright lights, fatigue, and emotional tension. As the disorder progresses, it occurs more frequently during the day. The spasms disappear during sleep, and some people find that after a good night's slumber, the spasms don't appear for several hours. Concentrating on a specific task often reduces the frequency of the spasms. As the condition progresses even further, the spasms may intensify so that when they occur, the patient is functionally blind. The eyelids may even remain forcefully closed for several hours.

CONVENTIONAL TREATMENT

Botulinum toxin (Botox) is an approved treatment for blepharospasm in the United States and Canada. Produced by the bacteria *Clostridium botulinum,* this toxin weakens the muscles by blocking the nerve impulses transmitted from the nerve endings of the muscles. When used to treat blepharospasm, it is injected in minute doses into muscles above and below the eyes.

The sites of the injections vary slightly from patient to patient and according to physician preference. The injections are usually given in the eyelid, the brow, and the muscles under the lower lid. They are administered through a very fine needle. The benefits begin one to fourteen days after the treatment and last for an average of three to four months. Long-term follow-up studies have shown the treatment to be very safe and effective, with up to 90 percent of patients obtaining almost complete relief from their blepharospasm.

The side effects of treatment with Botulinum toxin include drooping of the eyelids, blurred vision, and double vision. Excessive tearing may also occur. All these side effects are transient, caused mainly by excessive muscle relaxation. Providing the dose is kept small and the injections are given no less than three months apart, this method remains effective over a long period of time.

The effects of Botulinum toxin therapy may be increased with the use of some antibiotics or with other drugs that interfere with neuromuscular transmission. But drug therapy alone for blepharospasm is difficult. Different medications have different mechanisms of action and generally produce unpredictable and short-term benefits. One medication may work for some patients and not for others. When a medication that did work becomes ineffective, replacement with another drug sometimes helps. There is, therefore, no fixed or best regimen for this condition. Finding a satisfactory treatment regimen requires persistence on the part of both the physician and the patient. Some good medication options include amantadine (Symmetrel), baclofen (Lioresal), benztropine (Cogentin), bromocriptime (Parlodel), carbamazepine (Tegretol), clonazpam (Klonapin), diazepam (Valium), levodopa (Sinemet or Modopar), and trihexyphenidyl (Artane). This list is by no means complete, especially since there are new medications constantly being developed. The use of medication for blepharospasm always requires close supervision by a neurologist.

Another treatment option is surgery. However, before considering surgery, it is advisable to try potentially effective non-surgical therapies such as Botox injections. Functionally impaired patients with blepharospasm who cannot tolerate or do not respond well to medication or Botox are candidates for surgical therapy. At present, the removal of some or all of the muscles responsible for eyelid closure has proven to be the most effective surgical treatment for blepharospasm, though it is certainly also a last resort. Current experience has found that this procedure has improved visual disability in 75 to 80 percent of cases of blepharospasm.

Common treatment options for blepharospasm include:

● Botox

● Antibiotics or other drugs

● Surgery

● Acupuncture

● Relaxation techniques such as yoga and meditation

SELF-TREATMENT

One method of self-treatment for blepharospasm is stress reduction. Consider seeking out professional assistance to determine if you have excessive stress in your life and how you can best deal with it. Typical modalities used to treat stress are meditation, breathing techniques, biofeedback, visualization, yoga, and counseling. Acupuncture is also a viable alternative to traditional medical treatments. (For a complete discussion of acupuncture, see page 332.) Of course, some of these healing practices are not self-administered treatments in and of themselves, but the decision to adjust your life to a lower level of pressure and anxiety can be considered a self-directed avenue of treatment.

Because blepharospasm flare-ups have been linked to stress, try to reduce the stress in your life through counseling, breathing techniques, yoga, or simply taking more time for yourself.

Also, quinine—or tonic—water can act as a nerve-block. Consumption of such water can help with this condition. The gin is optional!

NUTRITIONAL SUPPLEMENTS

SUPPLEMENT	DIRECTIONS FOR USE	COMMENTS
Calcium	Take 1,000 mg daily.	Good for nerve function.
Folic acid	Take 400 mcg daily.	Good for proper nerve-cell production.
Phosphorus	Take 800 mg daily.	Good for proper nerve-cell growth.
Potassium	Take 2,500 mg daily.	Rebalances the nerves.
Vitamin-B complex	Take 100 mg daily.	Good for stress.
Vitamin B$_5$	Take 100 mg daily.	Improves the body's resistance to stress.
Vitamin C with bioflavonoids	Take 500 mg, every 3 hours, up to 4 times daily.	An antioxidant. Note: Use powdered buffered ascorbic acid.

HERBS AND HERBAL SUPPLEMENTS

HERB	DIRECTIONS FOR USE	COMMENTS
Lobelia	Apply as a compress.	Relieves muscle cramping. Caution: Do not take internally.
Valerian	Take as directed on the label; take at bedtime.	Good for relaxation.

HOMEOPATHIC REMEDIES

REMEDY	DIRECTIONS FOR USE	COMMENTS
Agaricus 6c	Place 3–4 pellets under the tongue, 3–4 times daily.	Good for eyelid twitching.
Belladonna 9c	Place 3–4 pellets under the tongue, 3–4 times daily.	Good for spasms.
Calcarea carbonica 6c and Magnesia phosphorica 6c	Place 3–4 pellets of each remedy under the tongue, 3–4 times daily.	Good for blepharospasm associated with mineral deficiency.
Hypericum p erforatum 6c	Place 3–4 pellets under the tongue, 3–4 times daily.	Good for blepharospasm affecting the eye only.
Ignatia amara 6c	Place 3–4 pellets under the tongue, 3–4 times daily.	Good for eyelid twitching.
Nux vomica 6c	Place 3–4 pellets under the tongue, 3–4 times daily.	Good for eyelid spasm after drinking coffee.
Physostigma 6c	Place 3–4 pellets under the tongue, 3–4 times daily.	Good for eyelid twitching.
Rheum 6c	Place 3–4 pellets under the tongue, 3–4 times daily.	Good for eyelid twitching.
Sulphur 6c	Place 3–4 pellets under the tongue, 3–4 times daily.	Good for eyelid twitching.

RECOMMENDATIONS

• Very often, a stressful situation will initiate an episode of blepharospasm. You may find that talking and releasing your feelings can make a significant difference in this condition.

• If the person with blepharospasm is your child, consider emotional counseling for them.

BLOOD VESSELS IN CORNEA

See Corneal Neovascularization, page 200.

BLOODSHOT EYES

Eye redness can come from a variety of conditions. Eye inflammations, infections, and irritations of all kinds can cause the blood vessels of the conjunctiva to dilate. The eyes then appear red, or bloodshot.

If your eyes are constantly bloodshot, look for an obvious cause, because redness is more a sign that something is amiss rather than a condition in and of itself. If your eyes also itch, you are probably allergic to something in your environment. If you have pain, the problem is likely to be an infection such as pinkeye (see page 303). If the redness occurs only in certain situations, such as while cleaning the oven or cutting onions, it is likely due to irritating fumes. If the problem persists or you suspect an infection that needs treatment, see your eye doctor.

A bloodshot appearance can also result from a deficiency of any of the following: vitamin B_2; vitamin B_6; the amino acid histidine; lysine; or phenylalanine. Once your body receives the nutrients it needs, the congestion in the blood vessels should disappear.

Unexplained redness can also be due to dry eyes. Without an adequate level of tears to supply oxygen to the cornea, the body will call on the blood vessels in the conjunctiva to supply the needed nutrients. This is the same process that occurs with over-wearing of contact lenses.

TREATMENT FOR BLOODSHOT EYES

- If you experience eye redness without any other symptoms, apply warm compresses.

- If redness is accompanied by itching, apply cool compresses.

- Until the problem improves, avoid visually intense activities such as reading and computer work.

- If you are unable to reduce the redness within a few days, see your eye doctor.

CONVENTIONAL TREATMENT

Most eye doctors look for the cause of the redness before recommending a treatment. As suggested above, there are dozens of causes for eye redness, and misdiagnosis can make the situation worse. For redness due to pinkeye, oftentimes no treatment is needed if proper hygiene is followed. This is because the cause of pinkeye is usually self-limiting, meaning that it will go away on its own. However, many doctors like to prescribe antibiotics and steroid combinations to be cautious. These medications are often over-prescribed, but patients frequently request the treatments because they feel that they do not have time to wait for the redness to go away on its own.

If it turns out that the redness is due to allergies, allergy medication could be recommended. There are so many effective over-the-counter allergy medicines available; the doctor might simply suggest one of those instead of issuing a formal prescription. And if vitamin deficiencies are the problem, either the eye doctor could recommend a nutritionist or, if he is knowledgeable in the area of nutrition, suggest a protocol of supplements. See the "Nutritional Supplements" section below for more on this approach.

If it is confirmed that you have no underlying medical condition, a new over-the-counter eye drop is available for eye redness. Called Lumify (Bausch + Lomb), it has a unique formula that can clear the redness in the eyes without the typical "rebound" phenomenon of other eye whitener products.

SELF-TREATMENT

If you experience redness in your eyes without any other symptoms (for example, burning, itching, discharge, or grittiness), then begin your self-treatment with warm compresses of plain water or of some of the herbs recommended below. If the compresses do not reduce the redness within a few days, consult an eye doctor. Do not use commercial eye-whitening drops, as they often tend to make the condition worse, which then requires additional drops.

Don't treat bloodshot eyes with eye-whitening drops as they can actually make the redness worse.

NUTRITIONAL SUPPLEMENTS

SUPPLEMENT	DIRECTIONS FOR USE	COMMENTS
Free-form amino-acid complex	Take as directed on the label.	Provides the proper overall nutrition to the tissues. Note: Use a formula containing both the essential and nonessential amino acids.
Vitamin A	Take 2,500 IU daily.	Good for conjunctiva cell support.
Vitamin-B complex	Take 100 mg, 3 times daily.	Deficiencies have been linked to bloodshot eyes.

HERBS AND HERBAL SUPPLEMENTS

HERB	DIRECTIONS FOR USE	COMMENTS
Eyebright	Apply as a compress or use as an eyewash.	Good for all eye conditions.
Ming mu shang qing pian (Brion)	Take 4 pills, 2 times daily.	Reduces "heat" in the body. Caution: Do not use during pregnancy.
Niu huang shang qing wan (Brion)	Take 10 pills daily.	Reduces "heat" in the body. Caution: Do not use during pregnancy.
Raspberry	Apply as a cool compress; apply for 10 minutes.	Make a tea out of the leaves; alleviates redness and irritation.
Shi hu ye guang wan (Brion)	Take 1 pill, 2 times daily.	Good for red or itchy eyes.

HOMEOPATHIC REMEDIES

REMEDY	DIRECTIONS FOR USE	COMMENTS
Aconite 6c	Place 3–4 pellets under the tongue, 3–4 times daily.	Alleviates redness caused by an eye injury.
Allium cepa 6c	Place 3–4 pellets under the tongue, 3–4 times daily.	Alleviates redness caused by a cold.
Apis mellifica 6c	Place 3–4 pellets under the tongue, 3–4 times daily.	Alleviates redness and reduces swelling.
Argentum nitricum 6c	Place 3–4 pellets under the tongue.	Alleviates redness caused by a cold.
Arsenicum album 6c	Place 3–4 pellets under the tongue, 3–4 times daily.	Alleviates redness caused by a cold.
Belladonna 6c	Place 3–4 pellets under the tongue, 3–4 times daily.	Alleviates redness caused by a cold.
Euphrasia officinalis 6c	Place 3–4 pellets under the tongue, 3–4 times daily.	Alleviates redness and reduces the size of blood vessels.
Glonoinum 6c	Place 3–4 pellets under the tongue, 3–4 times daily.	Alleviates redness.
Kali sulfuricum 6c	Place 3–4 pellets under the tongue, 3–4 times daily.	Alleviates redness accompanied by itching.
Natrum muriaticum 6c	Place 3–4 pellets under the tongue, 3–4 times daily.	Alleviates redness accompanied by discharge.
Nux vomica 6c	Place 3–4 pellets under the tongue, 3–4 times daily.	Alleviates redness accompanied by headache.
Sulphur 6c	Place 3–4 pellets under the tongue, 3–4 times daily.	Alleviates redness.

RECOMMENDATIONS

• If your eyes are bloodshot, avoid visually intense activities such as reading, computer work, and sewing. This will allow you to blink more often, thereby refreshing your eyes.

• If you make your own eyewash, be sure to strain the mixture until it runs clear to avoid getting particles in your eyes.

• Hot compresses are usually a good thing just before bed—they're very relaxing.

CATARACTS

A cataract (CAT-ah-rackt) is not a "film" over the eye, as is commonly thought. Instead, it is a clouding of the lens within the eye. This clouding can be partial or complete, so not all cataracts interfere with vision to a severe extent. However, the type of cataract that occurs with advancing age is generally progressive. Therefore, a cataract that today is small and not causing much of a problem will probably at some point become a large cataract that obscures vision. There are many possible causes for cataracts, including the use of certain medications (usually steroids), excessive UV light (see below), and poor nutrition.

Approximately 20 million people in the United States have their vision obstructed by cataracts, and 500,000 new cases are diagnosed annually. It is the most common surgical procedure annually in the US. Cataracts are not limited to the aged, although the so-called "senile" cataract is the most common type of cataract. Between the ages of sixty-five and seventy-four, about 23 percent of the population is expected to have a cataract. After the age of seventy-five, about 50 percent of people will have the condition.

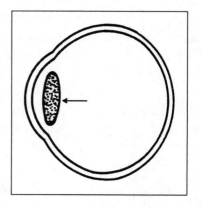

FIGURE 2.2.
An Eye Affected by a Cataract.

Cataracts can also be present at birth, although such a circumstance is pretty rare. This type of cataract is called a congenital cataract. It is sometimes caused by the mother having contracted German measles, mumps, chickenpox, or any of certain other infectious diseases during pregnancy. Rarely, congenital cataracts can also be inherited.

Some diseases and injuries, as well as a class of anti-inflammatory medications called steroids, as mentioned above, can also cause cataracts at any point in life. In addition, you can develop a cataract after being exposed to radiation (from having a large number of X-rays taken, for example), from being hit in the head by a high-voltage current (due to lightning or electrocution), from trauma to the eye or face (for example, an airbag in an auto accident), or from constant exposure to infrared light. The cataract caused by infrared light is called a glass blower's cataract, because glass blowers used to work with infrared light without eye protection.

In addition, recent research suggests that, also as mentioned above, many years of extreme exposure to UV light—which is part of sunlight but beyond the human visible spectrum—can also play a part in the development of cataracts. The crystalline lens inside the eye is a UV filter and absorbs most of the UV light entering the eye to prevent it from reaching the retina. Among the many environmental, lifestyle, and genetic risk factors associated with cataracts, exposure to UV radiation from sunlight and oxidative stress appears to be the most relevant in the development of this disease.

There have been a number of additional interesting studies done regarding cataract formation. Recent science suggests that there is a relationship between dietary carbohydrate intake and glycemic index in the development of cataracts. It seems that excessive intake of simple sugars and those sugars that raise blood-sugar levels to high, unhealthy levels contribute to the formation of cataracts. Yet another study suggests that cigarette smoking is linked to the formation of cataracts. The eye damage seems to be caused by certain chemicals that are transported internally to the lens while smoking. Secondhand smoke (smoke in the environment) does not have this effect.

There are further interesting study results that have come up. In Spain, a 1997 study found that women who took estrogen for more than four years had a reduced number of opacities in the lenses of their eyes. A 1999 study at Indiana University confirmed these results. Hopefully future research will explore the link between hormones and cataract formation.

Researchers believe that you may be able to avoid or at least postpone the formation of cataracts. A good pair of sunglasses, a balanced diet, limited exposure to X-rays, and avoidance of tobacco smoke can reduce your risk of developing this condition.

Are cataracts an inevitable consequence of advancing age, or are they the result of some action that can be changed? Researchers in the field of aging are asking this question about many conditions previously thought to be an unavoidable price of living a long life. The answer in the case of cataracts, as for most conditions, is that they probably are a combination of heredity, the aging process, and the environment. Years of exposure to UV light, radiation, and various environmental insults—such as smoking—eventually catch up with us as we age. At the same time, the eye's lens fibers begin to break down and are more vulnerable to stresses from the outside world. You may be able to prevent or postpone the development of a cataract by protecting your eyes from UV light with a good pair of sunglasses, eating a nutritious and balanced diet, limiting your exposure to infrared light and radiation from X-rays and other sources, and avoiding smoking.

CONVENTIONAL TREATMENT

When a cataract begins to interfere significantly with your vision and your life, it's usually time to consider surgery. Cataract surgery is the most common surgery in the United States today, with more than one million procedures performed every year. You may have heard that you have to wait until a cataract is "ripe" before it can be surgically removed. That was true years ago, but new surgical techniques have made it possible to remove a cataract at any time, as long as your doctor feels that you are in good enough physical condition to undergo the surgery. A good rule of thumb is that, as long as the cataract doesn't interfere with your lifestyle, there is no need to have it removed. Once it does start interfering, consider the surgical intervention.

Several different surgical techniques may be used. You and your surgeon can decide which one is best for you. Most times, cataract surgery can be done as an outpatient procedure. For more specifics on cataract surgery, see page 335.

SELF-TREATMENT

As suggested above, if you have a cataract, you may not necessarily need surgery—at least not right now. What you may be noticing with your cataract is that light is being refracted differently and doesn't look the same as it did before. You may see just a general sort of cloudy haze in your visual field, or you may see a dazzling air show of light bouncing off your cataract. What can you do to minimize these consequences of a cataract? Well, changes in how you see are almost always due to changes in the lighting around you. Learning how to control your environment to a certain degree will help.

When you are outdoors on a sunny day, wear a hat with a brim to reduce the dazzle effect of the bright sunlight. Sunglasses will help with this, too. Indoors, experiment with the room lighting. You'll find reading easier if you have a small reading lamp that you can move around and adjust for your comfort instead of a ceiling fixture that is bright and immovable. Also, you may want to keep the room lights low (but not off) when you watch television.

There's also a nutritional approach. Many studies have been conducted on nutrition and cataracts. It has been shown, for example, that diets low in vitamin B_2 can produce cataracts in animals. In horses, cataracts, which are a common cause of blindness in these animals, can be reduced when large amounts of vitamin B_2 are added to the diet. Galactose, a type of milk sugar, increases the need for vitamin B_2. In human infants who cannot utilize galactose normally, blindness from cataracts has been corrected by removing milk sugar from the diet and adding vitamin B_2. Also, a 1997 study found a significant reduction in cataracts in a group of nurses who took vitamin C supplements. It is apparent that, except in those cases of cataracts that are completely congenital, the major factor in the development of the disorder is nutrition.

If you have a cataract, you may be able to minimize its effects without surgery. Outside, wear a brimmed hat and dark sunglasses to reduce the "dazzle" effect of sunlight. Inside, try using small reading lamps that you can move around and adjust as needed.

Research has continued to link nutrition and cataracts into the twenty-first century. A study published in 2004 investigated the relationship between vitamin E and cataracts induced by ultraviolet B radiation (UVB). The conclusion was that vitamin E protects the lens against UVB-induced cataracts. Vitamin E protects as an antioxidant and/or indirectly through increasing levels of glutathione.

It is also suggested in a number of journals that concentrations of lutein and zeaxanthin in the lens contribute to its protection against UVB radiation. Another study strongly suggested that lutein supplementation diminished acute inflammatory responses after exposure to UVB. Data from a study published in the *Journal of Nutrition* indicated that lutein and zeaxanthin are far more potent than vitamin E for protecting the human lens' epithelial cells against UVB insult. Finally, a study published in the *Journal of Cataract and Refractive Surgery* found that grape seed extract effectively suppressed cataract formation in experimental cataracts.

The information from these studies certainly indicates that cataract formation has its foundation in nutrition. It certainly is worth considering the power of supplementation. Although the eye's lens can now be replaced with an artificial one, the best lens to have in your eye is the one with which you were born!

It is believed that except in cases of congenital cataracts, nutrition plays a major role in the development of this disorder. A healthy diet supplemented with key nutrients such as lutein helps protect the lens of the eye against the damaging effects of ultraviolet B radiation.

NUTRITIONAL SUPPLEMENTS

SUPPLEMENT	DIRECTIONS FOR USE	COMMENTS
Copper and manganese	Take 3 mg of copper and 10 mg of manganese daily.	Retard the growth of cataracts.
Glutathione	Take as directed on the label.	An excellent free-radical scavenger.
Grape seed extract	Take as directed on the label.	A powerful antioxidant.
L-lysine	Take as directed on the label.	Important in collagen formation; repairs the lens.
Selenium	Take 200 mcg daily.	A free-radical scavenger.
Superoxide dismutase (SOD)	Take as directed on the label.	A free-radical scavenger that is shown to be very effective at reducing cataract density.
Vitamin A	Take 2,500 IU daily.	Good for all eye conditions.
Vitamin-B complex and extra B_2 and B_5	Take 50 mg of vitamin-B complex, B_2, and B_5 daily.	Important for eye metabolism.
Vitamin C	Take 500 mg, 4 times daily.	A free-radical scavenger.
Vitamin E	Take 400 IU daily.	A free-radical scavenger.

Lutein and zeaxanthin	Take 15 mg lutein and 4 mg zeaxanthin daily.	Excellent antioxidants for lens health.
Zinc	Take 20 mg daily.	Protects against light-induced damage. Caution: Do not take more than 40 mg daily.

HERBS AND HERBAL SUPPLEMENTS

HERB	DIRECTIONS FOR USE	COMMENTS
Bilberry	Take 160 mg daily.	Boosts the circulation; supplies bioflavonoids, which remove toxic chemicals. Note: Use the extract form.
Eyebright	Use as an eyewash.	Maintains the elasticity of the lens.
Nei zhang ming yan wan (Brion)	Take 8 pills, 3 times daily.	Clarifies the vision. Caution: Contains aluminum, so limit its use.
Shi hu ye guang wan (Brion)	Take 1 pill, 2 times daily.	Valuable during the early stages of cataract formation.
Visioplex Eye Concentrate With Eyebright	Take 3 pills daily, as directed on the label.	Promotes the transfer of nutrients to the lens.

HOMEOPATHIC REMEDIES

REMEDY	DIRECTIONS FOR USE	COMMENTS
Calcarea fluorica 6c	Place 3–4 pellets under the tongue, 3–4 times daily.	Supports the connective tissue; restores the integrity of the elastic fibers.
Calcarea sulfurica 6c	Place 3–4 pellets under the tongue, 3–4 times daily.	Supports the connective tissue.
Causticum 6c	Place 3–4 pellets under the tongue, 3–4 times daily.	Good for the elastic fibers.
Cineraria (Natural Ophthalmics)	1–2 drops, 2 times daily.	Increases circulation, lymph drainage, and normal metabolism.
Magnesia carbonica 6c	Place 3–4 pellets under the tongue, 3–4 times daily.	Regulates the acidity of the body fluids.
Pulsatilla 6c	Place 3–4 pellets under the tongue, 3–4 times daily.	Good during the early stages of cataract formation.
Silicea 6c	Place 3–4 pellets under the tongue, 3–4 times daily.	Good for inflammation.
Sulphur 6c	Place 3–4 pellets under the tongue, 3–4 times daily.	Good for cortical cataracts.

RECOMMENDATIONS

● Avoid dairy products, saturated fats, and any fats or oils that have been subjected to heat, whether during cooking or processing. These foods promote the formation of free radicals, which can damage the lens. Use cold-pressed vegetable oils only.

● Consume nine or more portions per day of plant-based foods with high antioxidant content. These include but are not exclusive to spinach, broccoli, carrots, cantaloupes, and green peppers.

● An additional reason to eat spinach or kale is that it contains lutein—a carotenoid that has been shown to be effective in preventing cataracts.

● Avoid antihistamines; they are photosensitizing—that is, they increase your sensitivity to light—and can increase the likelihood of oxidation in the lens.

● Avoid steroid nasal sprays, as they can contribute to cataract formation.

● Diabetics are especially prone to cataracts. Fortunately, pure diabetic cataracts are reversible. Therefore, if you are a diabetic, careful monitoring of your blood-sugar level is critical.

CENTRAL SEROUS RETINOPATHY

Although the exact cause of central serous retinopathy (CSR) is not known, research suggests that its occurrence is related to high levels of stress. That's why an important part of CSR treatment is stress reduction. To deal with a current episode of CSR and prevent recurrence, consider using meditation, yoga, or another relaxation technique.

Central serous retinopathy (CSR) involves a collection of fluid under the retina that causes visual distortion. As the name suggests, the fluid affects the central (macular) vision—that is, it disturbs the central vision the most. CSR patients often complain of a blind spot, decreased or blurred vision, and distortion of shapes. The vision may be minimally to significantly affected, with the visual acuity ranging from 20/20 to 20/200.

CSR primarily affects adults aged twenty to forty-five. Men are affected ten times more frequently than women are. Many patients with CSR live under high levels of stress, lending to some speculation that lifestyle might be at least somewhat responsible. However, the exact cause of CSR is highly controversial. There appears to be an imbalance in the amount of fluid that enters the space under the retina and the amount that leaves it, resulting in a net accumulation there. Some experimental evidence suggests that high blood levels of epinephrine and selected hormones may be responsible.

Most CSR patients spontaneously recover their visual acuity within about six months. The average recovery time is three to four months. Many patients have some residual symptoms, such as distortion of shapes and disturbed color vision, contrast sensitivity, and night vision. Despite an overall good prognosis, 40 to 50 percent of patients experience one or more recurrences of the disorder.

CONVENTIONAL TREATMENT

No medical therapy has been proven to be effective against CSR. Laser treatment, used to block off some fluid leakage in the area, can shorten the duration of the disease but does not appear to alter the final visual acuity or the recurrence rate. Treatment with laser is controversial because of the potential complications and lack of apparent long-term benefits.

SELF-TREATMENT

The most practical thing that you can do for yourself if you develop CSR is to relax. Since the condition tends to be associated with high stress, reducing your stress level will be helpful. Consider meditation, yoga, or tai chi, all of which are effective against stress. Deep breathing techniques are also beneficial for bringing the mind and body to a calmer state. Externally, there is not much that you can do because the cause of CSR is internal. Eyewashes, eye drops, and other external treatments are all of limited value.

NUTRITIONAL SUPPLEMENTS

SUPPLEMENT	DIRECTIONS FOR USE	COMMENTS
Vitamin A	Take 2,500 IU daily.	Good for all eye conditions; supports the retina.
Vitamin-B complex	Take 75 mg daily.	Good for stress.
Vitamin B_6	Take 50–200 mg daily.	Reduces fluid retention.
Vitamin C	Take 2,000–5,000 mg daily.	Fortifies the blood vessel walls.
Vitamin E	Take 400 IU daily.	Reduces fluid retention.
Zinc and copper	Take 20 mg of zinc and 2 mg of copper daily.	Good in combination with vitamin A. Note: The copper supplementation balances the zinc supplementation.

HERBS AND HERBAL SUPPLEMENTS

HERB	DIRECTIONS FOR USE	COMMENTS
Alfalfa	Drink as a tea.	Good for relaxation and for chemical imbalance.
Chamomile	Drink as a tea.	Good for relaxation.
Gotu kola	Drink as a tea.	Good for relaxation.
Lady's slipper	Drink as a tea.	Good for relaxation.
Lobelia	Drink as a tea.	Good for relaxation. Caution: Do not take internally on an ongoing basis.
Passionflower	Drink as a tea.	Good for relaxation.
Valerian	Drink as a tea.	Good for relaxation.

HOMEOPATHIC REMEDIES

REMEDY	DIRECTIONS FOR USE	COMMENTS
Apis mellifica 6c	Place 3–4 pellets under the tongue, 3–4 times daily.	Alleviates swelling.

FIGURE 2.3
An Amsler Grid.

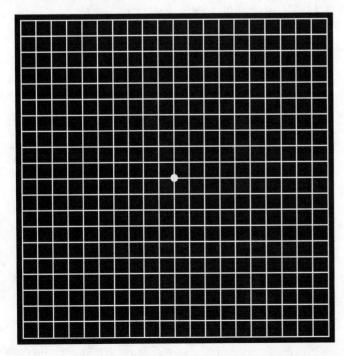

RECOMMENDATIONS

- Use an Amsler Grid to monitor your visual distortion. See left for a sample Amsler Grid. Cover one eye and, with the other eye, look at the dot on the grid. Note any distortions in the surrounding lines or shapes.

- Practice a relaxation technique such as tai chi, yoga, or meditation.

- Practice deep, relaxed breathing.

- Palming is a good technique for relaxing the muscles around the eyes. For a discussion of palming, see the "Vision Therapy" section, page 385.

CENTRAL VISION, DETERIORATION OF

See Macular Degeneration, page 273.

CHALAZION

A chalazion (sha-LAY-zee-ohn) is the next step up from a stye (see page 324) when it comes to seriousness. The word comes from the Greek word for hailstone. "Chalazion" is the singular form, and "chalazia" is the plural form.

Under normal circumstances, the meibomian (my-BOHM-ee-an) glands—glands in the eyelids that number twenty or thirty in each lid—secrete an oily substance that delays the evaporation of the tears and prevents drying of the eyes. But sometimes one or more of these glands gets plugged, and the resulting blockage causes a swelling known as a chalazion. Chalazia are therefore also known as meibomian cysts. The reason for the plugging is usually some kind of infection that makes the oily fluid thicker than it normally would be.

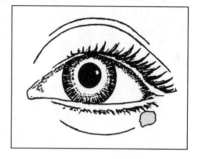

FIGURE 2.4
A Chalazion.

Chalazia are larger than styes and are located at some distance from the lid edge. They're usually not painful, whereas styes are often painful. If you're not sure whether you have a stye or a chalazion, tug the skin of the eyelid near the bump. If the skin moves and the bump doesn't, you have a chalazion. If the bump moves with the skin, you probably have a stye.

CONVENTIONAL TREATMENT

Many doctors will start with a treatment of an antibiotic eye drop to attack any bacteria that may be causing the condition. They should also recommend a hot compress to soften the chalazion and help it drain. While small chalazia might go away on their own, chalazia may occasionally grow large enough to obscure vision, at which point they can be opened and drained by a doctor. This is done under local anesthesia. It is, of course, more desirable to avoid surgery by treating the chalazia early on.

SELF-TREATMENT

As mentioned above, a small chalazion may disappear by itself. That usually occurs within six to eight weeks and can be helped by steam bathing, as you would do for a stye. In other words, a warm compress held to the affected eye, several times daily, with light massage on the lid, will help to resolve the condition. See the herbal treatments below for additional ideas regarding effective compresses.

FIRST AID FOR CHALAZIA

- Apply a warm wet washcloth to the affected eye as soon as possible after first noticing the problem. Use the compress several times a day.

- After using the compress, gently massage the chalazion lump with a clean finger.

- If the swelling does not respond to treatment, visit your eyecare professional.

HERBAL TREATMENT

HERB	DIRECTIONS FOR USE	COMMENTS
Eyebright	Use in a hot compress.	Helps open the pores for drainage.
Goldenseal	Use in a hot compress (external use only).	Good for eye infections.

HOMEOPATHIC TREATMENT

REMEDY	DIRECTIONS FOR USE	COMMENTS
Hepar sulphuris 6c	Place 4 pellets under the tongue, or dissolve them in water and use as an eyewash.	For abscesses, boils, and other skin eruptions or irritations.
Mercurius vivus 6c	Place 4 pellets under the tongue, or dissolve them in water and use as an eyewash.	For swollen glands, boils, and other skin eruptions or irritations.
Staphysagria 6c	Place 4 pellets under the tongue, 3 times daily.	For sticky eyelids.
Sulphur 6c	Place 4 pellets under the tongue, or dissolve them in water and use as an eyewash.	For redness on lids.
Thuja occidentalis	Place 4 pellets under the tongue, 3 times daily.	For sticky eyelids.

RECOMMENDATIONS

- Remember to not rub your eyes with dirty hands, which can lead to infections, including chalazia.

- Consider seeing an eye doctor for treatment of chalazia early in the process so that you can confirm your suspicions and do not require the more drastic treatment protocol of surgery in order to drain the cyst.

COLORBLINDNESS

For approximately 8 percent of men and half of 1 percent of women in this country (the numbers vary somewhat in different countries), something goes wrong with color perception; the color connection mechanism doesn't work properly. Such people are sometimes called "colorblind." Actually, the term "colorblind" is a misnomer, because nearly every person with this affliction has only a deficiency, not a total absence, in his ability to see a full range of colors. It's more accurate to use the term "color deficient."

The retina contains several million cones that are responsible for perception of color. There are three basic types of cones in the retina: one that processes blue (also called "S" cones); one that processes red (also called "L" cones); and one that processes green (also called "M" cones). When a person is color deficient, either a certain type of color cone is missing from the retinas or the cones are deficient in their ability to process color signals. When the red-receiving cones do not function properly or are absent, the person will have a defect in his perception of the color red. The technical term for "red blindness" is protanopia (PROH-tan-oh-pee-ah). When the green-receiving cones are not functioning or are absent, there will be "green blindness," which is called deuteranopia (DOO-ter-an-oh-pee-ah). Deficiencies in perceiving yellows and blues, called tritanopia (TRI-tan-oh-pee-ah), also occur, but they are extremely rare. When there are "partial" deficiencies in these cones, the conditions are called protanomoly, deuteranomoly and tritanomoly, respectively.

Most types of colorblindness occur when there is an excessive overlap of the M (green) and L (red) color cones in the eye, causing distinct hues to become indistinguishable. As a result, the number of shades of color a typical colorblind person can see may be reduced by as much as 90 percent. A company called "EnChroma" has developed lens technology that selectively filters out wavelengths of light at the precise point where this confusion or excessive overlap of color sensitivity occurs. The M and L cones are altered in such a way that there is a greater amount of difference in color discrimination along the so-called "confusion line" for that individual.

Although color deficiency can be acquired during a person's life because of certain diseases or as a side effect of certain drugs, it is more often genetically inherited and present from birth. Men are more likely to be color-deficient than are women because of the way in which color deficiency is inherited.

Color vision can be quickly and simply tested by your eye doctor. If it is determined that you have some form of color deficiency, fear not; color problems do not affect visual acuity. Even the most color-deficient person can have 20/20 vision. If you want to be an electrical worker or a pilot, you probably need excellent color discrimination, but a color deficiency can be coped with in most other occupations. Of course, colorblindness can be inconvenient. One of my patients told me that she always knew when her color-deficient co-worker had a disagreement with his wife; he would come to work in clothes that clashed.

CONVENTIONAL TREATMENT

EnChroma glasses are designed to improve color vision of people with forms of anomalous trichromacy, which are estimated to comprise four out of five cases of color blindness. The most common types are Protanomaly and Deuteranomaly, which are forms of partial red-green color blindness. In the most extreme cases, the complete absence of one of the cone photopigments, called protanopia or deuteranopia, are considered dichromats who may see limited results due to the complete inability to see red and green color differences. Reduced color discrimination of shades of blue and yellow is called tritanomaly, or tritanopia which is not a type of what is commonly referred to as red-green color blindness, but is also a form of color vision deficiency. EnChroma glasses are designed to address only forms of red-green color blindness and are not intended to assist the vision of people with tritan-type deficiency.

Since color deficiency involves no actual eye or vision disease or aberration in the clarity of eyesight, its treatment is very limited. Most often it consists of making a note in the patient's record, making sure that he is aware of the problem, and counseling him to be cautious of taking jobs that require accurate color matching. We will list the contact information on the EnChroma system in Recommended Suppliers on page 411.

RECOMMENDATIONS

• Although there have been no definitive studies on vitamin A and color deficiency, it is always important to be sure that the cones of the retina are well supplied with this important vitamin.

• If you are a parent, be sure to have your child's (especially boy's) color vision checked as early as possible. The best time would be at the eye exam just before entering kindergarten.

COMPUTER VISION SYNDROME

Because computer work is such a highly demanding task on the visual system, vision problems and symptoms are very common. Most studies indicate that computer operators report more eye-related problems than do office workers who perform most of their work on paper. A study by the National Institute of Occupational Safety and Health showed that 88 percent of computer users complained of computer-related eyestrain. The symptoms generally affecting computer users are now collectively known as computer vision syndrome (CVS).

CVS most often occurs when the viewing demand of the task exceeds the visual abilities of the computer user. The American Optometric Association defines CVS as that "complex of eye and vision problems related to near work which are experienced during or related to computer use." The symptoms can vary, but they usually include eyestrain, headaches, blurred vision (distance and/or near), disturbed accommodation, neck pain and/or backache, light sensitivity, double vision, disturbed color vision, and eyes that are dry and irritated. More recently, the AOA has modified its definition and name of the condition because we are now viewing digital images in many forms. They now call the condition digital eyestrain (DES) and define it as: A group of eye- and vision-related problems that result from prolonged computer, tablet, e-reader, and cell phone use.

The causes of CVS/DES are a combination of individual visual problems, poor work habits, and poor office ergonomics. Many people find that computer use exacerbates any marginal vision disorders—ones that do not cause symptoms when performing less visually demanding tasks. Such people must address their work environment as well as their visual condition when treating CVS/DES. If you are a full-time computer user, further study into CVS/DES is likely to be worth your time, so it would be appropriate to consult an ergonomic professional who has extensive knowledge in this area. The information here simply hits the "high points" and gives basic help to the casual computer user who needs to reduce the effects of CVS/DES.

Since the advent of tablet displays and the use of LED lights to create the images, there has been a concerned raised about the amount of blue-wavelength light coming from the screen. It is true that LED lights do emit more light on the high-energy blue light end of the color spectrum and blue light is the highest energy light reaching the retina. However, the amount of light coming from the display in minimal compared to the

REDUCING THE SYMPTOMS OF COMPUTER VISION SYNDROME

● When working at a computer, blink often because this rests and re-wets the eyes.

● Breathe fully, because taking complete breaths is important in relaxing the muscles, including the eye muscles.

● Take breaks from the computer. Use the 20/20/20 rule—every 20 minutes, take 20 seconds and look 20 feet away.

major source of blue light we receive, which is the sun. Someone would have to spend about thirteen hours in front of an LED backlit display screen in order to receive the amount of blue light coming from the sun in fifteen minutes. Some authorities claim that the blue light is responsible for several maladies, including poor sleep quality (especially using a tablet display prior to sleep), eyestrain, and possibly age-related macular degeneration (AMD). Briefly, the only one of these issues of concern that has any validity is poor sleep quality. Blue light is responsible for the "waking" response when light from daylight wakes us up. This response is due to the suppression of melatonin production when blue light enters the eyes. The other issues of eyestrain (mostly due to over-accommodation at a near viewing distance) and AMD (no studies confirm the cause of the disease) have not been validated.

CONVENTIONAL TREATMENT

Most likely, an eye doctor will prescribe a specific type of glasses to help reduce the eyestrain caused by the computer work. What the doctor will recommend is a pair of glasses designed to help you see the computer monitor without having to over-focus your eyes. See "Occupational Progressive Lenses" on page 358 for more information on this type of visual aid.

Unfortunately, many doctors overlook a key factor in managing CVS/DES: making adjustments to the workspace to help improve the conditions that are contributing to your vision problems. If a computer monitor is too high in your visual field, you may have to lift your eyes or head to see it properly, especially if you wear bifocals. Putting the monitor off to one side can cause neck problems. Reading glasses that were designed for seeing things 16 inches away may cause blurriness when a monitor is 25 or more inches away, so you might lean toward the monitor, creating a back problem. Proper ergonomics should be addressed along with proper visual correction.

SELF-TREATMENT

Since there are many different environmental and visual corrections that can be made to achieve the proper balance for computer use, giving overall recommendations is difficult. However, I have often recommended a "3-B" approach to reducing eyestrain from computer use. The three Bs are "blink, breathe, and break."

Blinking is extremely important for maintaining clarity of vision and eye health. It spreads tears over the eye and cleans the surface. These new tears also facilitate oxygen transmission to the cornea, allowing the cornea to stay clear and healthy. Research has shown that we blink less when we read, and even less when we work at computers (up to one-third less). I could recommend that you remember to blink, but that is sort of silly, since your mind has too many other things to remember and blinking is generally automatic. However, just being aware of the importance of blinking will leave you better off. Another idea is to put a small sticky note with the word "blink" on the corner of your monitor as a reminder.

Breathing controls the stress level of many muscles. Imagine a weight lifter attempting to lift a very heavy weight. He inhales deeply and holds his breath while lifting the weight. Once he has achieved the lift, he quickly exhales. This is a simple illustration of how we hold our breath while confronting stressful conditions. Computer use actually can be very stressful. Awkward posture, glaring lights, unreasonable deadlines, low humidity, and other stresses can affect you while you are using a computer. Breathing regularly and deeply can help to alleviate the resulting symptoms.

The eyes are designed to see mostly at distance and occasionally at near point. However, today we do much more near-point work, especially since computers showed up on our desks at work. We must take more breaks to ease the stress on the focusing system. This is why I created the "20-20-20" Rule: Every 20 minutes, take 20 seconds and look 20 feet away. Varying your viewing distance is critical to maintaining comfortable vision. Another way to resolve computer-related eyestrain is to remember a "30-30-30" Rule: Don't work closer than 30 cm for more than 30 minutes at time, and keep the center of your screen 30 degrees below your distance line of sight. And remember, when taking a visual break, don't do needlepoint or read or do any other near-point activity. For eye techniques to use during breaks and for general improvement of the visual abilities, see "Vision Therapy" on page 385.

In dealing with the "blue light" issue mentioned above, the best thing you can do to help yourself is to eat the best diet you can, which should include richly colored vegetables. I previously mentioned the carotenoids lutein and zeaxanthin. These molecules accumulate in the very center of the macula and are yellow in color. They are specifically designed to absorb blue light. It has been shown that patients who experience AMD have lower levels of these carotenoids. Thus, it makes sense to increase these in the diet, which is challenging to do. This is where supplements come in. Most full spectrum supplements should contain adequate amounts of lutein and zeaxanthin. This will make yellow-tinted computer glasses unnecessary.

NUTRITIONAL SUPPLEMENTS

SUPPLEMENT	DIRECTIONS FOR USE	COMMENTS
Vitamin A	Take 2,500 IU daily.	Good for all eye conditions.
Vitamin-B complex	Take 75 mg daily.	Good for stress.
Vitamin C	Take 3,000 mg daily.	An antioxidant that is good for stress.
Vitamin E	Take 300 IU daily.	An antioxidant.
Lutein	Take 10-20 mg daily	Excellent antioxidant and absorbs blue light.
Zeaxanthin	Take 4-6 mg daily	Similar to lutein.
CapsiClear	Take one pill daily	Helps with dry eyes and lowers eye pressure.
Astaxanthin	Take 6 mg daily	Supports eye muscles.

HERBS AND HERBAL SUPPLEMENTS

HERB	DIRECTIONS FOR USE	COMMENTS
Eyebright	Take 3–4 drops daily or apply as a compress.	Good for the eye tissues.
Goldenseal	Apply as a compress.	Soothing for the tissues. Caution: Do not take internally. Do not use during pregnancy.

HOMEOPATHIC REMEDIES

REMEDY	DIRECTIONS FOR USE	COMMENTS
Euphrasia officinalis 6c	Place 3–4 pellets under the tongue, 3–4 times daily.	Alleviates redness.
Nux vomica 6c	Place 3–4 pellets under the tongue, 3–4 times daily.	Good for eyestrain associated with overwork.
Ruta graveolens 6c	Place 3–4 pellets under the tongue, 3–4 times daily.	Good for eyestrain followed by headache; heals the tendons and ligaments.
Sulphur 6c	Place 3–4 pellets under the tongue, 3–4 times daily.	Alleviates redness following near-point work.

RECOMMENDATIONS

• Lower your monitor so that when you hold your head in the normal position, you can look straight ahead and see just over the top of it.

• Make the background illumination of the screen and the illumination of your immediate work area approximately equal. To achieve this, you might need to dim the brightness of your screen somewhat, but don't forget to increase the contrast.

• The best screen colors to use are black letters on a white background. This combination simulates paper and ink and provides the highest contrast between the letters and the background.

• Make sure the screen does not have any glare. To check for this, turn the computer off and look for any reflections of lights or lightly colored articles in the screen.

• Make sure there is no other light hitting your eyes, either directly from a window or lamp, or by reflection off a shiny surface.

Adjust your computer monitor as necessary to avoid or eliminate computer-related eyestrain. Proper positioning of the monitor, increased contrast, and other relatively minor adjustments can make a big difference to your eyes.

CONJUNCTIVA, BLEEDING UNDER

See Subconjunctival Hemorrhage, page 327.

CONJUNCTIVITIS

See Pinkeye, page 303.

CONVERGENCE EXCESS

Convergence is the process in which the two eyes turn in toward one another in order to view an object that is less than 20 feet away. In convergence excess, the eye muscles that control this process are not coordinated, and the eyes turn inward too far. However, convergence excess does not actually occur in the eye muscles but rather in the brain, since that is where the signals to converge originate.

There are a number of possible causes of convergence excess. The most common is an over-stimulation to focus or "accommodate." The two systems of convergence and accommodation are tied together in the brain. Therefore, when we accommodate, we converge; and when we converge, we accommodate. If there is too much stimulus to accommodate, the eyes will be forced to overconverge. This creates a stressful situation and makes it difficult to read comfortably.

CONVENTIONAL TREATMENT

The most popular conventional treatment for convergence excess is prescribed reading glasses. Glasses prescribed for this disorder are intended to reduce the need of the eyes to over-focus. This allows the eyes to realign more easily. Glasses are often very effective at achieving the desired results of straight eyes and comfortable vision. The good news is that these glasses are often needed just for times when the amount of reading (and other close work) is excessive—for example, a law student or other professional school graduate who reads for extended periods of time would want to use the glasses throughout the academic year. The glasses are designed to reduce the stress on the eyes. When the reading load is reduced, the glasses may not be necessary. Note that the recommendation is for *prescribed* reading glasses, not off-the-rack types, which are not targeted to your specific needs.

SELF-TREATMENT

Excessive reading and other close work can cause convergence excess, an overly inward turning of the eyes. Reading glasses and short breaks can reduce the need for your eyes to over-focus.

There are a number of techniques that you can do as part of a vision therapy program to treat your own convergence excess. For sample techniques, see the "Vision Therapy" section, which begins on page 385. In addition, in most cases of convergence excess, relaxation is an important part of the treatment. Among the relaxation techniques I recommend are meditation and tai chi, both of which are extremely effective at reducing stress. More effective results could be achieved by working with an optometrist who oversees an office-based vision therapy program. See Resource Organizations on page 413 to find a vision therapy optometrist.

NUTRITIONAL SUPPLEMENTS

SUPPLEMENT	DIRECTIONS FOR USE	COMMENTS
Vitamin-B complex	Take 75 mg daily.	Good for nerve function.
Vitamin C	Take 3,000 mg daily.	Good for stress.
Astaxanthin	6 mg daily.	Keeps ocular muscles relaxed.

RECOMMENDATIONS

• Make sure your near-point vision is tested during your next eye examination.

- Take breaks when reading or doing extensive close work. Generally, try to close your eyes for a short time every twenty to thirty minutes, in order to relax them.

CONVERGENCE INSUFFICIENCY

As explained previously in the "Convergence Excess" section, the two eyes must turn toward one another while viewing an object within 20 feet. This process is called convergence. If, for some reason, the eye muscles are not able to smoothly or efficiently achieve adequate convergence to view the desired object, the visual system will experience convergence insufficiency.

The main symptom of convergence insufficiency is tiring of the eyes when doing near-point work. This can manifest as a preference to read while trying to go to sleep (in other words, using reading as a method to bring on sleep) or as difficulty remaining focused on the reading material. If you have convergence insufficiency you may get headaches or eyestrain, or often lose your place while reading, among other possible symptoms.

CONVENTIONAL TREATMENT

There are a few different treatments for convergence insufficiency. One is eyeglasses, usually used just for reading. The lenses of these glasses might have some power to reduce the focusing requirement of your eyes, but they may also contain prism. Prism helps to displace the image laterally so that the eyes don't have to converge as much. This might be good for relieving the symptoms of convergence insufficiency, but it does not really cure the disorder. If you are satisfied with the glasses and the glasses relieve your symptoms, however, you may not need to do anything else.

In some cases, the doctor will recommend a program of vision therapy. The aim of therapy for convergence insufficiency is to teach you to better coordinate your eyes so that they can converge more efficiently. This is more than just eye-muscle exercising. It's actually a form of visual biofeedback that can enhance your ability to see more effectively. (For a complete discussion of vision therapy, see page 385.) Also, since some of the nerves that control convergence travel through the spinal column, chiropractic adjustment may have an effect on convergence ability. Therefore, some eyecare professionals might recommend a chiropractic evaluation.

SELF-TREATMENT

As mentioned above, vision therapy might be a very productive approach to reducing convergence insufficiency. There are a number of techniques usually used in vision therapy that you can do by yourself. Moreover, they are among the easiest and most effective techniques to do. Included are the Brock string technique and convergence stimulation. For descriptions of these techniques, see the "Vision Therapy" section, which begins on page 385.

NUTRITIONAL SUPPLEMENTS

SUPPLEMENT	DIRECTIONS FOR USE	COMMENTS
Vitamin-B complex	Take 75 mg daily.	Good for nerve function.
Astaxanthin	6 mg daily	Keeps eye muscles relaxed.

RECOMMENDATIONS

• Make sure your near-point vision is tested during your next eye examination.

• Test your convergence ability with this technique: Hold your fingertip or a pencil straight out in front of your face at arm's length. Slowly move the finger or pencil toward your nose, following it with both of your eyes. Watch it until it splits in two. It should be closer than 4 inches away when you begin to see double.

CORNEA, BARREL-SHAPED

See Astigmatism, page 164.

CORNEA, CONE-SHAPED

See Keratoconus, page 259.

CORNEAL ABRASION

A corneal abrasion is a scrape on the cornea, most often from a foreign body such as a grain of sand, a piece of dirt, or an ill-fitting contact lens. Patients with scraped or scratched corneas often tell the doctor that something is under their upper eyelid. Oftentimes, the foreign body is no longer present, but the patient feels some discomfort when the eyelid passes over the scrape. Usually, it is the first few layers of the cornea that are affected, and since these layers have the most nerve endings, the prominent sensation is pain.

Most corneal abrasions heal within a few days, although injuries from a plant material such as wood or a very dirty substance may take longer. It is extremely important to have a professional evaluation if you get any organic material into your eye. The material could cause a fungal infection, which is much worse than a simple scratched eye.

CONVENTIONAL TREATMENT

Scratches on the cornea usually cannot be seen with the naked eye. Your eye doctor will examine the injury under magnification and may also use a green stain called *fluorescein* (FLOOR-es-seen) to make the abrasion visible. You may be given a prescription for a topical antibiotic, in the form of an ointment or drops, to help prevent an infection.

In the past, doctors routinely patched eyes with corneal abrasions, but many now feel the eye is better off healing without a patch. One reason is that a patch keeps the eye warm, which increases the chance of an infection developing. Also, it's easier to monitor the eye's healing and apply medications if your eye is not covered. On the other hand, a patch makes the healing eye more comfortable.

SELF-TREATMENT

If you suffer a corneal abrasion, your eye will generally tear profusely when the injury first occurs. This tearing might wash out the foreign body that caused the abrasion, but that object might have become trapped in your eye. If the latter is the case and you or someone else can see the foreign body, you can try to remove it with a cotton swab or facial tissue. Make sure that the swab or tissue is clean and wet, and be very gentle!

FIRST AID FOR CORNEAL ABRASION

● Gently pull your upper eyelid away from the eyeball by grasping the lashes, then shake the eyelid from side to side.

● Flush the eye with a sterile saline solution, if available, or cool clean water.

● Avoid blinking excessively.

● If the pain is severe, take a pain reliever.

● Call your eye doctor as soon as possible.

The first thing you should do, though, is to look down and gently grasp the upper eyelashes between your thumb and forefinger. Gently pull the lid away from the eyeball and "shake" it in a side-to-side motion. This will hopefully dislodge the foreign body if it is stuck. Be careful not to shake the lid hard enough to pull out any of the lashes. You can try washing your eye with a sterile saline solution or commercial eyewash. However, do not use commercial eye-whitening drops. Always make sure you use a sterilized eyewash cup or a very clean hand when washing out your eye. This is not the same procedure as the one recommended for a chemical splash into the eye. (See page 144.) Although this condition can be self-limiting, you must use caution to prevent an infection.

Good hygiene is a must when treating your eyes. Wash your hands well and make sure that anything else you use, such as an eyewash cup, is absolutely clean.

NUTRITIONAL SUPPLEMENTS

SUPPLEMENT	DIRECTIONS FOR USE	COMMENTS
Artificial tears	Take 1–2 drops, 3–4 times daily, for 2 days.	Flushes the tear film as the cornea heals.
Vitamin C	Take 500 mg, 3 times daily, for several days.	Builds collagen tissue.

HERBS AND HERBAL SUPPLEMENTS

HERB	DIRECTIONS FOR USE	COMMENTS
Bayberry, eyebright, and goldenseal	Use as an eyewash, 2 times daily.	Good for all eye conditions. Caution: Do not take goldenseal internally. Do not use goldenseal during pregnancy.
Comfrey	Use as an eyewash.	Promotes healing.
White willow bark	Take 400 mg, as needed.	Good for pain.

HOMEOPATHIC REMEDIES

REMEDY	DIRECTIONS FOR USE	COMMENTS
Aconite 6c	Place 3–4 pellets under the tongue, 3–4 times daily.	Good for general eye discomfort.
Aurum 6c	Place 3–4 pellets under the tongue, 3–4 times daily.	Good for pain.
Belladonna 6c	Place 3–4 pellets under the tongue, 3–4 times daily.	Good for pain.

REMEDY	DIRECTIONS FOR USE	COMMENTS
Bryonia 6c	Place 3–4 pellets under the tongue, 3–4 times daily.	Good for pain.
Chamomilla 6c	Place 3–4 pellets under the tongue, 3–4 times daily.	Good for pain.
Cinchona officinalis 6c	Place 3–4 pellets under the tongue, 3–4 times daily.	Good for pain.
Hypericum perforatum 6c	Place 3–4 pellets under the tongue, 3–4 times daily.	Good for nerve injury.
Lycopodium 6c	Place 3–4 pellets under the tongue, 3–4 times daily.	Good for pain.
Mercurius vivus 6c	Place 3–4 pellets under the tongue, 3–4 times daily.	Good for corneal abrasions accompanied by discharge.
Natrum muriaticum 6c	Place 3–4 pellets under the tongue, 3–4 times daily.	Good for pain.
Nitricum acidum 6c	Place 3–4 pellets under the tongue, 3–4 times daily.	Good for pain.
Sanguinaria 6c	Place 3–4 pellets under the tongue, 3–4 times daily.	Good for pain.
Staphysagria 6c	Place 3–4 pellets under the tongue, 3–4 times daily.	Good for corneal abrasions associated with anger.
Spigelia 6c	Place 3–4 pellets under the tongue, 3–4 times daily.	Good for pain.

RECOMMENDATIONS

• To aid the recovery of a corneal abrasion, get plenty of rest, including a good night's sleep.

• Take an over-the-counter pain medication if the homeopathic remedies aren't effective enough or if your eye is still very uncomfortable.

• Use a cool compress to calm the eye and to reduce the inflammation.

• If your eye doesn't feel "normal" again in twenty-four to thirty-six hours, see your eye doctor. Both optometrists and ophthalmologists are qualified to deal with corneal abrasions that don't respond to self-treatment.

CORNEAL ABRASION, NONHEALING

See Recurrent Corneal Erosion, page 313.

CORNEAL CROSS LINKING

See Keratoconus, page 256.

CORNEAL LESION

See Corneal Ulcer, page 202.

CORNEAL NEOVASCULARIZATION

Yes, this is quite a mouthful to pronounce. And corneal neovascularization (NEE-oh-vas-cue-ler-eh-ZAY-shun), also called angiogenesis (meaning "birth" of new blood vessels), is a potentially serious problem of which you should be aware. First, let's learn some details on a healthy cornea, so that this disorder can be clearly defined below. The cornea is normally a clear membrane that contains no blood vessels. It receives its oxygen and nourishment from the tear film, which covers the front surface of the eye, as well as the aqueous humor in the anterior chamber behind the cornea. There are, however, blood vessels in the conjunctiva, the thin tissue covering the eye. These blood vessels travel to the edges of the cornea and then turn back to feed the other parts of the eye. As long as the cornea continues to receive an adequate supply of oxygen from the tears, it does not need any blood vessels to grow through it.

What happens if there is a significant decrease in the oxygen flow to the cornea? The body responds by growing new blood vessels into the cornea. This new growth of blood vessels is called neovascularization, which literally means "new blood-vessel growth." Even a slight amount of blood-vessel growth into the edges of the cornea indicates that the amount of oxygen reaching the cornea has decreased. This most commonly occurs with the over-wearing of contact lenses.

A small amount of growth is not normally considered significant or a threat to eyesight. However, if left unchecked, the growth will continue until blood vessels have grown throughout the cornea. This will cause the clear cornea to become clouded and to block light from passing through, causing blindness. The possibility of blindness should be enough to encourage all contact lens wearers to heed their doctors' instructions on wear and care of lenses and to get regular check-ups. Once vessels have grown in the cornea, they are there for good, although they can become dormant.

CONVENTIONAL TREATMENT

There is really only one conventional treatment recommended for corneal neovascularization: to remove your contacts! Depending on how severe the condition is and for how long you wear your lenses, this discontinuation may be temporary. A doctor will evaluate the extent of the corneal neovascularization and offer specific suggestions. As emphasized above, blood vessels that have grown into the cornea are permanent. If you remedy the situation that is causing the problem and more oxygen is again diffused to the cornea in the proper manner, your body will not need to send blood into those new vessels and the vessels will become dormant. Be warned, however, that if the amount of oxygen reaching the cornea is decreased again, the vessels will fill with blood very quickly, and the process will start over.

SELF-TREATMENT

The best way to avoid corneal neovascularization is to take proper care of your contact lenses. If you use daily-wear soft lenses, be sure to remove them nightly, clean them properly or throw them away if they are daily-disposable lenses, and follow your doctor's recommendations. If you sleep with your contacts on—that is, if you use "extended wear" lenses—be sure to remove them at least weekly and give them a very thorough cleaning. The best way to assure that you always wear clean lenses is to use disposable lenses, which are thrown away regularly, according to your doctor's instructions. Disposable lenses have a reputation for being the healthiest for the eye because there is less chance for debris to build up on them and block oxygen transmission. However, they are also the most prone to patient abuse by wearing them too long. So your eyesight is literally in your own hands!

Whatever type of contact lens you use, make sure to continually check in with your doctor and follow her recommendations. In addition, review the information in "Contact Lenses" on page 338.

Follow your doctor's advice regarding your contact lenses. By wearing your lenses no longer than advised and cleaning or replacing them as directed, you will help avoid potentially serious eye problems.

NUTRITIONAL SUPPLEMENTS

SUPPLEMENT	DIRECTIONS FOR USE	COMMENT
Vitamin A	Take 2,500 IU daily.	Good for all eye conditions.
Vitamin C	Take 2,000 mg daily.	Maintains eye stability.
Vitamin E	Take 300 IU daily.	Fortifies the blood-vessel walls.

HERBS AND HERBAL SUPPLEMENTS

Herb	Directions for Use	Comments
Eyebright	Use as an eyewash.	Good for all eye conditions.

HOMEOPATHIC REMEDIES

Remedy	Directions for Use	Comments
Aconite 6c	Place 3–4 pellets under the tongue, 3–4 times daily.	Alleviates redness.
Apis mellifica 6c	Place 3–4 pellets under the tongue, 3–4 times daily.	Alleviates swelling.

RECOMMENDATIONS

• Don't wait until your contact lenses start to irritate your eyes before getting them evaluated. Instead, schedule regular annual check-ups at your ophthalmologist's or optometrist's office. Subtle changes in the eye are painless and can cause damage before you are aware of it.

• Check with your doctor at the first sign of redness in your eyes.

CORNEAL RING

See Arcus Senilis, page 163.

CORNEAL SCRATCH

See Corneal Abrasion, page 197.

CORNEAL ULCER

An ulcer of any kind is a very serious condition. It usually starts as a break in the surface tissue, which is called an abrasion. If unchecked, this leads to progressive erosion and death of the tissue. The main symptoms of a corneal ulcer are extreme pain, tearing, and redness. If you experience these symptoms and see what looks like a small white dot on the cornea, you probably have an ulcer, or at least a corneal infiltrate. An untreated corneal infiltrate can lead to an ulcer.

The most common cause of corneal ulcers today is over-wear of contact lenses. The constant contact between the lens and the corneal surface combined with poor lens hygiene and/or long wearing time can lead to a break in the surface of the cornea. Once a break occurs, there is an increased likelihood that bacteria, which are normally dormant in the tears, will infect the tissue and create an ulcer.

One condition that may be mistaken for an ulcer is a fungal infection. These disorders appear similar to the untrained eye so the proper treatment may be delayed. This is no time to play doctor yourself, so if there is any question as to whether or not you might have a corneal ulcer, get yourself to an eye doctor quickly!

If you are experiencing eye pain, tearing, and redness, or if you see a small white dot on your cornea, you may have a corneal ulcer. This serious condition requires immediate treatment by an eyecare professional.

CONVENTIONAL TREATMENT

The first course of treatment for a corneal ulcer is an antibiotic, which is designed to kill bacteria. Depending on the severity of the condition and the type of bacteria, the medication may be used as often as every fifteen minutes during the first few hours. In addition, the eye may be patched to reduce excess irritation.

The doctor may want to see you every day to gauge the effectiveness of the treatment. A corneal ulcer could be caused by several different types of organisms, so continual monitoring of the situation is critical. Newer antibiotics are more effective against more organisms. A change of medication may be necessary to cover all possibilities.

SELF-TREATMENT

The best thing you can do if you have a corneal ulcer is to follow your doctor's advice exactly. Ulcers can cause permanent vision loss if they are not dealt with quickly and effectively, so pay attention to all of your doctor's instructions. Keep excessive makeup away from the eye area, and be sure not to touch the eye area with unwashed fingers. Once the main episode has resolved and the healing process has begun, you can use some supplemental support, as described below, to speed up the healing.

NUTRITIONAL SUPPLEMENTS

Supplement	Directions for Use	Comments
Folic acid	Take 5 mg, 3 times daily.	Aids tissue healing.
Vitamin A	Take 5,000 IU daily.	Good for all eye conditions.
Vitamin B$_2$	Take 400 mg daily.	Aids nerve healing.
Vitamin C	Take 3,000 mg daily.	Aids tissue healing.
Vitamin E	Take 400 IU daily.	Aids tissue healing.

HERBS AND HERBAL SUPPLEMENTS

Herb	Directions for Use	Comments
Eyebright	Take 1–2 drops, 4–5 times daily.	Good for overall eye healing. Note: Begin taking *after* you have finished taking your antibiotic drops.

HOMEOPATHIC REMEDIES

Remedy	Directions for Use	Comments
Aconite 6c	Place 3–4 pellets under the tongue, 3–4 times daily.	Alleviates pain and inflammation in the early stages of corneal ulcer formation.
Apis mellifica 6c	Place 3–4 pellets under the tongue, 3–4 times daily.	Good for inflammation.
Calcarea sulfurica 6c	Place 3–4 pellets under the tongue, 3–4 times daily.	Reduces light sensitivity.
Euphrasia officinalis 6c	Place 3–4 pellets under the tongue, 3–4 times daily.	Good for all eye conditions.
Mercurius corrosivus 6c	Place 3–4 pellets under the tongue, 3–4 times daily.	Good for pain.

RECOMMENDATIONS

● If you experience sharp pain and discomfort in or around the eyes, see your eye doctor immediately. A corneal ulcer is one of the possible causes.

● Generally, if you wear contact lenses, do not wear the lenses if there are any signs that a corneal ulcer might be present.

● If you wear contact lenses and are diagnosed with a corneal ulcer, wait until your eye doctor says it is okay for you to return to wearing them.

CROSSED EYES

See Strabismus, page 320.

CSR

See Central Serous Retinopathy, page 182.

CVS

See Computer Vision Syndrome, page 189.

DIABETIC RETINOPATHY

Diabetic retinopathy (ret-tin-OP-a-thee) is a complication of diabetes mellitus. In diabetes mellitus, the body is unable to either produce enough insulin or, in some cases, to use the insulin it produces. That causes sugar (glucose) to stay in the blood instead of entering the cells of the body, where it is needed. Most often, the disorder can be controlled through diet and medication, which normalize the blood-sugar level and the way the cells utilize the sugar. For reasons that are not completely understood, diabetes, even when controlled, also affects the blood vessels, especially in the kidneys and eyes.

There are two types of diabetes mellitus: type I, formerly called juvenile diabetes because it strikes mainly children and young adults; and type II, formerly called adult-onset diabetes because it strikes mainly adults. In type I diabetes, the body's immune system destroys the insulin-producing beta cells in the pancreas. Therefore, type I diabetics must give themselves insulin—either by injection or pump—on a daily basis to keep their blood sugar from rising to dangerous levels, which can cause coma and death. The classic symptoms of type I diabetes are frequent urination, excessive thirst and hunger, and weight loss. The disorder affects about 700,000 Americans.

Type II diabetes mellitus has nothing to do with the immune system. It is caused by a combination of insulin resistance and improper secretion of insulin. In the beginning, it usually can be controlled with diet, exercise,

If you have been diagnosed with diabetes, be sure to have yearly check-ups with an optometrist or ophthalmologist who is experienced with the disorder and its progression. If diabetic retinopathy does occur, laser surgery can provide effective treatment.

and oral medications. Eventually, however, 40 percent of type II diabetics require insulin injections. The symptoms—including blurred vision; frequent or recurring infections of the skin, gums, or bladder; and tingling and numbness in the hands or feet—appear more gradually than do the symptoms of type I diabetes, so many people with type II diabetes only become aware that they have the disorder when they develop one of its life-threatening complications.

Early in the onset of diabetes, before the blood sugar is brought under control, diabetics often experience blurred vision. This is because the high blood sugar causes changes in the lens within the eye. Blurred vision may, in fact, be the first sign of diabetes. After the proper insulin dosage is determined and the disease is stabilized, the blurred vision from the lens change resolves, although it may recur if the blood sugar rises again.

Diabetic retinopathy usually occurs about ten to twelve years into the disorder, but it can occur earlier. It involves dilation of and small hemorrhages in the blood vessels of the retina. These can occur without any symptoms, unless the macula is affected. If the macula is affected, you may see spots or streaks in your vision that correspond to the blood-vessel leaks in the retina. If left unchecked, these hemorrhages and fluid leaks will eventually spill into the vitreous of the eye. Once in the vitreous, they can scar and pull on the retina, often causing retinal detachment and blindness. Diabetes is the second leading cause of adult blindness. It is important to note, however, that not all diabetics develop diabetic retinopathy.

CONVENTIONAL TREATMENT

If you have diabetes, you should be checked yearly by an optometrist or ophthalmologist experienced with the disorder. Your eyecare practitioner should perform a dilated eye exam and be qualified to follow the progression of the disease and be able to counsel you on appropriate care. When it comes time for treatment of diabetic retinopathy, you will need to see an ophthalmologist, who will have to perform surgery. The hemorrhages of diabetic retinopathy can be stopped with a laser through a painless outpatient procedure that takes about half an hour to complete.

Exactly what does the medical laser do? It is directed at the retina, where it "spot welds" the hemorrhages. The laser administers hundreds to thousands of flashes of light to the affected eye. Anesthesia is unnecessary, although your eyes will be dilated and you may feel somewhat "dazzled" afterwards. The areas where the laser strikes will not see clearly anymore, so this procedure will not be performed if those hemorrhages are near the macula.

SELF-TREATMENT

The best treatment for diabetes and, therefore, diabetic retinopathy is to prevent them from beginning in the first place. Watching your diet is the number one controllable factor to prevent type II diabetes. In fact, over 75 percent of all overweight people have their weight problem due to excess insulin in the body. The follow-up concern is low blood sugar, or hypoglycemia. Excess insulin production and over-active insulin receptor sites cause low blood sugar. The Institute of Nutritional Science has specialized in Syndrome X (or now prediabetes)—a catchall term for a group of problems that share a common cardinal cause, namely excess insulin in the bloodstream—and the related problems of obesity, hypoglycemia, and diabetes, and offers a three-phase program for both managing and preventing this devastating cycle of disease.

Natural alternatives to controlling blood-sugar levels have come a long way in recent years. Chromium, vanadium, alpha-lipoic acid, and select herbal extracts in key combinations have shown to lower insulin and blood-sugar levels both safely and effectively. Chromium naturally helps to lower blood sugar by sparing glucose usage. Vanadium has a direct effect on the insulin receptor sites of the body, making them much more effective. The end result is lowered insulin requirements. The key in managing conditions such as hypoglycemia and type II diabetes is lowering insulin levels.

If you are significantly overweight and low-calorie diets have not worked well for you in the past, consider finding out if your weight problem is due to excess insulin production in response to carbohydrate ingestion. There is also a hereditary factor linked to diabetes, so if you have a parent with diabetes, you are automatically at high risk and should be especially careful to eat a healthy diet and get regular medical check-ups. If you are already affected with diabetes, there is evidence that staying in good diabetic control—that is, keeping the blood-sugar level normal through a healthy diet and healthy insulin production—minimizes the long-term, as well as short-term, complications of the disorder. A consultation with a nutritionist is critical.

If you have been diagnosed with diabetes, be sure to have yearly check-ups with an optometrist or ophthalmologist who is experienced with the disorder and its progression. If diabetic retinopathy does occur, laser surgery can provide effective treatment.

NUTRITIONAL SUPPLEMENTS

SUPPLEMENT	DIRECTIONS FOR USE	COMMENTS
Alpha-lipoic acid	Take 200 mg daily.	Increases cellular uptake of glucose.
Chromium picolinate	Take 400–600 mcg daily.	Improves insulin efficiency.
Magnesium	Take 500 mg daily.	Protects against arterial spasm.
Manganese	Take 4 mg daily.	An enzyme activator.
Potassium	Take 300 mg daily.	Maintains proper fluid balance.
Selenium	Take 100 mcg daily.	Suppresses development of new blood vessels.
Vanadium	Take 100 mg daily.	Improves insulin sensitivity.
Vitamin A	Take 2,500 IU daily.	Recommended for diabetics, who often have difficulty converting beta-carotene to vitamin A.
Vitamin B complex	Take a multivitamin that includes a B complex.	Boosts circulation.
Vitamin C	Take 1,000–3,000 mg daily.	Reduces the chance of vascular problems developing. Note: Use powdered buffered ascorbic acid, if possible.
Vitamin D	Take 1,000 IU daily.	Necessary for proper blood clotting.
Vitamin E	Take 400 IU daily.	Aids tissue healing.

HERBS AND HERBAL SUPPLEMENTS

HERB	DIRECTIONS FOR USE	COMMENTS
Comfrey	Drink as a tea.	Strengthens the blood.
Dandelion	Drink as a tea.	Boosts the activity of the pancreas.
Ginseng	Drink as a tea.	Normalizes the blood.
Gymnema sylvestre	Drink as a tea.	Helps the pancreas produce insulin.
Yarrow	Drink as a tea.	Controls bleeding.

HOMEOPATHIC REMEDIES

REMEDY	DIRECTIONS FOR USE	COMMENTS
Lachesis 6c	Place 3–4 pellets under the tongue, 3–4 times daily.	Restores vascular integrity.

Natrum sulfuricum 6c	Place 3–4 pellets under the tongue, 3–4 times daily.	Supports pancreatic function.
Phosphorus 6c	Place 3–4 pellets under the tongue, 3–4 times daily.	Improves metabolism of the vascular tissue.
Syzygium jambolanum 6c	Place 3–4 pellets under the tongue, 3–4 times daily.	Supports sugar metabolism.
Uranium nitricum 6c	Place 3–4 pellets under the tongue, 3–4 times daily.	Acts as a glucose stabilizer.

RECOMMENDATIONS

• Have your blood-sugar level checked regularly, especially if diabetes runs in your family.

• If you notice any fluctuations in your vision, either day-to-day or within the day, request that you be tested for diabetes.

• Since diabetes is a systemic disease, even the control of diabetic eye changes is initially done using general treatments such as diet and exercise.

• Once you are diagnosed with diabetic retinopathy, you should have a dilated eye exam once a year, and more often if recommended by your doctor.

DIGITAL EYESTRAIN

See Computer Vision Syndrome, page 189.

DIPLOPIA

See Double Vision, page 209.

DOUBLE VISION

The eyes act as a team, working together to create one distinct picture from two separate images. This process, which is referred to as fusion, occurs at the back of the brain. If the eyes experience a breakdown of coordination, they will aim at different points in space, and the two images they receive will be dissimilar. Two different images will be transmitted to one single brain cell, and this brain cell will attempt to see them both. The final result will be a condition commonly referred to as double vision.

Double vision, also known as *diplopia* (dih-PLO-pee-ah), is not desirable, so the brain will actually suppress, or tune out, one of the images. This will have the beneficial effect of the brain receiving one image again. However, the visual system will lose some of its function because it will be seeing with just one eye instead of both. (For a complete discussion of suppression, see page 328.)

Looking at the disorder from this perspective, you might think that double vision is the worst of all possible situations. (It can be, if it happens while you're driving!) Yet, there are times when double vision is actually a good thing. Let me explain. If you have a lazy eye or crossed eyes, the brain will usually suppress one of the images your eyes see. In order to correct the problem, you are then likely to be assigned a vision therapy program. Through the therapy, your doctor will attempt to get both of your eyes working at the same time, even though they may still be pointing in different directions. As you start to develop the capacity for the eyes to work together, double vision will occur. In this instance, double vision is a step in the right direction.

Then there are worst case scenarios. If you experience double vision when looking out of just one eye, there could be something seriously wrong. Seeing double images from just one eye is rare and might indicate something as simple as astigmatism (usually a large amount of it). On the other hand, it could be a sign of something more complicated, such as a retinal problem or cataract.

CONVENTIONAL TREATMENT

The treatment for double vision depends on the cause of the condition, and the causes range from convergence insufficiency, convergence excess, and accommodative insufficiency to strabismus, trauma, intracranial tumor, and even cataracts. Assuming there is no pathological reason for the double vision, the cause is likely poor coordination of the eyes. This coordination difficulty actually does not occur in the eye muscles, but in the brain. Therefore, a vision therapy program to improve eye coordination is really more of a "brain training" program than eye-muscle exercises. See page 385 for more on vision therapy.

If vision therapy proves ineffective, your doctor may prescribe glasses with prism. Prism relocates the image of one eye so that the two eyes see the same image at the same location. However, prism most often is used in conjunction with a vision therapy program.

Sometimes, if no other treatment is effective, patching one eye will achieve single vision. Wearing a patch, however, is not an ideal solution because it is superficial and temporary. If you are in a vision therapy program designed to encourage the use of both of your eyes, then patching one of the eyes doesn't really make sense. Patching is normally reserved for cases of lazy eye, when the vision in one eye needs to be enhanced. (See the in-depth discussion of lazy eye on page 264).

In extreme cases of double vision that cannot be corrected by any other means, surgery to reposition the eye muscles is sometimes necessary. However, surgery is useful only in getting the eyes more closely aligned and very often requires a number of procedures, none of which may be totally successful. Remember that the muscles are controlled by the brain, so if the muscles are manually repositioned, the brain may not be able to successfully control them anymore. In some cases, though, success has been achieved with a combination of surgery and follow-up vision therapy that reinforces the effects of the surgery. I recommend surgery as a last resort, to be used only if all other attempts at fusion fail.

Vision therapy can often eliminate double vision by better coordinating the eyes. In extreme cases, though, surgery may be necessary.

SELF-TREATMENT

If your double vision is a symptom of a pathological or traumatic condition, see the appropriate section in Part Two for the self-treatment options for that condition. In addition, see "Vision Therapy" in Part Three (page 385) for a vision therapy program to do at home to augment your doctor's program.

NUTRITIONAL SUPPLEMENTS

SUPPLEMENT	DIRECTIONS FOR USE	COMMENTS
Manganese	Take 4 mg daily.	Stimulates the nerve-muscle connection.
Vitamin-B complex	Take 75 mg daily.	Good for nerve function.

HOMEOPATHIC REMEDIES

REMEDY	DIRECTIONS FOR USE	COMMENTS
Agaricus 6c	Place 3–4 pellets under the tongue, 3–4 times daily.	Good for double vision resulting from overwork.

REMEDY	DIRECTIONS FOR USE	COMMENTS
Arnica montana 6c	Place 3–4 pellets under the tongue, 3–4 times daily.	Good for double vision resulting from injury.
Aurum 6c	Place 3–4 pellets under the tongue, 3–4 times daily.	Good for double vision accompanied by a flushed feeling and congestion.
Gelsemium sempervirens 6c	Place 3–4 pellets under the tongue, 3–4 times daily.	Good for double vision accompanied by general muscle spasm or headache.

RECOMMENDATIONS

● If you ever see double, note whether the two images are side-by-side or above one another.

● After determining whether your vision doubles vertically or horizontally, do the following self-assessment: While keeping both eyes open, cover one eye with your hand and note which image disappears. Report these findings to your doctor.

DROOPING EYELIDS

When your eyes are open, does one eyelid hang lower than the other? Both eyelids should provide about the same amount of coverage over the eyeball. If they cover significantly different amounts of the eyes, you could be suffering from a condition known as *blepharoptosis* (blef-er-oh-TOE-sis), which is more commonly referred to as ptosis. And true to its other name, blepharoptosis is simply the drooping of the upper eyelid to lower than its normal position. When the edge of the upper eyelid falls and covers the top part of the pupil, it blocks the upper part of the vision. In severe cases, the head may have to be tilted backward or the eyelid lifted with a finger in order to see out from under the drooping lid.

In most cases, a drooping upper eyelid results from the aging of previously normal structures. Typically, the tendon that attaches the *levator* (leh-VAY-tor) muscle to the eyelid becomes stretched, causing the eyelid to fall too low. The levator muscle is the major muscle responsible for elevating the upper eyelid. In these cases, since the levator muscle still has its normal strength, surgical correction of the drooping eyelid involves repair of the stretched tendon. It is not uncommon for a person to develop a drooping upper eyelid following cataract surgery. In such cases, the surgical procedure is apparently the last straw that causes a weak tendon to finally give way and cause the eyelid to drop.

Blepharoptosis that is present from birth is called congenital ptosis. This form of ptosis may be mild, with the lid only partially covering the pupil, or severe, with the lid completely covering the pupil. While the cause of congenital ptosis is often unclear, the most common reason for this condition is improper development of the levator muscle. Children who suffer from congenital ptosis may also have lazy eye, strabismus, refractive errors, astigmatism, or blurred vision. In addition, they may have an undesirable facial appearance because of the drooping lid.

A certain aging process often appears similar to ptosis, but is really different. After the age of fifty, the skin of the upper eyelids may begin to sag significantly, creating a condition in which the lids appear to droop. This condition is known as *blepharochalasis* (blef-ah-roh-kal-AY-sis). In rare occurrences, a lid that has blepharochalasis coupled with a significant amount of body fat will droop because of the excessive weight of the fat.

Another condition that may cause one to think the eyelids are drooping—when actually the opposite is occurring—is Graves' disease. This disorder causes the eyeball to protrude from the eye socket, which often happens in one eye sooner than the other eye. Therefore, it appears that one eye is more prominent than the other. If you haven't been paying much attention to your appearance, you may think that the unaffected eye has a drooping eyelid. See page 240 for a discussion of Graves' disease.

Ptosis—most commonly known as drooping eyelids—is usually a result of the normal aging process. But since there can be other causes, some of which are serious, it's a good idea to consult your eye doctor and determine the source of the problem.

CONVENTIONAL TREATMENT

If an eyelid droops minimally due to the aging process, medical treatment is not called for. But blepharoptosis is another story. For acquired ptosis, the doctor must first determine the cause of the problem. If the cause is muscle or nerve disease, the doctor will treat the disease first. If the cause is a tumor, the doctor may remove the tumor. If the cause is something else, the doctor will often suggest surgery to correct the ptosis. The surgical procedure might involve work on the tendon associated with the levator muscle, as detailed in the segment above, or it might involve shortening the levator muscle or connecting it to the brow muscles. Surgery to correct ptosis is most commonly performed by ophthalmic plastic and reconstructive surgeons who specialize in diseases and conditions affecting the eyelids, lacrimal (tear) system, orbit (bone cavity around the eye), and adjacent facial structures.

A new medication has been developed to address this disorder. UPNEEQ (oxymetazoline hydrochloride ophthalmic solution) 0.1% is a prescription eye drop used to treat acquired blepharoptosis. The most common adverse reactions with UPNEEQ (occurring in 1 to 5 percent of patients) were eye inflammation, eye redness, dry eye, blurred vision, eye pain at time of use, eye irritation, and headache. Consult your physician to determine if this product is right for you.

Congenital ptosis is also treated surgically, with the specific operation based on the severity of the ptosis and the strength of the levator muscle. If the ptosis is not severe, the surgery is generally performed when the child is between three and five years of age—during the preschool years. However, if the ptosis interferes with the child's vision, surgery is performed at an earlier age to allow the vision to develop properly.

SELF-TREATMENT

Self-treatment of ptosis is appropriate when the condition is caused by muscle weakness, which can be helped by exercises. In most cases of drooping eyelids, though, the problem must be treated by an eyecare professional.

The self-treatment of ptosis depends on the cause of the condition. If the problem is a torn or stretched tendon, no type of self-treatment can help. However, if the problem is a muscle weakness, and the nerve connection to the muscle is complete, the ptosis can sometimes be overcome using exercises. Your eye doctor can best determine the cause of this condition.

NUTRITIONAL SUPPLEMENTS

SUPPLEMENT	DIRECTIONS FOR USE	COMMENTS
Manganese	Take 4 mg daily.	Stimulates the nerve-muscle connection.
Vitamin-B complex	Take 75 mg daily.	Good for nerve function.

HOMEOPATHIC REMEDIES

REMEDY	DIRECTIONS FOR USE	COMMENTS
Causticum 6c	Place 3–4 pellets under the tongue, 3–4 times daily.	Aids muscle "heaviness" and facial paralysis.
Gelsemium sempervirens 6c	Place 3–4 pellets under the tongue, 3–4 times daily.	Good for drooping eyelids associated with fever or nerve conditions; also good for muscle weakness and anxiety.
Rhus toxicodendron 6c	Place 3–4 pellets under the tongue, 3–4 times daily.	Good for rheumatic and muscle pain.
Sepia 6c	Place 3–4 pellets under the tongue, 3–4 times daily.	Good for drooping eyelids associated with headache.

RECOMMENDATIONS

• Because there are a number of possible reasons why an eyelid would droop, it is important to discuss a drooping eyelid with your eye doctor. Whether the drooping is part of a normal aging process or the symptom of something more serious should not be determined without professional consultation.

• Low-lying lids may be related to conditions such as stroke or brain aneurysm, Horner syndrome, myasthenia gravis, loss of the ability to move eye muscles, eye infection, and eye tumors. Ask your doctor if you have any of these conditions.

• If it is decided that the drooping eyelid can be helped with eye exercises instead of surgery, your eye doctor can refer you to a vision therapist or she might be able to counsel you on ocular muscle exercises herself, depending on her areas of specialty and her background.

DRY EYE DISEASE

Dry eye disease is due to a problem with either the quantity or the quality of the tear film of the eye. It leads to the symptoms of dryness, redness, burning, grittiness, or excessive tearing of the eyes. The eyes may also be very light sensitive. At one time, dry eye disease was not considered a disease but a group of symptoms that develop as a result of another condition. For example, it would be attributed to an allergy or arthritis, the use of a particular medication, or environmental factors such as low humidity or computer use. We now know that it is a specific disease process—an inflammation—and can be exacerbated by these other conditions.

To understand dry eye disease, we must first understand the function and components of the tear film. There are three layers of the tear film on the cornea. The outermost is the oily layer. It is produced by the meibomian glands, which are located primarily in the eyelids. The oily layer reduces tear evaporation. The second layer is the watery layer, the middle layer that is the major part of the tear film. The watery layer is produced by the lacrimal (LAK-rih-mal) glands in the conjunctiva. The innermost layer, which is called the mucin (MEW-sin) layer, is a mucous layer and is produced by the cells in the cornea. Any or all of these layers can be affected in the case of dry eye disease.

Probably the most common of all eye problems, dry eyes affect 33 million American adults.

Dry eye disease is probably the most common of all the eye problems. A recent Harris Poll indicated that dry eyes affect 33 million American adults. At the same time, 89 percent of Americans are unfamiliar with the condition. And many of those who have been told they suffer from dry eye disease do not understand how their eyes can run with tears yet their problem was diagnosed as dry eye. Dry eyes may be excessively wet because the tear glands pump extra amounts of watery tears onto the eyes to compensate for the dry condition. (Note that eyes that are constantly watery may also have a blocked tear duct.)

Adults who have arthritis or another autoimmune disorder are more likely to have dry eye disease. Dry eyes accompanied by dry mouth (difficulty swallowing), joint stiffness in the morning, vaginal dryness, gastric reflux, and muscle weakness can be signs of Sjögren's (SHOW-grins) syndrome, an autoimmune condition that occurs most commonly among women over the age of forty. In Sjögren's syndrome, the body's immune system mistakes the moisture-producing glands for foreign invaders. The immune system then attacks and destroys these glands, causing the hallmark symptoms of dry eyes and dry mouth. Sjögren's syndrome can also damage vital organs of the body with symptoms that may plateau, worsen, or go into remission. Some people experience only the mild symptoms of dry eyes and mouth, while others go through cycles of good health followed by severe illness.

There are other possible causes of dry eye disease. The eyes produce about 40 percent less moisture with advancing age. So, a normal aging process could be the source behind this disorder. Moreover, certain medications may also interfere with tear production. For a list, see the "Self-Treatment" section on page 219. In addition, drooping lower eyelids and/or excessive computer use (accompanied by less blinking) may expose the surface of the eyes to the air, increasing evaporation and symptoms. It is best to discuss your symptoms and lifestyle with your eyecare professional, who can then help you identify the cause and alleviate the symptoms.

CONVENTIONAL TREATMENT

The first treatment that doctors tend to recommend for dry eyes is the application of artificial tears. There are many types of eye-drop preparations. It is best to avoid those with preservatives, which can eventually make a dry eye condition worse. Most preservative-free eye drops come in individual-dose vials, which can be conveniently carried in the pocket or purse. It is very important that you do not allow the unpreserved drops to stay exposed to air for too long. Be sure to discard them if the drops have been exposed to air for more than one day. Since there are no preservatives, the solution is prone to contamination and, once contaminated, can cause a serious eye infection. Another option to consider is the thickness of the eye drops. Some of the more viscous (thicker) eye drops remain on the eye longer, but your vision is likely to be foggy for the first few minutes after application. So you will have decisions to make regarding what type of eye-drop preparations to purchase.

What if your dry eye disease is due to Sjögren's syndrome? Unfortunately, there is no known cure for Sjögren's syndrome, but there are ways to treat the symptoms. Nonsteroidal anti-inflammatory drugs (NSAIDs), steroids, and disease-modifying medications are often used, and moisture-replacement therapies can ease the symptoms of dryness. Studies indicate that the male hormone androgen may restore lacrimal gland function and relieve chronic dry eye symptoms. However, androgen can have side effects, such as virilism—the growth of facial hair and the manifestation of other male characteristics—when used by women. Further studies are being conducted to identify an androgen compound that does not have these side effects.

Another recent advance in the medical treatment of dry eye disease is a prescription medication called Restasis. This is an immunosuppressant and can knock down the inflammatory response that can lead to dry eyes. However, the treatment most often takes three months to become effective and is very costly. A newer product, called Xiidra (ZIE-drah) is also available by prescription. This one has a metallic taste as a side effect. Eyesuvis is another prescription medication that is a corticosteroid. Most of these medications cost in the hundreds of dollars without insurance. A more recent addition to this list is Cequa (SEE-kwah), which is a different formulation of Restasis. Always discuss these medications with your eyecare practitioner.

One of the most common methods for treating dry eye is to plug the hole in the "tear sink." There are tear-drainage canals on the edges of the upper and lower eyelids, near the nose area. Inside these drainage openings are tiny pumps that suck away the fluid from the surface of the eyes. The lacrimal gland behind the eyelid produces the tears; the eyelid spreads the tears across the eye's surface, much like a windshield wiper; and the drain at the bottom permits the fluid to drain away. If the drain is plugged, more fluid stays on the surface of the eye. When other methods of treating dry eye disease prove unsatisfactory, closure of the tear drains may be indicated.

However, recent studies have shown that there might be an inflammatory factor that causes the dryness. If this is the case, then just keeping more poor-quality tears on the surface of the eye will likely create a worsening situation.

There are also some newer in-office procedures for treating dry eyes. Lipiflow is a technique where the doctor places heating "pads" under each lid and these pads gently massage and heat the eyelids. This is designed to soften the fluids inside the glands and get them flowing better. The process is somewhat uncomfortable but not painful, and the results typically last about six to eight months, depending on the underlying condition.

Another procedure is called intense pulsed light therapy (IPL) is used for a number of purposes, including removal of skin lesions, and treatment for rosacea and other skin conditions. This procedure is FDA-approved for skin conditions and has had some success in eye care. Eye doctors have also used IPL to treat meibomian gland blockages as well as to reduce ocular inflammation and bacterial colonies that result in dry eyes. During an IPL session, your eye doctor will apply infrared light directly to the eyelids with a handheld device. This light wavelength can reduce inflammation and loosen meibomian gland blockages.

A similar treatment is called low level light therapy (LLLT). This treatment utilizes a thin beam of electromagnetic waves of a single frequency and red light to promote tissue healing and pain relief. It has been used to enhance the integrity of the meibomian glands inside the eyelid.

An at-home treatment for cleaning the edges of your eyelids is called NuLids. It uses an eyelid-cleaning brush that works by gently stimulating and rejuvenating the meibomian glands and is an effective alternative treatment for dry eye disease. The self-regulating design halts the movement of the NuLids soft tip if too much pressure is applied to the eye. Treatment takes just one minute.

Yet another new procedure is electric-pulse tear production. This treatment is mainly used for patients that suffer with a specific type of meibomian gland dysfunction known as "aqueous deficient." Unlike many other treatments, this treatment is done through the nose rather than the eyes. Your eye doctor will insert a tiny probe into each nostril, which will deliver small electrical currents to the nerves lining the inside of your nose. The electrical pulses will stimulate the nerves, telling the brain that it needs to increase tear production. Because it involves electrical currents, this treatment is not meant for patients who have pacemakers or defibrillators.

SELF-TREATMENT

You can relieve some of the symptoms of dry eye disease by making changes to your lifestyle. First, if you smoke, it is important to quit. Cigarette smoke causes dry spots to develop on the surface of the eye 40 percent more quickly than when the lids are held open. Also, check your medications. Some medications can cause dry eyes as a side effect. These medications include antihistamines such as Benadryl and Coricidin; atropine; beta blockers such as Timoptic, Betoptic, Betagan, and Ocupress; cancer medications such as methotrexate; chlorothiazide; codeine; decongestant eye drops such as Visine, Murine, Prefrin, and Clear Eyes; decongestants such as Sudafed; diazepam; morphine; Patanol, prescribed for allergic conjunctivitis; scopolamine; tranquilizers such as Elavil and Valium; and vitamin-A analogs such as isotretinoin. The artificial sweetener aspartame, supplemental vitamin B_3, and cannabis can also cause dry eyes.

Next, check your dietary habits. The body requires the consumption of the essential oils—which are fats—for lubrication of the joints and the eyes, as well as for restoration of normal lubrication to the body. There are good fats and bad fats. The undesirable fats, called saturated fats, are found in meats, fried foods, butter, dairy products, and margarine. The good fats, especially the omega-3 oils, are polyunsaturated and are found in cold-water fish, flaxseeds, and walnuts. There has been a large amount of debate on the nutritional aspects of treating dry eyes, but we now know that the omega-3 and omega-6 essential fatty acids, in the right combination, can effectively treat this condition. For more on these fatty acids, see page 66 of the "Nutrition and Vision" section of Part One.

There are additional steps you can take to assuage your dry eyes. Quite simply, blink your eyes. When you blink, you squeeze out tears from the glands in your eyelids. Waiting twenty to thirty seconds between blinks may cause the tear film to break, which can lead to dehydration of the surface of the eye. We normally blink about twenty times a minute, depending on the viewing situation.

Moreover, reduce, replace, or avoid eye makeup. Eye makeup has been shown to thin out the oily layer of the tear film—the outer layer that keeps the eyes from becoming dehydrated. Also, in its container, eye makeup can harbor bacteria. So it should be replaced frequently. Gentle removal of all eye makeup every night is essential.

If you wear glasses, check the nose pads on your eyeglasses. If your lower eyelids are pushed down by the nose pads of your glasses, you may

RELIEVING DRY EYE DISEASE

- Quit smoking.

- Check your medications, as dry eyes are a side effect of some drugs.

- Check your diet to make sure you are getting enough essential fatty acids.

- Avoid eye makeup.

- Make sure that the nose pads on your glasses do not push your lower eyelids down.

- Use humidifiers in your home.

- Position your computer so you look down on the monitor.

- Wear sunglasses with side shields.

- Avoid smog and fumes.

- Blink your eyes as often as possible.

experience increased evaporation of tears. In such a situation, have an optician adjust the pads. And if you wear soft contact lenses, consider their role in your dry eyes. Soft contact lenses often promote the evaporation of tears from the surface of the eye. In severe dry eye cases, contact lenses cannot be worn.

What can you do to make your home environment kinder to your dry eyes? Use humidifiers. This is especially important if you live in a dry, desert area. Also, reposition your computer monitor. Position it so that your eyes aim downward when you look at the monitor. This will allow you to keep your eyes partially closed, reducing the surface area of the eye exposed to the air. (For a complete discussion of computer vision syndrome, see page 189.)

A few helpful pointers can be applied to outdoor lifestyle. Wear wrap-around sun goggles outdoors. Sunglasses (and even clear goggles) with side shields can help to reduce the evaporation of moisture from the eye by as much as 40 percent. And avoid smog and fumes. They not only cause dry and irritated eyes, but they also inactivate the enzyme that acts as an antibacterial agent in the tear fluid.

NUTRITIONAL SUPPLEMENTS

SUPPLEMENT	DIRECTIONS FOR USE	COMMENTS
Black currant seed oil	Take 3,000 mg daily at bedtime.	Supplies essential fatty acids, which promote circulation.
Coenzyme Q_{10}	Take 80 mg daily.	A powerful antioxidant.
Fish oil	Take 3 tbsp daily.	High in vitamin A; re-moisturizes the eye tissues.
Vitamin A	Take 2,500 IU daily in tablet form, or apply drops directly to the eye.	Maintains the moisture in the eye tissues.
Vitamin B_6	Take 50 mg daily.	Regulates kidney function.
Vitamin C	Take 7,500 mg daily.	An antioxidant.
CapsiClear	One tablet daily	Reduces inflammation in the tears.

HERBS AND HERBAL SUPPLEMENTS

HERB	DIRECTIONS FOR USE	COMMENTS
Chamomile	Use warm as an infusion or cool as an eyewash.	Supports the eye tissues.

REMEDY	DIRECTIONS FOR USE	COMMENTS
Goldenseal	Use warm as an infusion or cool as an eyewash.	Supports the eye tissues. Caution: Do not take internally for more than 1 week. Do not use during pregnancy.
Ming mu di huang wan (Brion)	Take 10 pills, 3 times daily, or drink as a tea.	Builds "yin" in the kidneys, and "cools" the liver.
Qi ju di huang wan (Brion)	Take 8 pills, 3 times daily, or drink as a tea.	Builds "yin" in the kidneys, and "cools" the liver.
Shi hu ye guang wan (Brion)	Take 1 pill, 2 times daily.	Good for all eye conditions.

HOMEOPATHIC REMEDIES

REMEDY	DIRECTIONS FOR USE	COMMENTS
Aconite 6c	Place 3–4 pellets under the tongue, 3–4 times daily.	Alleviates dryness.
Alumina 6c	Place 3–4 pellets under the tongue, 3–4 times daily.	Alleviates dryness.
Arsenicum album 6c	Place 3–4 pellets under the tongue, 3–4 times daily.	Alleviates dryness.
Belladonna 6c	Place 3–4 pellets under the tongue, 3–4 times daily.	Good for dry eyes associated with fever and redness.
Dry Eye Formula (Natural Ophthalmics)	Take 1–2 drops daily as needed for relief.	Found in two different formulas— one for men and one for women.
Euphrasia officinalis 6c	Place 3–4 pellets under the tongue, 3–4 times daily.	Good for dry eyes associated with wind and gas in the environment.
Optique 1 6c (Boiron)	Take 1–2 drops daily as needed for relief.	A good general remedy.
Pulsatilla 6c	Place 3–4 pellets under the tongue, 3–4 times daily.	Alleviates dryness.
Similisan No. 1 6c	Take 1–2 drops daily as needed for relief.	Good for red, dry eyes.
Sulphur 6c	Place 3–4 pellets under the tongue, 3–4 times daily.	Alleviates dryness and reduces redness.
Veratrum album 6c	Place 3–4 pellets under the tongue, 3–4 times daily.	Alleviates dryness.
Zincum metallicum 6c	Place 3–4 pellets under the tongue, 3–4 times daily.	Alleviates dryness.

RECOMMENDATIONS

- If you have dry eyes, contact your eye doctor before changing your diet. In addition to your specific eye condition, your medical history, prescription medications, and allergies all need to be taken into account.

- Avoid consuming margarine, fried foods, and saturated fats in general.

- Use preservative-free eye drops.

- Check your medications for any that may cause dry eyes as a side effect.

- Wear wrap-around, blue-light blocking sun goggles when you go outdoors.

EYE PRESSURE, ELEVATED

See Glaucoma, page 233.

EYELID GLAND, PLUGGED

See Chalazion, page 185.

EYELID INFLAMMATION

See Blepharitis, page 167.

EYELID SPASM

See Blepharospasm, page 170.

EYESTRAIN

Eyestrain can be a symptom of a deeper problem. If your eyes feel fatigued or uncomfortable, consult your eye doctor.

Eyestrain is a term that doesn't really exist in the minds of many eye doctors. The term that professionals use for this type of discomfort is *asthenopia* (as-then-OH-pee-ah). Asthenopia is defined in visual science dictionaries as eye discomfort or fatigue attributed to an uncorrected refractive error, an eye-muscle disorder, the prolonged use of the eyes, or something similar.

The above definition for asthenopia is rather broad and vague, but in general, eyestrain can be thought of as just about any discomfort involving the eyes. The complaint of eyestrain really means little because we doctors must delve more deeply into the specific complaints to determine the cause of the problem. Most people have their own personal definition of eyestrain, and therefore the use of this term is not very helpful when it comes to diagnosing and treating a problem. In any case, ocular discomfort is something that should be checked out by an eyecare professional. So it is important to discuss it with your eye doctor if you feel that your eyes are strained or fatigued.

CONVENTIONAL TREATMENT

Since eyestrain can result from a variety of causes, the treatment varies with the source of the problem. The conventional treatments for eyestrain that are used most often, however, are eyeglasses and vision therapy.

The glasses used to relieve eyestrain have what are called plus lenses. For a discussion of plus lenses, see "Minus Lenses and Plus Lenses" on page 355. If the eyes and/or visual system are not able to perform their functions correctly and efficiently, plus lenses can take over some of the workload and allow the eyes to function with less strain or effort. If your eyes do not react correctly to these lenses, a program of vision therapy can help you learn how to better coordinate your eyes and see more effectively. (For a discussion of vision therapy, see page 385.)

SELF-TREATMENT

There are many things that you can do for yourself to reduce eyestrain. Most often, eyestrain is the result of excessive use of the eyes for near-point tasks. Therefore, simply taking adequate breaks from your near-point chores will allow your eyes to relax, thus relieving much of the tension. (Remember the "20-20-20" Rule: Every 20 minutes, take 20 seconds and look 20 feet away). If you use a computer, taking these breaks is especially important.

Another way to resolve computer-related eyestrain is to remember a "30-30-30" Rule: Don't work closer than 30 cm for more than 30 minutes at time, and keep the center of your screen 30 degrees below your distance line of sight. For a complete discussion of computer vision syndrome, see page 189.

Since eyestrain is often the result of excessive near-point tasks, give yourself frequent breaks when working on a computer, reading a book, doing needlework, or performing other near-point activities. Look away from your work, or simply close your eyes to give them some much-needed rest.

Eye fatigue can also be considered a form of eyestrain. If you find your-self tiring after short periods of reading or doing any type of close work, you may have a condition called "convergence insufficiency" (see page 195). A course of vision therapy—either with an in-office or home-based program—might be very helpful. If you learn eye exercises that you can do at home, you can virtually treat yourself for this problem.

Also, ask yourself whether your eyes feel *irritated*, not just strained. If your eyes become irritated with continued use, try an eyewash or lubri-cating drops to refresh them. Remember *do not* use an eye drop that is for whitening the eyes—such drops have chemicals in them that actually tend to make redness worse.

It is very important to note that eyestrain can also be a result of insuf-ficient nutrition. Calcium deficiency, magnesium imbalance, and sodium excess can cause muscle and nerve problems, which may manifest as eye mis-coordination and eyestrain. See the recommendations below for some nutritional support for eye muscles.

NUTRITIONAL SUPPLEMENTS

SUPPLEMENT	DIRECTIONS FOR USE	COMMENTS
Vitamin A	Take 2,500 IU daily.	Good for all eye conditions.
Vitamin-B complex	Take 50–100 mg daily.	Improves intraocular cellular metabolism.
Vitamin B$_2$	Take 25 mg, 3 times daily.	Alleviates eye fatigue.
Vitamin C	Take 500 mg, 3 times daily.	An antioxidant.
Vitamin E	Take 400 IU daily.	An antioxidant.
Astaxanthin	Take 6 mg daily	Supports eye muscles.
CapsiClear	Take one pill daily	Helps dry eyes.

HERBS AND HERBAL SUPPLEMENTS

HERB	DIRECTIONS FOR USE	COMMENTS
Bayberry	Take in supplement form as directed on the label, or drink as a tea.	Boosts the circulation around the eyes.
Cayenne	Take in supplement form as directed on the label, or drink as a tea.	Boosts the circulation around the eyes.

SUPPLEMENT	DIRECTIONS FOR USE	COMMENTS
Eyebright	Take in supplement form as directed on the label, drink as a tea, or use as an eyewash.	Rejuvenates the eye tissues.
Goldenseal	Take 200 mg daily . for 1 week	Rejuvenates the eye tissues. Caution: Do not take internally for more than 1 week. Do not use during pregnancy.
Raspberry	Take in supplement form as directed on the label, or drink as a tea.	Boosts the circulation around the eyes.

HOMEOPATHIC REMEDIES

REMEDY	DIRECTIONS FOR USE	COMMENTS
Nux vomica 6c	Place 3–4 pellets under the tongue, 3–4 times daily.	Good for eyestrain associated with overwork.
Ruta graveolens 6c	Place 3–4 pellets under the tongue, 3–4 times daily.	Good for eyestrain followed by headache; promotes healing of the tendons and ligaments.
Sulphur 6c	Place 3–4 pellets under the tongue, 3–4 times daily.	Alleviates redness following near-point work.

RECOMMENDATIONS

● Include broccoli, raw cabbage, carrots, cauliflower, green vegetables, squash, sunflower seeds, and watercress in your diet. These foods promote eye health.

● Taking $1/4$ tsp or 1,000 mg of cod-liver oil per day may also be helpful.

● Eliminate sugar and white flour from your diet.

● Get plenty of sleep. Fatigue can contribute to eyestrain.

FARSIGHTEDNESS

Farsightedness, also called *hyperopia* (high-per-OH-pee-ah), is one of the refractive errors of the eye. Farsightedness, nearsightedness, and astigmatism are all known as refractive errors because they cause distortions in the way light is refracted—that is, deflected from a straight path—as it passes through the eye. If you are farsighted, the image of an object 20 or more feet away is focused behind your retina (if the lens is relaxed) and looks blurred. Farsightedness happens when the eye is too short or the cornea too flat, or from some combination of these and other factors. Because the light coming through the eye is not "bent" or refracted enough, the eye has to compensate for this lack of power. This will cause the eye to increase the effort needed to see far away, and that in turn translates to more effort when viewing close objects as well.

Farsightedness is not exactly the opposite of nearsightedness. The main difference between them is that in farsightedness, the eye can accommodate, or refocus, to adjust for the misplacement of the light, while in nearsightedness, any accommodation of the eye makes the image more blurred. Because of this difference, the farsighted eye may be able to see clearly at a distance, but must work harder to do so. This makes it more difficult to test the farsighted eye because there may not be any blurring of the image. In addition, a farsighted eye may fatigue easier, a symptom that a quick eye chart screening may not be able to detect.

If you are farsighted, a combination of prescription eyeglasses and vision therapy can help you with near-point chores while improving your visual abilities. It is also important to change your focusing distance on a regular basis.

CONVENTIONAL TREATMENT

The conventional treatment for farsightedness is simply eyeglasses, usually mostly worn for reading and near-viewing tasks. Most often, these glasses have lenses that approximate the shape of the lens within the eye, thus relieving the internal lens from overworking. This may sound like the glasses act as a "crutch" that will make the eye lazy and not work enough. However, there are different degrees of farsightedness and different reasons to wear glasses, so one general statement cannot apply to all conditions. In other words, sometimes that "crutch" is necessary for a person to function effectively, albeit for a short period of time.

Oftentimes, people (mostly children) have difficulty reading due to farsightedness or a similar condition affecting focusing ability. If you have this problem, you may be advised to utilize a combination of reading glasses and vision therapy to improve your visual abilities to perform more efficiently. For a complete discussion of vision therapy, see page 385.

SELF-TREATMENT

If the cause of your farsightedness is a physically short eyeball, there is likely nothing that can be done to *change* your vision, meaning to truly correct it.

However, keeping your focusing mechanism in good functional condition will help you. One way to do that is to alter your focusing distance on a regular basis. Avoid focusing at a close distance for an extended period of time, and make sure you blink frequently.

NUTRITIONAL SUPPLEMENTS

SUPPLEMENT	DIRECTIONS FOR USE	COMMENTS
Vitamin A	Take 2,500 IU daily.	Good for all eye conditions.
Vitamin C	Take 2,000 mg daily, evenly spread out over the course of the day.	Maintains the flexibility of the lens.

HERBS AND HERBAL SUPPLEMENTS

HERB	DIRECTIONS FOR USE	COMMENTS
Eyebright	Take as directed on the label.	Good for all eye conditions.

HOMEOPATHIC REMEDIES

REMEDY	DIRECTIONS FOR USE	COMMENTS
Argentum nitricum 6c	Place 3–4 pellets under the tongue, 3–4 times daily.	Good when doing intense near-point work.

RECOMMENDATIONS

• If you notice that it takes a second or two to refocus when you look from far to near, then you may be farsighted. Contact your eye doctor, and schedule a complete examination.

• Farsightedness is different from presbyopia, which is *not* considered a type of farsightedness. The latter condition manifests after the age of forty. However, if you are farsighted and over forty, you may notice presbyopia developing earlier than it does in people with normal vision. Essentially, if you're farsighted and have to focus a lot, then presbyopia will creep in earlier due to the excessive focusing requirement that over-taxes the focusing muscles.

• School vision screenings rarely check for farsightedness, so make a complete eye examination for your school-aged child an annual event.

FARSIGHTEDNESS, AGE-RELATED

See Presbyopia, page 308.

FLOATERS

Patients often talk about seeing small dark spots in front of their eyes that seem to move as their eyes do. These spots may look like dots, squiggles, strands, or any of hundreds of other different shapes, and they are very common. They exist because, before birth the eye develops with the help of blood vessels growing through the center of it. During the last three months of fetal life, these blood vessels dissolve, but sometimes they don't disappear completely. So, what you see after birth are small strands of old blood vessels floating in the vitreous of the eye. These remnants are called floaters. I often use the analogy of seeing banana pieces suspended in a bowl of clear Jello.

Floaters can also occur when protein fibers from the gel in the vitreous clump together. They may be more obvious when you look at bright areas, such as a blank light-colored wall or the white pages of a book. You may even see floaters when your eyes are closed, especially if you're under a bright light or lying in the sun. Why? Because the strands can float closer to the retina and toward the macula (the center of your vision). When the bright light shines into your eyes, a shadow is cast on the retina and you perceive the floater.

Although floaters do not normally increase in number with age, oftentimes they seem to become more apparent. The reason for this is that the vitreous of the eye becomes less gel-like and slightly more fluid with age. This allows the floaters to move more freely and to get into your line of sight more frequently. While floaters can be a very natural and common occurrence, there are times when you should report them to your doctor. See "When to Call the Doctor for Floaters" at right.

CONVENTIONAL TREATMENT

Floaters themselves are harmless, and there is no practical treatment for them. One word of caution, however: if you become aware of a lot of floaters that appear all of a sudden or are associated with flashes of light in your vision, see your eye doctor immediately to make sure there is nothing seriously wrong.

Some ophthalmologists have taken up a procedure that is somewhat controversial but has had limited success with floaters. In this procedure, an ophthalmologist aims a special laser at the floaters in the vitreous, which may break them up and make them less noticeable. If the floaters are large and disturbing the vision, it might be useful to reduce the size of these floaters within the eye. However, while some people who have this treatment report improved vision, others notice little or no difference. Risks of laser therapy include damage to your retina if the laser is aimed incorrectly. Laser surgery to treat floaters is typically reserved for extreme cases.

SELF-TREATMENT

When you become aware of floaters in your field of vision, just try to quickly look away and then back at what you were viewing. This is often enough to move the floaters out of the way—at least until they float back into your field of vision later on! Another thing you may want to do is to add antioxidants to your diet. They help to preserve the integrity of the vitreous by reducing free radicals.

RECOMMENDATIONS

• Make sure you report any floater activity to your doctor. As detailed above, note if the spots appeared suddenly and if flashes of light are associated with them.

• Consider discussing an antioxidant regimen with your eye doctor or nutritionist. Remember, not all healthcare practitioners are adequately educated in nutrition and supplementation, so be sure to seek out professionals who can properly address your needs and provide you with quality recommendations.

FLUID UNDER THE RETINA

See Central Serous Retinopathy, page 182.

FOCUSING PROBLEM

See Accommodative Insufficiency, page 153.

WHEN TO CALL THE DOCTOR FOR FLOATERS

The presence of a few floaters is generally considered normal. However, there are certain situations that warrant concern and the immediate attention of an eye doctor:

• If you see "dozens" of floaters all of a sudden, meaning there is a significant increase in the number of floaters evident in your eye. This could indicate some type of retinal inflammatory condition.

• If you see floaters with flashes of light. This might be an indication of a retinal detachment.

GIANT PAPILLARY CONJUNCTIVITIS

**SYMPTOMS
OF GPC**

- Itchy eyes

- White mucus
discharge that
collects on the lids

- Contacts that slide
around and feel dry

- A milky deposit on
the contacts

Giant papillary conjunctivitis (GPC) is a type of pinkeye that usually occurs in contact lens wearers. (For a more general discussion of pinkeye, see page 303.) GPC is a chronic low-grade allergic reaction in the conjunctiva of the upper lid. Many people who wear conventional soft contacts and don't clean or replace them frequently enough will encounter GPC. The disorder can also develop over time from the irritation caused by a surgical suture or other foreign body.

GPC is not a threat to vision or to the long-term health of the eyeball, but it can be a nuisance. In contact lens wearers, it usually appears after lenses have been worn for a long time, and it is often not associated with any other problems. The symptoms include the following: itching, often more in one eye and worse with the contact lenses on; a white mucus discharge that collects at the lids, especially when you're awake; contacts that slide around and feel dry, especially when you blink; and a milky deposit, sometimes a ring-like and chalky stain, which appears on the contacts and won't come off. The symptoms often continue to worsen until you can no longer wear your contact lenses. When you quit wearing the lenses, the symptoms diminish gradually and then eventually get better. To evaluate your condition, your doctor must look under your upper lids, turning them inside out using a cotton applicator to see the inner linings of the lids. Everted lids feel funny, but not painful, when this is done correctly.

When looking with magnification at an eye affected by GPC, the lid membrane is bumpy instead of glassy smooth or finely grained. The lumps are papillae—ashy gray bumps that are "giant" only in comparison with other common conditions. The papillae are sticky, and, as mentioned in the symptoms above, they secrete whitish mucus that collects in the lids and makes contact lenses misbehave.

CONVENTIONAL TREATMENT

In most cases, the treatment of GPC involves discontinuing the use of the contact lenses to allow the eye to recover. The contacts may need to be avoided for several days or weeks. Severe cases may take even longer to resolve. Sometimes the lenses may need to be professionally cleaned and polished to remove the deposits that triggered the allergic reaction. Often, the lenses must be discarded. Changing the type of lenses worn may help;

daily disposable lenses are much less prone to contributing to this condition. Also, switching to a contact lens solution that does not contain preservatives might help. Prescription eye drops can further help to alleviate the symptoms, especially the itchiness. Over-the-counter eye drops are generally not recommended, however, because they are not sufficiently effective.

Follow-up care with your eye doctor is important. GPC is difficult to control. If the condition is not treated properly and steps are not taken to prevent a recurrence, it can become a chronic condition. It may even prevent the further use of contact lenses.

SELF-TREATMENT

If you wear contact lenses, be sure to pay attention to your doctor's instructions. As the lenses age, it is important to maintain a proper care schedule. That means proper cleaning and storage. If an enzyme cleaner is recommended (it usually is for non-disposable lenses), do not skimp on its use. Weekly use of an enzyme cleaner will assure that protein, which has been shown to be one of the possible causes of GPC, does not build up on the lenses.

However, considering the state-of-the-art disposable contacts lenses that are available, no soft-lens wearer should suffer from GPC. Over the years, disposable contact lenses have become much more reasonable in price. For most people, they are the best choice because the lenses can easily be replaced before build-up of dirt and proteins becomes severe enough to be harmful to the eye. There are now daily disposable lenses which are replaced every day.

To avoid GPC, take proper care of your contact lenses. Good cleaning and storage practices will help ensure that irritating proteins and dirt do not accumulate on lenses. An even better option is disposable lenses that can be replaced every day.

NUTRITIONAL SUPPLEMENTS

SUPPLEMENT	DIRECTIONS FOR USE	COMMENTS
Vitamin A	Take 2,500 IU daily.	Maintains the moisture in the eye tissues.
Vitamin-B complex	Take 50–100 mg daily.	Improves the intraocular cellular metabolism.
Vitamin C	Take 2,000–3,000 mg daily.	Protects the eye from further inflammation.
Zinc and copper	Take 20 mg of zinc and 2 mg of copper daily.	Enhances the immune response. Note: The copper supplementation is needed to balance the zinc supplementation.

HERBS AND HERBAL SUPPLEMENTS

HERB	DIRECTIONS FOR USE	COMMENTS
Eyebright	Use as an eyewash.	Good for all eye conditions.
Goldenseal	Apply as a compress.	Soothing for the mucous membranes. Caution: Do not take internally for more than 1 week. Do not use during pregnancy.

HOMEOPATHIC REMEDIES

REMEDY	DIRECTIONS FOR USE	COMMENTS
Allium cepa 6c	Place 3–4 pellets under the tongue, 3–4 times daily.	Relieves mucus discharge.
Apis mellifica 6c	Place 3–4 pellets under the tongue, 3–4 times daily.	Alleviates swelling.
Mercurius corrosivus 6c	Place 3–4 pellets under the tongue, 3–4 times daily.	Relieves discharge.
Pulsatilla 6c	Place 3–4 pellets under the tongue, 3–4 times daily.	Relieves discharge associated with emotions.

RECOMMENDATIONS

• Change your contact lenses often. Fresh, new lenses promote GPC far less than older ones do.

• Switch to a different type of lens. Some soft-lens materials aggravate GPC more than others do, and hygiene is always a contributing factor. If you wear reusable lenses, the problem usually goes away if you switch to disposable or frequently replaced lenses.

To relieve the itching associated with GPC, apply a cold compress to your eyes several times a day.

• If you have GPC or have suffered from it in the past, modify your lens-wearing schedule; wear your contacts only occasionally. On the night before a special occasion, get them out and change the solution they've been in.

• A cold compress used several times per day will help to relieve the itching associated with GPC.

• Since GPC is a form of pinkeye, the same treatments and recommendations offered in the "Pinkeye" section are effective. See page 303.

- If your eyes feel dry, use your recommended contact lens lubricant. Dirt collects much more easily on dry lenses than on moist lenses, and it can lead to irritation of the upper-eyelid tissue.

GLAUCOMA

Glaucoma (glaw-KO-mah) is a condition in which the optic nerve loses its integrity and eventually dies. It is most often associated with pressure inside the eye (intraocular pressure) being markedly elevated, which prevents blood from reaching, nourishing, and circulating through the eye. If the pressure remains high for an extended period of time, it causes the eventual death of the optic nerve. Glaucoma is deceptive and dangerous. Most sufferers have few or no symptoms of the disease, which occurs in 1 to 2 percent of the over-forty population and is the most common cause of blindness in the United States. A family history of glaucoma or diabetes, a previous eye injury or surgery, or the use of eye drops containing steroids, are considered risk factors for developing glaucoma. This condition is also much more common in African Americans than in Caucasian Americans.

In a normal eye, the aqueous humor is produced inside the eye and drained into the bloodstream at a constant rate so that you always have a fresh supply and always the correct amount. It drains out of the eye into the bloodstream through a little canal between the iris and the cornea. With glaucoma, either too much aqueous humor is produced, or the drainage mechanism has broken down and the fluid can't escape quickly enough. Either way, the increased pressure interferes with the blood circulation to and from the eye, and the result is damage to the optic nerve with increasing loss of vision. Peripheral vision is the first area of vision loss. Unless it is caused by a specific injury or a tumor in one eye, glaucoma usually affects both eyes, but the two eyes may not succumb at the same rate.

Sometimes the doctor can see the blockage in the drainage channel. In this case, the glaucoma is called narrow- or closed-angle glaucoma. More often, however, the channel appears to be normal despite the elevated pressure. In such cases, the glaucoma is called open-angle.

About 15 percent of glaucoma patients know they have a problem. They have an acute form of glaucoma characterized by extreme eye pain, redness, dilated pupils, blurred vision, and halos around lights. These people, in reality, are lucky because they usually get themselves to an eye doctor promptly. In the remaining 85 percent of glaucoma patients, the disease is chronic and insidious. The symptoms are subtle and may not even be noticed until significant vision has been lost. Contrary to popular conception, there is no feeling of pressure in the eye with the chronic type of glaucoma.

Fortunately, the test for glaucoma, which checks for increased eye pressure, is very simple and can be easily done in the office by your optometrist or ophthalmologist. In the most common version done today, a puff of air is blown at your eye by a machine, although other methods are also used. In the "puff" test, the air depresses slightly and measures how much pressure it takes to flatten it to a certain point. Whichever test the doctor uses, be sure you have this test done every time you have an eye check-up. Another indication of glaucoma is a change in your peripheral vision or an enlarging blind spot. Unfortunately, people rarely notice these changes early on; rather, eye doctors usually detect them during examinations. Your eye doctor should check for these indicators regularly.

There is also a condition known as normal-tension glaucoma, whereby the eye pressure remains in the normal range yet there is peripheral vision loss and damage to the optic nerve. It is difficult to distinguish from primary optic atrophy (loss of integrity of the optic nerve). This is a very difficult condition to identify, as well as to treat. This shows how important complete and regular eye examinations can be.

As is true for many conditions, there is no single cause of glaucoma. Prolonged stress and an inadequate diet over a long period of time, as well as a genetic inheritance are considered by many authorities to be the main causative factors in glaucoma. Prolonged stress leads to adrenal exhaustion, and exhausted adrenals are no longer able to produce aldosterone, which stabilizes the salt balance in the body. When too much salt is lost from the body, the tissue fluids build up and often will push into the eyeball, increasing the intraocular pressure, forcing the lens forward, and closing off the drainage tubes.

There are additional possible causes. It is suspected that a general stiffening of the sclera and other parts of the eye plays a role in the development of the disorder in people over forty. Other causes are a serious eye injury, eye surgery, some medications (especially steroids), and an eye tumor, to name a few. When glaucoma develops in a child during the first year of life, it is almost always due to an inherited malformation of the aqueous humor drainage canal.

Glaucoma can be very dangerous, and most sufferers do not experience any symptoms until there is significant vision loss. That's why it's important to have a test for glaucoma every time you have an eye check-up.

CONVENTIONAL TREATMENT

Glaucoma can be treated with medications, with surgery, or with both drugs and surgical procedures. Treatment with medication involves the use of one or more products—some topical and some systemic, some old and some relatively new. Because each family of medications works through a different mechanism and has its own advantages and drawbacks, it makes sense to briefly discuss each one below. However, the role of any glaucoma medication is to lower eye pressure.

Beta-blockers became the standard first line of treatment for glaucoma over the past forty years. Examples of the beta-blockers are betaxolol (Betoptic), carteolol (Ocupress), levobunolol (Betagan), metipranolol (Optipranolol), timolol hemihydrate (Betimol), and timolol maleate (Timoptic). Most patients take beta-blockers without any problems. However, these medications should be used cautiously by patients who have breathing disorders such as asthma, bronchitis, emphysema, or chronic obstructive pulmonary disease, and by patients who have certain heart problems such as congestive heart failure or a pulse rate of less than sixty beats per minute. Occasionally, depression, confusion, and impotence have been reported by people who are taking such medications.

Although there is no cure for glaucoma, early diagnosis and treatment can prevent the loss of eyesight.

With the newer forms of glaucoma medications available, the drugs known as the miotics are rarely used anymore. But because of their history in association with treating glaucoma, they are worth discussing. Examples of the miotics are carbachol (Isopto and Miostat) and pilocarpine (Ocusert, Pilocar, and Pilostat). The pupil of the eye becomes small, or miotic, in patients who take the drops. When the pupil is miotic, less light is able to get into the eye, which causes the vision to dim, especially at night and in patients with cataracts. Also, the vision may vary between clear and blurry, especially when the drops are used by younger patients. In addition, it is very common to have a brow- or headache during the first several days of taking the miotic. However, this discomfort usually disappears within five to ten days. The stronger miotics—for example, phospholine iodide—occasionally cause excess sweating, stomach cramps, or nausea. Pilocarpine, which is the most common miotic agent, comes in the form of eye drops, an ocular insert similar to contact lenses, and a convenient one-dose-a-day ointment. Your doctor can help you decide if this type of medication is the best choice for you.

A new formulation of a lower concentration of pilocarpine is being marketed as a treatment of presbyopia, or age-related loss of accommodation. Marketed under the name *Vuity*, it relies on the same effect of pilocarpine to reduce the pupil size, which will extend the "depth of focus" to allow clearer vision at the reading distance. There are limitations to this new drop, which we will discuss under the category of presbyopia on page 308.

The epinephrine medications, which come in eye-drop form, commonly cause stinging, tearing, and burning when they are first placed on the eye. They also often cause the eye to become red or bloodshot several hours after application, although at first they actually whiten the eye. Examples of the epinephrines are epinephrine (Epifrin and Glaucon) and dipivefrin (Propine). Some patients develop true allergies to these medications, occasionally after taking them for years without any problems. Propine, which is more expensive than the basic epinephrine eye drop, is less likely to have these annoying side effects. Patients may also find that epinephrine drops cause their pupils to dilate. These drops should be used cautiously by patients whose blood pressure is difficult to control or who have an irregular heartbeat or rapid pulse rate.

The alpha-agonists are a newer class of medications developed to control eye pressure. Examples of the alpha-agonists are apraclonidine (Iopidine) and brimonidine (Alphagan). Generally, the alpha-agonists are used only by those patients whose eye pressure cannot be controlled with any of the other glaucoma medications. The side effects may include stinging, tearing, and burning when the drops are first placed on the eye, as well as redness or a bloodshot appearance. These side effects are similar to those of the epinephrine class of glaucoma medications. Additionally, the eyelids may open up slightly. Some elderly patients whose eyelids normally droop find this cosmetic side effect desirable rather than unwanted! It is important to note that Alphagan P is a reformulation of the original Alphagan. Alphagan P was developed to achieve comparable effectiveness to that of Alphagan and to improve Alphagan's side-effect profile, particularly as it pertains to ocular allergy.

The carbonic anhydrase inhibitors are eye-pressure-reducing medications that come in pill form. Examples of this class of medicine are acetazolamide (Diamox), dorzolamide (Trusopt), and methazolamide (MZM and Neptazane). As you might expect, systemic side effects are more common with these pill forms than with the glaucoma eye drops. About half the patients who take carbonic anhydrase medicines must stop because of the side effects, which include tingling in the hands and feet, poor appetite and poor taste of food, stomach upsets and diarrhea, fatigue, and depression. Less common side effects are kidney stones and, very rarely, a serious form of anemia that prevents the body from fighting infection, which could prove fatal. The carbonic anhydrase inhibitors are a type of sulfa medication and should be avoided by patients who have known allergies to these substances. A more recent development of an eye drop, dorzolamide (Trusopt), should have fewer side effects than the carbonic anhydrase inhibitors in oral forms.

Latanoprost (Xalatan) is the first of the prostaglandin-agonists, which are the latest class of glaucoma medications. It works by opening the so-called accessory drainage pathway in the eye. The medicine is administered as one drop on the affected eye at bedtime. Examples of other prostaglandin-agonists are bimatoprost (Lumigan) and travoprost (Travatan). Each of these medicines may have local and systemic side effects. For example, bimatoprost has one unusual side effect: In some people with hazel, green, or bluish-brown eyes, the eye color is permanently changed to brown, even if the medication is discontinued. This side effect appears to be only cosmetic, with no known ill effects on the eye. It is this side effect that gave it another "life" as Lastisse. Yes, this product is based on a side effect of a glaucoma medication. Prostaglandin-agonists may help to reduce the eye pressure in patients who are already taking the maximum doses of other anti-glaucoma eye drops if they are not effective enough. However, adherence to the medication protocol can be confusing and expensive. And if side effects do occur, the patient must be willing either to tolerate them or to communicate with the treating physician to improve the drug regimen.

Another prostaglandin category is a Rho kinase inhibitor, such as Rhopressa (netarsudil). Another class of glaucoma medication is nitric oxides, such as Vyzulta (latanoprostene bunod).

Now that we've covered the various types of prescription medications available for the treatment of glaucoma, we can move onto additional methods of treatment. Much has been made in recent years of the use of marijuana to treat glaucoma. One side effect of marijuana is the lowering of the intraocular pressure. Yes, it does the job, but the effects are only temporary. There are many other medications that achieve this desired effect more easily and with less of the euphoric side effect. It is also important to consider the negative effect on the lungs when it comes to smoking marijuana.

Surgery for glaucoma is an option for some individuals. Often the surgery involves the creation of new channels through which the aqueous fluid can escape from the eye. In another procedure, a laser is used to burn little spots into the area around the iris. As these burns heal, they form scars that pull the tissue in toward them. This contracting of the tissue around the burns opens up the meshwork of the eye and reduces the overall intraocular pressure by increasing the drainage of the aqueous fluid. The laser procedures for glaucoma are still being improved and are typically reserved for those patients who do not respond to the other types of glaucoma therapy.

SELF-TREATMENT

Because of the uncertainty surrounding the causes of the various types of glaucoma, there is no one self-treatment that is appropriate for everyone. However, there are some general guidelines that seem to help most of the people who are afflicted with the disorder.

Since one cause of glaucoma may be adrenal exhaustion, it is important to give the adrenal glands nutritional support. For a list of supplements that have been found useful in the treatment of glaucoma, see the table below. Also, avoid consuming refined carbohydrates, such as white bread, which are taxing to the adrenal glands. In general, any disturbance in the metabolism may lead to an increase in eye pressure. Many of these supplements should be taken in conjunction with the medication the doctor prescribes.

Exercise and yoga have also been shown to be effective at reducing eye pressure. Be sure to check with your primary healthcare provider before starting an exercise program. It is important to practice a regimen that does not exacerbate any pre-existing health conditions.

NUTRITIONAL SUPPLEMENTS

SUPPLEMENT	DIRECTIONS FOR USE	COMMENTS
Choline and inositol	Take 1,000–2,000 mg of a combination supplement daily.	Important B vitamins for the eyes.
Fish Oil	Take 1,000 mg daily.	Increases aqueous outflow.
Glutathione	Take 500 mg, 2 times daily.	A powerful antioxidant.
Manganese	Take 4 mg daily.	An enzyme activator.
Pycnogenol	Take 80 mg daily.	Reduces eye pressure; increases blood flow to optic nerve.
Rutin	Take 50 mg, 3 times daily.	Works with vitamin C to reduce eye pressure.
Vitamin A	Take 2,500 IU daily.	Aids in mucopolysaccharide metabolism; mucopolysaccharides are long molecular chains of sugar used by the body in the building of connective tissues.
Vitamin B$_5$	Take 100 mg, 3 times daily.	A stress vitamin needed for the adrenal glands.

SUPPLEMENT	DIRECTIONS FOR USE	COMMENTS
Vitamin C	Take 5,000–10,000 mg daily.	Reduces eye pressure.
Vitamin E	Take 400 IU daily.	Protects retina and optic nerve.

HERBS AND HERBAL SUPPLEMENTS

HERB	DIRECTIONS FOR USE	COMMENTS
Bilberry	Take as directed on the label.	Acts as an antioxidant.
Er ming zuo ci wan (Brion)	Take 8 pills, 3 times daily, or drink as a tea.	Reduces congestion.
Eyebright	Take in supplement form as directed on the label, or drink as a tea.	Good for all eye conditions.
Ginkgo biloba	Take as directed on the label.	Slows vision loss.
Ming mu di huang wan (Brion)	Take 10 pills, 3 times daily, or drink as a tea.	Clarifies the vision.
Nei zhang ming yan wan (Brion)	Take 8 pills, 3 times daily.	Clarifies the vision. Caution: Contains aluminum, so limit its use.
Rose hips	Take in supplement form as directed on the label, or drink as a tea.	A source of vitamin C.
Shi hu ye guang wan (Brion)	Take 1 pill, 2 times daily.	Reduces eye pressure.
Mirtogenol (Life Extension)	Take as directed	Helps other glaucoma medications work better.

HOMEOPATHIC REMEDIES

REMEDY	DIRECTIONS FOR USE	COMMENTS
Belladonna 6c	Place 3–4 pellets under the tongue, 3–4 times daily.	Relieves the colored halo around lights.
Nux vomica 6c	Place 3–4 pellets under the tongue, 3–4 times daily.	Good for high eye pressure.
Phosphorus 6c	Place 3–4 pellets under the tongue, 3–4 times daily.	Relieves the colored halo around lights.
Pulsatilla 6c	Place 3–4 pellets under the tongue, 3–4 times daily..	Relieves the colored halo around lights.
Sulphur 6c	Place 3–4 pellets under the tongue, 3–4 times daily.	Good for glaucoma with pain.

RECOMMENDATIONS

- It is critical to have your eye pressure checked regularly to monitor the progress of your glaucoma. In addition, be very careful to heed your eye doctor's instructions.

- Since the peripheral vision is affected first, be sure to have that tested periodically, too.

- Be careful when drinking large amounts of fluids. Lower amounts are recommended if you are considered a "borderline" glaucoma suspect.

- Avoid tobacco smoke, nicotine, alcohol, and all caffeine.

- A large study in 2004 suggests that a diet consisting of more omega-6 than omega-3 polyunsaturated fats may offer some protection against developing glaucoma. Note that the omega-6 EFAs do not refer to hydrogenated fats so common in commercial baked goods, chips, and the like. See page 66 in Part One for more information on these nutrients.

- Nitric oxide, which is produced in the body, also helps to relieve eye pressure. Foods that promote the creation of nitric oxide include beets, garlic, dark chocolate (in small amounts), leafy greens, nuts, seeds, citrus fruit, pomegranates, and watermelon.

GPC

See Giant Papillary Conjunctivitis, page 230.

GRAVES' DISEASE

Graves' disease is one of the more common types of hyperthyroidism. It is a disorder in which the thyroid gland produces too much thyroid hormone, resulting in an overactive metabolism. All of the body's processes speed up, so the symptoms may include nervousness, irritability, a constant feeling of being hot, increased perspiration, insomnia, and fatigue. If you are a woman of menopause age, these symptoms may sound familiar as they are similar to menopause symptoms, so be sure your doctor checks your thyroid as a part of your yearly exam. Graves' disease patients often also present the symptoms of goiter (enlarged thyroid gland), exophthalmos (bulging eyeballs, generally caused by lid retraction), tachycardia (rapid heartbeat), weight loss, hyperactive reflexes, drooping eyelids, and tremor. However, the thyroid gland may be of a normal size in a small number of patients. The eye symptoms may include pain, excessive tearing, blurred vision, and double vision. Other eye findings may be swelling around the eyes, optic nerve inflammation, and enlargement of the extraocular muscles.

These additional eye findings have now been categorized as thyroid eye disease (TED). This has allowed a pharmaceutical company to develop a new drug called Tepezza. It has been shown to reduce eye bulging, lessen double vision, provide relief from pain and swelling around the eye, and improve the appearance of the eyes. With Tepezza, some people began to have less eye bulging in as few as six weeks, with improvements continuing for the full course of eight treatments. The most common side effects of Tepezza include muscle cramps or spasms, nausea, hair loss, diarrhea, feeling tired, high blood sugar, hearing problems, taste changes, headache, and dry skin. Discuss this medication with your physician.

The thyroid gland is the body's internal thermostat. It regulates the body's temperature by secreting two hormones that control how quickly the body burns calories and uses energy. If the thyroid gland secretes too much hormone, hyperthyroidism results. If it secretes too little, hypothyroidism results. Many cases of hyper- and hypothyroidism are believed to result from an abnormal immune response. The exact cause is not understood, but the immune system produces antibodies that invade and attack the thyroid, disrupting the hormone production.

The age of onset of Graves' disease is most commonly between thirty and forty years old. Females are affected seven times more often than men. Although not specifically an eye disorder, its effects on the eyes can be quite extensive. Therefore, it is included in this part of the book.

> Although Graves' disease is not specifically an eye disorder, but a disorder of the thyroid gland, its effects on the eyes can be extensive. The preferred method of treatment is medication, but surgery can also be an option.

CONVENTIONAL TREATMENT

Graves' disease can be treated with surgery or medication. The surgery for Graves' disease involves the removal of thyroid tissue to reduce the overall hormone output to a normal level. Surgery, however, is not the preferred method of treatment because of the complications that may be caused by the general anesthesia and the possibility of nerve damage. Furthermore, too little or too much thyroid tissue frequently is removed.

The medications used to treat Graves' disease are called antithyroidal medications. These medications, such as methimazole (Tapazole) and propylthiouracil (Propylthiouracil Tablets), act by blocking the formation of thyroid hormone. The therapeutic actions of these agents begin as soon as four to twelve hours after administration. Levothyroxine (Synthroid) treats hypothyroidism and also is used to treat or prevent goiter associated with hyperthyroidism, which can be caused by hormone imbalances.

The antithyroidal medications may also alter the thyroid-immune system mechanisms that are central to the cause of Graves' disease. They control the symptoms of hyperthyroidism in 90 percent of patients. Permanent remission is achieved in 10 to 30 percent of patients. Unfortunately, the relapse rates are high, many about 50 percent, even in patients who were treated for more than two years. The relapse rates are even higher, at nearly 90 percent, in patients who were treated for less than two years.

The side effects of the antithyroidal medications include fever, rash, itching, and neutropenia (decrease in the white blood cell count). Rare but serious side effects are arthritis, blood vessel inflammation, and hepatitis. The risk of side effects increases as the dose of the medication increases. Treatment with these medications is certainly something that must be monitored carefully and frequently by a doctor.

Eyelid surgery is one option. Because the eyelids are usually more widely open in Graves' disease, some patients may have difficulty closing their eyelids, leaving the eyeballs more exposed, which causes excessive tearing and irritation. Surgical repositioning of the eyelid may help reduce the irritation.

Sometimes scar tissue from Graves' ophthalmopathy can cause one or more eye muscles to be too short. This pulls your eyes out of alignments, leading to double vision. Eye muscle surgery may help correct double vision by cutting the affected muscle from the eyeball and reattaching it farther back. The goal is to achieve single vision when you read and look straight ahead. In some cases, you may need more than one operation to get these results. These procedures are performed by an eye specialist called an ophthalmologist.

When eyesight is threatened, a type of surgery called orbital decompression can be done. In this procedure, a bone between the eye socket (orbit) and sinuses is removed to allow more space for the swollen tissues. When the procedure is successful, it improves vision and provides room for your eyes to return to their normal position. There is a risk of complications, including double vision that persists or appears after surgery.

All these surgical interventions should be performed at a medical center with expertise in this area, as they require a team approach and correct timing to ensure best likelihood of success and minimize risks.

It is important that thyroid blood levels be maintained in the normal range. After treatment of an overactive thyroid, there is a high risk of becoming hypothyroid (an underactive gland). Adequate thyroid replacement is essential to help keep Graves' disease from getting worse.

SELF-TREATMENT

Because Graves' disease is a metabolic disturbance, it is imperative that you watch your diet closely. Be sure to eat plenty of cruciferous vegetables, such as broccoli, Brussels sprouts, cabbage, cauliflower, kale, mustard greens, peaches, pears, rutabagas, soybeans, spinach, and turnips. These foods are potent modulators of the innate immune response system with potent antiviral, antibacterial, and anti-cancer activity.

To help with your eye symptoms, use eyewashes and artificial tears to maintain eye moisture. If your eyes tend to dry out at night, lightly tape them closed. Use surgical paper tape; it is designed for use on the body and will not stick harshly to your eyelashes. You may also try to do the following:

• Apply cool compresses to your eyes. The extra moisture may provide relief.

• Wear sunglasses. When you have Graves' disease your eyes are more vulnerable to ultraviolet rays and more sensitive to sunlight. Wearing sunglasses helps protect them from both sun and wind.

• Use lubricating eye drops. Eye drops, like artificial tears, may help relieve dryness and scratchiness. Be sure to use eye drops that do not contain redness removers. A lubricating gel can be used before bed to prevent the cornea from drying out because your eyelids may not cover the entire eye when sleeping.

• Elevate the head of your bed. Keeping your head higher than the rest of your body may reduce swelling and may help relieve pressure on your eyes.

• If double vision is a problem, glasses containing prisms may be prescribed by your doctor. However, prisms don't work for all people with double vision and your doctor may recommend surgery as a more effective option.

• Swelling in the eyes may be improved by treatment with steroids (such as hydrocortisone or prednisone).

To help with your eye symptoms, use eyewashes and artificial tears to maintain eye moisture. If your eyes tend to dry out at night, lightly tape them closed. Use surgical paper tape; it is designed for use on the body and will not stick harshly to your eyelashes.

NUTRITIONAL SUPPLEMENTS

SUPPLEMENT	DIRECTIONS FOR USE	COMMENTS
Multivitamin and mineral complex	Take as directed on the label.	People with Graves' disease need increased amounts of all the vitamins and minerals.
Vitamin-B complex	Take 50 mg, 3 times daily, with meals.	Benefits thyroid function.
CapsiClear	Take one pill daily	Supports a healthy tear film.

HERBS AND HERBAL SUPPLEMENTS

HERB	DIRECTIONS FOR USE	COMMENTS
Alfalfa	Take as directed on the label.	A good source of vitamin K; good for relaxation.
Burdock	Take as directed on the label.	A good source of iron.
Eyebright	Use as an eyewash.	Maintains eye moisture.
Gotu kola	Take as directed on the label.	Good for relaxation.
Kelp	Take as directed on the label.	An infection fighter.
Licorice	Take as directed on the label.	Good for stress.

HOMEOPATHIC REMEDIES

REMEDY	DIRECTIONS FOR USE	COMMENTS
Aconite 6c	Place 3–4 pellets under the tongue, 3–4 times daily.	Good for anxiety.
Arsenicum album 6c	Place 3–4 pellets under the tongue, 3–4 times daily.	Good for anxiety.
Belladonna 6c	Place 3–4 pellets under the tongue, 3–4 times daily.	Good for restlessness.
Iodium 6c	Place 3–4 pellets under the tongue, 3–4 times daily.	Restores iodine intake by the thyroid gland.
Thyroidium 6c (Boiron)	Place 3–4 pellets under the tongue, 3–4 times daily.	Regulates the metabolism.

RECOMMENDATIONS

- Avoid dairy products for at least three months when you have a flare up of eye symptoms due to Graves' disease. Also avoid stimulants, including coffee, tea, nicotine, and soft drinks.

- Be wary of treatment with radioactive sodium iodine, which is often recommended for this condition. It has been known to cause severe side effects.

- Do not rush into surgery. Instead, try to improve your diet first.

HEADACHE

The most common complaint among optometric patients is headache. It is very often the first sign of a vision-related problem. However, almost everyone experiences headache at one time or another. Common causes are stress, tension, anxiety, allergies, constipation, coffee consumption, hunger, sinus pressure, muscular tension, hormone imbalance, trauma, nutritional deficiency, alcohol consumption, drug use, smoking, fever, and, of course, eyestrain. Experts estimate that about 90 percent of all headaches are tension headaches, and 6 percent are migraines. Tension headaches, as the name implies, are caused by muscular tension. Migraines result from, most likely, a disturbance in the blood circulation to the brain. Another relatively common type of headache is the cluster headache. This is a severe, recurring headache that strikes about 1 million Americans.

Vision-related headaches most often are located toward the front of the head, although there are a few exceptions. They usually occur at the middle or end of the day, are not present upon awakening in the morning, and do not produce visual auras such as flashing lights. These headaches often strike in a different pattern on the weekend than during the week. Some people do not experience them at all on the weekend. They also affect one side of the head more than they do the other, and may be accompanied by a number of more general symptoms.

Because of the symptoms that accompany headaches, it is important that your doctor obtain a thorough history to determine the type of headache from which you suffer. Be aware of the time of the headache's onset, specific location of the pain, frequency, duration, severity, and precipitating factors such as stress and certain foods. Also note such associated symptoms as nausea, vomiting, light sensitivity, and sound sensitivity.

SYMPTOMS OF VISION-RELATED HEADACHES

- The pain is usually located toward the front of the head.

- The pain tends to occur midday or at the end of the day.

- The pain affects one side of the head more than the other.

It is important to discuss more thoroughly the subject of migraines, since they are associated with numerous eye symptoms. The migraine headache is a disorder consisting of localized symptoms that may or may not actually be associated with headaches. The eye symptoms are similar to those of many other diseases, so you should seek professional care in order to properly diagnose and treat the disorder. Migraines have a number of phases that exhibit definite symptoms. The first is called the prodromal or premonitory phase, during which you might suffer irritability, depression, light sensitivity, and/or sound sensitivity. These symptoms may show up as early as two days before the actual headache. The second phase is called the aura phase and consists of visual symptoms such as flashing lights, halos around lights, zigzagging of lines, and distortion of shapes and colors. This phase typically evolves over twenty minutes and is commonly, but not always, followed by a headache. The headache may throb, be located on one or both sides of the head, and last from four to seventy-two hours. The final phase is called the post-dromal phase, which brings a washed out and exhausted feeling.

Because migraine headaches have a visual aspect to them, eye doctors are often consulted. To summarize, possible visual effects of migraines include but are not limited to the following: light sensitivity; blurred vision; auras; blind spots; flashes of colored lights; and tunnel vision. Many who suffer from these symptoms have been able to gain relief through one or more treatment options, which are discussed below.

CONVENTIONAL TREATMENT

The medical establishment has trained us to expect some type of medication to cure almost every malady. This is no truer than with the common headache. The largest-selling over-the-counter medications in this country today are aspirin and the newer forms of pain relievers. The latter include the non-steroidal anti-inflammatory drugs (NSAIDS), which form a billion-dollar business. Advil, Aleve, and Motrin are the most common of these. So, if you call your doctor about a headache, you might be given the classic recommendation: "Take two aspirin and call me in the morning."

If you have been diagnosed with migraine headaches, several suggestions are commonly offered. For "mild" migraines, most doctors just recommend an over-the-counter NSAID or Acetaminophen (Tylenol). While both can be effective, long-term use is discouraged due to stomach-related side effects. For more moderate to severe headaches, there are two general classes of prescription drugs: triptans and ergots.

The triptans reduce inflammation by constricting the blood vessels. This stops the headache. The triptan with the longest history of use is sumatriptan (Imitrex). Sumatriptan is available in the United States as an injection, oral tablet, and nasal spray. Zolmitriptan (Zomig) and rizatriptan (Maxalt) are newer triptans that are available as oral tablets and as tablets that melt in the mouth. Naratriptan (Amerge), almotriptan (Axert) and frovatriptan (Frovalan) are available only as oral tablets.

Triptans should be used early after the migraine begins, before the onset of pain or when the pain is mild. Using a triptan early in an attack increases its effectiveness, reduces side effects, and decreases the chance of recurrence of another headache during the following twenty-four hours. Used early, triptans can be expected to abort more than 80 percent of migraine headaches within two hours.

Ergots, like triptans, are medications that abort migraine headaches. Examples of ergots include ergotamine preparations (Ergomar, Wigraine, and Cafergot) and dihydroergotamine preparations (Migranal and DHE-45). Ergots, like triptans, cause constriction of blood vessels, but ergots tend to cause more constriction of vessels in the heart and other parts of the body than the triptans, and their effects on the heart are more prolonged than the triptans. Therefore, they are not as safe as the triptans. The ergots also are more prone to cause nausea and vomiting than the triptans are. The ergots can cause prolonged contraction of the uterus and miscarriages in pregnant women.

> Recurring headaches are often caused by a specific food trigger, so when you get a headache, review the foods you have eaten over the last few hours. Common triggers include wheat, chocolate, MSG, sulfites, sugar, fermented foods, marinated foods, cheese, alcohol, and vinegar.

SELF-TREATMENT

There are many options for self-treating a headache. Most of them involve discovering the source of the condition that led to the headache, then treating that condition. People who suffer from frequent headaches may be reacting to certain foods or food additives, such as wheat, chocolate, monosodium glutamate (MSG), sulfites, sugar, fermented foods (such as cheese, sour cream, and yogurt), alcohol, vinegar, or marinated foods. Other possible causes are anemia, bowel problems, brain disorders, teeth grinding, high blood pressure, low blood sugar, sinusitis, spinal misalignment, toxic overdose of vitamin A, deficiency of vitamin B, or a nose, throat, or eye disorder. As suggested above, when you get a headache, review all of the dietary and physical activities over the previous several hours to see if there is a recurring theme that triggers the headache.

A number of simple self-treatments can help alleviate a headache. The next time you have a headache, try the following:

- Lie down and remain quiet for a few minutes.

- Massage your scalp and temples.

- Apply a cold wash–cloth to the painful area.

- If you are not a regular caffeine drinker, take a small amount of caffeine.

Many times, lying down and remaining quiet for a short period of time will alleviate a headache, especially a tension headache. You might consider using acupressure points on various parts of your head (see page 332) if your headache is visual in origin. Massaging the area around your head is also helpful to reduce muscle tension. You might also try a cold washcloth over the painful spot to reduce the excessive blood flow to the area. If you are *not* a regular coffee drinker, sometimes taking a small amount of caffeine will affect the blood vessels enough to relieve the headache. However, if you drink coffee regularly, it is unlikely that this treatment will be effective. Migraine headaches should be evaluated by a professional healthcare practitioner since they are most often associated with other physical symptoms and related to blood flow within the body.

NUTRITIONAL SUPPLEMENTS

SUPPLEMENT	DIRECTIONS FOR USE	COMMENTS
Bromelain	Take 500 mg, as needed.	An enzyme that helps to regulate the inflammatory response.
Calcium with vitamin D	Take 1,500 mg of calcium daily.	Relieves muscular tension. Note: The calcium dosage in the capsule should be balanced with vitamin D.
Coenzyme Q_{10}	Take 30 mg, 2 times daily.	Improves cellular energy production.
Evening primrose oil	Take 500 mg, 3–4 times daily.	Supplies essential fatty acids, which promote circulation.
Glucosamine sulfate	Take as directed on the label.	A natural alternative to aspirin and NSAIDs.
Magnesium	Take 1,000 mg daily.	Relieves muscular tension.
Potassium	Take 100 mg daily.	Maintains the proper balance between sodium and potassium.
Vitamin-B complex	Take 50 mg, 3 times daily.	Good for nerve function. Note: It is better to take the entire B complex than just isolated B vitamins.
Vitamin B2	Take 400 mg	Take for 3 months to reduce migraine symptoms. For adults only!
Vitamin C	Take 2,000–8,000 mg daily, in divided doses.	A free-radical scavenger that is good for reducing damage due to stress.
Vitamin E	Take 400 IU daily.	Boosts the circulation.

HERBS AND HERBAL SUPPLEMENTS

Herb	Directions for Use	Comments
Burdock	Take as directed on the label.	An excellent detoxifier.
Er ming zuo ci wan (Brion)	Take 8 pills, 3 times daily.	Good for headaches accompanied by ear-ringing.
Fenugreek	Take as directed on the label.	Good for headache.
Feverfew	Take as directed on the label.	Good for headache. Caution: Do not use during pregnancy.
Goldenseal	Take as directed on the label.	Soothing for the tissues. Caution: Do not take internally for more than 1 week. Do not use during pregnancy.
Lavender	Rub essential oil on the temples.	Good for headaches accompanied by stomach upset.
Lobelia	Use as directed on the label.	Good for tension headaches. Caution: Do not take internally.
Long dan xie gan wan (Brion)	Take 6 pills, 2 times daily.	Reduces inflammation and "heat."
Marshmallow	Take as directed on the label.	An anti-inflammatory.
Mint	Rub essential oil on the sore area.	Calms the nerves.
Niu huang shang qing wan (Brion)	Take 10 pills daily.	Reduces "heat" and toxins in the body. Caution: Do not use during pregnancy.
Qi ju di huang wan (Brion)	Take 8 pills, 3 times daily, or drink as a tea.	Good for headaches resulting from a "yin" deficiency.
Rosemary	Take as directed on the label.	Boosts the circulation.
Skullcap	Take as directed on the label.	Relieves spasm.
Thyme	Take as directed on the label.	Good for sinus headaches.
White willow bark	Take as directed on the label.	Good for pain.
Xiao yao wan (Brion)	Take 8 pills, 3 times daily.	Good for a wide range of symptoms.

HOMEOPATHIC REMEDIES

Remedy	Directions for Use	Comments
Aconite 6c	Place 3–4 pellets under the tongue, 3–4 times daily.	Good for throbbing headaches.

Remedy	Directions for Use	Comments
Remedy	Directions for Use	Comments
Arsenicum album 6c	Place 3–4 pellets under the tongue, 3–4 times daily.	Good for head colds.
Belladonna 6c	Place 3–4 pellets under the tongue, 3–4 times daily.	Good for colds, flu, sore throats, and similar problems.
Bryonia 6c	Place 3–4 pellets under the tongue, 3–4 times daily.	Relieves pressure inside the head.
Gelsemium sempervirens 6c	Place 3–4 pellets under the tongue, 3–4 times daily.	Good for headaches that form a band around the head.
Nux vomica 6c	Place 3–4 pellets under the tongue, 3–4 times daily.	Good for headaches at the back of the head or over the eyes, for sharp pains in the eyes and eyestrain resulting from overwork.
Ruta graveolens 6c	Place 3–4 pellets under the tongue, 3–4 times daily.	Supports the tendons and ligaments.
Sulphur 6c	Place 3–4 pellets under the tongue, 3–4 times daily.	Relieves hot, burning sensations at the top of the head.

RECOMMENDATIONS

● Eat a well-balanced diet. Avoid chewing gum, ice cream, iced beverages, and salt. Chewing gum puts more pressure on your jaw and therefore can be problematic when headaches "pound" your head. The other items will specifically affect blood flow to the head.

● When experiencing a headache, avoid excessive sunlight if you are light sensitive.

● Practice deep-breathing exercises. A lack of oxygen can cause headaches.

● If you use a computer, take breaks often. For more treatments and recommendations, see "Computer Vision Syndrome" on page 189.

● Always seek and treat the cause of a headache. Long-term reliance on aspirin and other painkillers can make chronic headaches worse by interfering with the brain's natural ability to fight them, as well as increasing the likelihood of stomach problems.

● Poor vertebral alignment, often caused by flat feet or wearing high heels, can cause a reduced blood flow to the brain. Chiropractic adjustment can be helpful.

HIGH BLOOD PRESSURE, EYE PROBLEMS RELATED TO

See Hypertensive Retinopathy, below.

HORDEOLUM

See Stye, page 324.

HYPEROPIA

See Farsightedness, page 225.

HYPERTENSIVE RETINOPATHY

Hypertensive retinopathy is a pathological condition of the retina. This disorder is directly caused by long-standing high blood pressure. Because many of the blood vessels of the eye lie within the structure of the retina, any condition that affects the blood vessels can in turn affect the retina.

It is beyond the scope of this book to discuss all of the causes of high blood pressure, which is also called hypertension. If you are diagnosed with hypertension, be sure to work with your doctor on the best program to reduce the effects of the disease. However, it is certainly worth looking more closely at hypertension's effect on the eyes, and how to control the disorder in general. High blood pressure most often has no symptoms. The warning signs associated with advanced hypertension include headache, sweating, a rapid pulse, shortness of breath, dizziness, and visual disturbances.

High blood pressure is usually divided into two categories—primary and secondary. Primary hypertension is high blood pressure that is not due to any other underlying disorder. The precise cause of primary hypertension is unknown, but a number of definite risk factors have been identified. These include cigarette smoking, stress, obesity, as well as excessive use of stimulants such as coffee or tea, drug abuse, high sodium intake, and the use of oral contraceptives.

When the blood pressure rises as a result of another health problem, such as a hormonal abnormality or an inherited narrowing of the aorta, it is called secondary hypertension. Secondary hypertension may also result

A pathological condition of the retina, hypertensive retinopathy is caused by long-standing high blood pressure. If you have hypertension, work with your doctor to reduce the effects of this disease before it can have an impact on your eye health.

from the blood vessels being chronically constricted or having lost their elasticity due to a build-up of fatty plaque on their inside walls, a condition known as atherosclerosis. Atherosclerosis and arteriosclerosis (thickening of the artery walls due to aging or calcium deposits) are common precursors of hypertension, and viewing the blood vessels inside the eye can assess both of these conditions.

In hypertensive retinopathy, the fluids gradually seep out of the blood vessels that have been weakened by hypertension. They then seep into the spaces within the structure of the retina. This blood eventually clots, and the retina forms scar tissue as a result of the irritation due to the clots. The scar tissue pulls on the structure of the retina, causing blindness in extreme cases. If the condition progresses too far, the blindness can be permanent; if treated early, the remaining vision can be at least maintained.

CONVENTIONAL TREATMENT

The standard treatment for hypertensive retinopathy is directed at both resolving the basic problem (the high blood pressure) and preventing the progression of the disease. Preventing the development of hypertension should be a primary goal of everyone who is at risk for the disease—that is, everyone who has the risk factors discussed above or has a family history of this disorder.

The first thing that must be done to treat hypertensive retinopathy is to recognize that the disorder exists. Only an eye doctor looking into the eye and viewing the blood vessels in the retina can accomplish this. Signs of the condition can show up early in the disease process, so treatment of the disease can reduce the severity of the eye complications.

There are more than a hundred different blood-pressure-lowering medications presently available. Most of these belong to one of six major classes: beta-blockers; diuretics; alpha-blockers; calcium channel blockers; angiotensin-converting enzyme (ACE) inhibitors; and angiotensin antagonists. Within each class are several medications that are very similar to each other. Many physicians start with either a beta-blocker or a diuretic because these are the medications that have been the most widely used in the trials demonstrating that lowering of the blood pressure reduces the risk of stroke and heart attack. In other words, they are the tried-and-true medications. Of the newer agents, the calcium channel blockers and ACE inhibitors are very popular, and they may have fewer side effects than the beta-blockers and diuretics. However, it remains to be seen if the newer medications are as good as the beta-blockers and diuretics when it comes to preventing stroke and heart attack.

Not every medication works well for every patient. It would be wonderful if your doctor could tell you which medication will work the best for you and produce the least side effects, but unfortunately, no doctor can do this. There are some medications that you cannot or should not take if you have certain medical conditions. For example, beta-blockers make asthma worse. Beyond that, selecting the most appropriate medication is, in good part, a hit-or-miss process.

As far as managing damage to the eyes, blood leakage is often detected using a procedure called fluorescein angiography. It involves injecting a dye into the blood vessels and then taking pictures of the retina in a timed sequence. As the dye begins to fill the arteries, the point of leakage can be observed. If there are several points of leakage, a scanning type of treatment can be effective at targeting the multiple areas. Once the problem areas are identified, laser treatment is used on the retina to seal off the leakages in the blood vessels. Usually, spot laser treatments are the protocol, as they can target very specific points.

A newer procedure for visualizing the retina is called optical coherence tomography (OCT). This imaging technique gives the doctor a "side-view" (also called a cross-section) of the retina so they can see where the problems may lie. An advancement of this procedure is called "OCT-A," where the "A" stands for Angiography. OCT-A has emerged as a non-invasive technique for imaging the small blood vessels of the retina and the choroid.

SELF-TREATMENT

Whether or not you take medication, there are several things that you can do yourself to lower your blood pressure. First, lose weight. Of all the non-drug methods of lowering blood pressure, losing weight is definitely the most effective. On average, a 10-pound loss of weight lowers the blood-pressure reading by as much as five points. Then, exercise more. Exercise certainly helps to boost weight loss, but it is also beneficial in its own right. The usual goal is at least thirty minutes of aerobic exercise, three times per week. Importantly, weightlifting and bodybuilding are not recommended. These put too much pressure on the vascular system and can initially make the problem worse.

There are also some dietary and supplemental approaches you should take. If you are a regular drinker, cut down on your alcohol intake. More than one or two drinks per day raises the blood pressure. In addition, reduce

WHAT YOU CAN DO TO LOWER BLOOD PRESSURE

- Lose excess weight
- Exercise
- Reduce alcohol consumption
- Lower salt intake
- Increase potassium intake
- Reduce stress
- Quit smoking

your salt intake. However, this doesn't work for everyone, and it is more likely to be effective if you are more than forty-five years old and have definite hypertension. In younger people and those with borderline hypertension, losing weight is much more important. Also, increase your potassium intake. Fruits and vegetables are good sources of potassium and are also low in sodium.

Stress reduction is another approach you can take to reduce hypertension and therefore the risk of hypertensive retinopathy. In general, however, stress-reduction techniques such as biofeedback, yoga, and relaxation have been found to be only marginally successful. And on the subject of lifestyle changes, it is definitely important to quit smoking. If you smoke, quitting may be the best thing you ever do. It won't have much effect on your blood pressure, but it will greatly reduce your risk of having a stroke or heart attack. Also, if you do smoke, you're likely to be wasting your time reading this book! Tobacco smoke will easily negate many of the positive recommendations I can make. Incidentally, smoking reduces the size of the blood vessels and increases pressure through them.

> Simply quit smoking, and you'll reduce your risk of not only eye disease but also stroke and heart attack.

NUTRITIONAL SUPPLEMENTS

SUPPLEMENT	DIRECTIONS FOR USE	COMMENTS
Calcium and magnesium	Take 1,500–3,000 mg of a combination supplement daily.	Deficiencies have been linked to hypertension.
Coenzyme Q_{10}	Take 100 mg daily.	Improves heart function and lowers blood pressure.
L-carnitine, L-glutamic acid, and L-glutamine	Take 500 mg of a combination supplement, 2 times daily, on an empty stomach.	Helps to prevent heart disease.
Lecithin	Take 1,200 mg, 3 times daily.	Emulsifies fat in the body and lowers blood pressure.
Omega-3 essential fatty acid	Take 1,000–2,000 mg each day.	Has an anti-inflammatory effect.
Selenium	Take 100 mcg daily.	Deficiency has been linked to heart disease.
Vitamin C	Take 1,000–3,000 mg daily.	Improves adrenal function and reduces blood clotting.
Vitamin E	Take up to 400 IU daily.	Improves heart function.

HERBS AND HERBAL SUPPLEMENTS

HERB	DIRECTIONS FOR USE	COMMENTS
Cayenne	Take as directed on the label.	Boosts the circulation.
Fennel	Take as directed on the label.	An anti-inflammatory.
Garlic	Take 250 mg, 3 times daily.	Effective at lowering the blood pressure.
Hawthorn	Take as directed on the label.	Boosts the circulation.
Hops	Take as directed on the label.	Promotes relaxation of the smooth muscles.
Lady's slipper	Take as directed on the label.	Good for relaxation.
Parsley	Take as directed on the label.	Relieves mucus discharge.
Passion flower	Take as directed on the label.	Good for relaxation.
Rosemary	Take as directed on the label.	Stimulates the skin.
Skullcap	Take as directed on the label.	Relieves smooth-muscle spasm.
Valerian	Take as directed on the label.	Calms the nerves.

HOMEOPATHIC REMEDIES

REMEDY	DIRECTIONS FOR USE	COMMENTS
Crataegus oxycantha 6c	Place 20 drops of tincture in 4 oz of water, and drink. Use daily for 3 months.	Regulates the blood pressure.
Lachesis 6c	Place 3–4 pellets under the tongue, 3–4 times daily.	Increases vascular integrity.
Natrum muriaticum 6c	Place 3–4 pellets under the tongue, 3–4 times daily.	Good for increased salt intake.

RECOMMENDATIONS

• Consider lifestyle counseling, a program to revamp your way of living. Lifestyle counseling will address your eating habits, exercise routine, stress level, work habits, and more.

• People with high blood pressure often have sleep apnea—temporary cessation of breathing while sleeping. If you have this condition, consult your physician.

• Avoid artificial sweeteners, which contain phenylalanine. Many contain warnings on their packages. Phenylalanine may cause a severe increase in blood pressure in people taking MAOIs (such as phenelzine, tranylcypromine, pargyline, and selegiline). This severe increase in blood pressure (also called "hypertensive crisis") can lead to a heart attack or stroke. For this reason, individuals taking MAOIs actually should avoid all foods and supplements that contain phenylalanine.

• Have your blood pressure checked at least every four to six months. If necessary, buy your own blood-pressure monitor. Also, many pharmacies have self-test equipment available for public use.

HYPERTHYROIDISM

See Graves' Disease, page 240.

INVOLUNTARY EYE MOVEMENTS

See Nystagmus, page 292.

IRIS, INFLAMMATION OF

See Iritis, below.

IRITIS

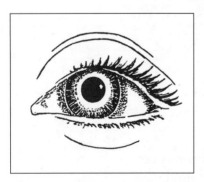

FIGURE 2.5
An Eye Affected by Iritis.

Iritis (eye-RITE-iss) is an inflammation of the iris. Sometimes it also involves the inflammation of the ciliary body, which is behind the iris. Specifically, inflammation of the ciliary body is termed uveitis (YOU-vee-eye-tis).

In iritis, microscopic white blood cells from the inflamed area and excess protein that leaked from the small blood vessels inside the eye float in the aqueous fluid between the iris and the cornea. If there are a lot of floating cells, they may become attached to the back of the cornea or settle at the bottom of the area. See Figure 2.5 for an illustration of an eye affected by iritis. The shading around the iris designates a pinkish area due to the inflammation below the level of the sclera.

In many cases, iritis is related to a disease or infection in another part of the body. Diseases such as arthritis, tuberculosis, and syphilis can contribute to its development. Infection in some parts of the body, such as the tonsils, sinuses, kidneys, gallbladder, and teeth, can also cause inflammation of the iris. In other cases, iritis may follow an injury to the eye or accompany an ulcer or foreign body on the cornea. Often, the exact cause of the disorder remains unknown. And even when the disorder is treated early, it often recurs. In most cases, however, it eventually disappears completely.

The symptoms of iritis usually appear suddenly and develop rapidly over a few hours or days. Iritis commonly causes extreme pain, tearing, light sensitivity, and blurred vision. Redness often occurs. Some patients experience floaters—small specks or dots moving in the field of vision. In addition, the pupil may become smaller in the affected eye.

A thorough eye examination is considered an emergency when the symptoms of iritis occur, as inflammation inside the eye can affect the sight and could possibly lead to blindness. Since iritis can be associated with another disease, an evaluation of your overall health is sometimes necessary for proper diagnosis and treatment. In some cases, blood tests, skin tests, and X-rays may be conducted, and other specialists may be consulted to help determine the cause of the inflammation.

SYMPTOMS OF IRITIS

- Tearing
- Light sensitivity
- Blurred vision
- Redness
- Pain
- Floaters
- Smaller pupil

CONVENTIONAL TREATMENT

The conventional treatment of iritis is often directed at finding and removing the cause of the inflammation. That might involve fully treating another disorder. In addition, eye drops and ointments are recommended to relieve the pain, quiet the inflammation, dilate the pupil, and reduce any scarring that may occur. Both steroids and antibiotics may be prescribed either topically or internally.

A case of iritis can last six to eight weeks. During this time, you must be observed carefully for side effects from the medications and any complications. Cataracts, glaucoma, corneal changes, and secondary inflammation of the retina may occur as a result of the iritis or the medications.

SELF-TREATMENT

Self-treatment is not recommended for this disorder. Since iritis is an inflammation inside the eye, the condition is potentially sight-threatening. Proper diagnosis and prompt treatment are essential. To minimize vision loss, you should have a complete eye examination as soon as you notice any symptoms. If diagnosed in the early stages, iritis usually can be controlled with eye drops before any loss of vision occurs. The application of hot packs may also provide relief from the symptoms, but only after medical treatment has begun.

NUTRITIONAL SUPPLEMENTS

SUPPLEMENT	DIRECTIONS FOR USE	COMMENTS
Boron	Take 3 mg daily.	Supports the connective tissue.
Bromelain	Take as directed on the label.	Assists in the production of prostaglandins.
Evening primrose oil	Take as directed on the label.	Assists in the production of anti-inflammatory prostaglandins.
Salmon oil	Take as directed on the label.	Assists in the production of anti-inflammatory prostaglandins.
Superoxide dismutase (SOD)	Take as directed on the label.	An excellent antioxidant.
Vitamin E	Take 400 IU daily.	An antioxidant.

HERBS AND HERBAL SUPPLEMENTS

HERB	DIRECTIONS FOR USE	COMMENTS
Belladonna	Take as directed on the label.	Dilates the pupil to reduce possible scarring inside the eye.
Cat's claw	Take as directed on the label.	Good for pain. Caution: Do not use during pregnancy.
Feverfew	Take as directed on the label.	Good for pain and soreness; combine with ginger for even better results. Caution: Do not use feverfew during pregnancy.
Ginger	Take as directed on the label.	Good for pain and soreness; combine with feverfew for even better results.

HOMEOPATHIC REMEDIES

REMEDY	DIRECTIONS FOR USE	COMMENTS
Aconite 6c	Place 3–4 pellets under the tongue, 3–4 times daily.	Good for iritis in the early stages.
Allium cepa 6c	Place 3–4 pellets under the tongue, 3–4 times daily.	Good for reducing inflammation.

REMEDY	DIRECTIONS FOR USE	COMMENTS
Apis mellifica 6c	Place 3–4 pellets under the tongue, 3–4 times daily.	Alleviates swelling.
Calcarea fluorica 6c	Place 3–4 pellets under the tongue, 3–4 times daily.	Good for inflammation accompanied by light sensitivity.
Euphrasia officinalis 6c	Place 3–4 pellets under the tongue, 3–4 times daily.	Good for all eye conditions.
Mercurius corrosivus 6c	Place 3–4 pellets under the tongue, 3–4 times daily.	Alleviates pain and inflammation.
Rhus toxicodendron 6c	Place 3–4 pellets under the tongue, 3–4 times daily.	Good for inflammation accompanied by muscle paralysis.

RECOMMENDATIONS

• If you are diagnosed with iritis, keep your eyes "quiet"—that is, avoid light, wind, dust, sun, and other irritants.

• Taking an aspirin or NSAID will help to reduce the inflammation associated with iritis. Confirm this with your physician.

• If you wear contact lenses, you should remove them for the entire course of treatment of this disease.

KERATOCONUS

The word *keratoconus* (carrot-oh-CONE-us) is formed from two Greek words—"kerato," meaning cornea, and "konos," meaning cone. Keratoconus (KC), or conical cornea, is a condition in which the normally spherical shape of the cornea has become deformed. A cone-like bulge is present, causing significant visual impairment. The distortion in vision has been compared to viewing a street sign through a car windshield during a driving rainstorm. KC's progression is generally slow and can stop at any stage, from mild to severe. As the disease progresses, the cornea bulges and thins, becoming irregular and sometimes developing scars.

Keratoconus, a cone-like bulge in the normally spherical shape of the cornea, can cause significant visual distortion. Usually, this disorder shows up at puberty or during the late teens.

KC is not one of the common eye diseases, but it is by no means rare. It has been estimated to occur in 1 out of every 2,000 persons in the general population. The disease usually shows up in young people at puberty or during the late teens. It is found in all of the parts of the United States and the rest of the world. It has no known significant geographic, cultural, or social pattern. One line of thought on the cause of KC is eye rubbing. Thus, if you see someone (especially a child) rubbing his eyes very hard for extended periods of time, it is prudent to see what the source of the problem might be.

The first indication of KC is a blurring and distortion of vision, which the doctor may indicate as a large increase in the amount of astigmatism. If caught in the early stages, KC may be corrected with glasses; frequent changes in the astigmatism prescription are necessary. The thinning of the cornea usually progresses slowly for five to ten years and then tends to stop. We now know that the progression is often due to the vulnerability of the flexible, young cornea, so aging actually helps to reduce the changes in corneal shape.

Occasionally, the change is rapid, and in the advanced stage, the patient may experience a sudden clouding of vision in one eye that then clears over a period of weeks or months. This is called acute hydrops (HIGH-drops) and is due to the sudden infusion of fluid into the stretched cornea. This begins the advanced stage of the disease process. It is at this time that the vision changes significantly and the current mode of vision correction (contacts or glasses) may no longer be effective. In advanced cases of KC, superficial scars form at the apex of the corneal bulge, resulting in more vision impairment. It is as this stage that a surgical correction is called for.

CONVENTIONAL TREATMENT

In the earliest stages of KC, ordinary eyeglasses may correct the mild nearsightedness and astigmatism that are experienced. As the disease advances, gas permeable contact lenses or a new hybrid lens (see Contact Lenses on page 338) are the only options to correct the vision adequately. Most of the time, contact lenses are a permanent remedy.

Contact lenses must be fitted with great care, and most KC patients need frequent check-ups and changes in their prescriptions in order to achieve good vision and comfort. In some instances, the use of one lens on top of another (piggybacking a gas permeable lens on top of a soft lens) is an alternative solution when upgrading the prescription doesn't work anymore. Technological advances in both gas permeable and soft lenses are being made constantly, offering more and more options to KC patients. For example, a combination soft/gas permeable lens was developed to provide the clarity of a gas permeable lens with the comfort of a soft lens. It has proven to be helpful even in advanced cases of KC. This is why the wearing of contact lenses is the preferred method of managing KC until surgery is necessary.

Most recently, a new procedure has started being studied in the United States. This involves the application of riboflavin (vitamin B_2) and then shining UV light onto the cornea. The procedure, called "corneal cross-linking," has become the standard for treating advanced KC. In fact, many doctors are recommending it at earlier stages to hopefully stall the progression of the disease.

In only about 10 percent of KC cases, a corneal transplant becomes necessary. In this process, much of the central cornea of the KC patient is removed and is replaced with a healthy donor cornea. For a complete discussion of corneal transplants, see page 353.

From a medical standpoint, the most important thing you can do is to keep in touch with your eye doctor and follow his instructions. Be alert to any changes in your eye condition and in your vision. If you experience blurring, scratchiness, irritation, tearing, or discharge, contact your eye doctor as soon as possible. These symptoms signal a problem with your eyes' tolerance of the contact lenses or the need for refitting.

SELF-TREATMENT

Eventually, you will learn to live with your KC, whether or not you need surgery. People react differently to the news that they have KC, and you may find a group discussion to be enlightening and reassuring. Perhaps there is no better psychological therapy than sharing your experience with others in similar circumstances. In addition, lack of knowledge often creates fear, so it is best to become as informed as possible about the disorder. The National Keratoconus Foundation maintains a registry of KC patients and organizes self-help groups in various communities. To contact the organization, see the Resource Organizations section, which begins on page 413, for the address and phone number.

The National Keratoconus Foundation offers information on the disorder, organizes self-help groups, has a referral service, and otherwise assists those with KC. See page 416 for contact information.

NUTRITIONAL SUPPLEMENTS

SUPPLEMENT	DIRECTIONS FOR USE	COMMENTS
Vitamin A	Take 2,500 IU daily.	Good for all eye conditions.
Vitamin C	Take 2,500–3,000 mg daily.	Builds collagen, which makes up the corneal tissue.
Riboflavin	Take 200 mg daily.	Strengthens collagen, which makes up the corneal tissue.

RECOMMENDATIONS

- Studies in stem cell research are currently being conducted to address this disease process. Keep informed on the latest findings by using the Internet and talking with your healthcare professionals. Adult stem cells exist at the edges of the cornea, so new research is looking into using them to grow new corneal tissue.

- In most cases, keratoconus is not inherited and occurs in individuals with no family history of the disorder. The condition can also occur in families. In some cases, keratoconus is inherited in an autosomal dominant pattern, which means one copy of the altered gene in each cell is sufficient to cause the disorder.

- Seasonal allergies are known for causing extreme itchiness in the eyes. This can exacerbate an already frustrating eye situation in the person with KC, so resolving the allergic response is important.

LATTICE DEGENERATION

Lattice degeneration is a condition in which small areas of the retina are thinner than normal. These thin areas are more prone to developing retinal holes or tears than the areas of normal thickness. Therefore, although we do not know for sure if lattice degeneration is congenital or develops during life, we do know that it slightly increases the risk of retinal holes and tears. As a result, it increases the risk of retinal detachment. No one progresses directly from lattice degeneration to retinal detachment, but sometimes a retinal tear or hole will develop in or near the area of lattice degeneration and progress to retinal detachment.

Lattice degeneration usually has no symptoms, but occasionally it is associated with sudden flashes of light inside the eye, usually at night, when the eyes move quickly. This is due to the jelly-like vitreous of the eye tugging on the retina in the area of the degeneration. The flashes are more likely if there is a hole or tear in the retina associated with the degeneration. However, in older people a vitreous detachment is also likely a cause of flashing lights. Only a dilated eye exam can determine if the condition is lattice degeneration or vitreous detachment, the latter of which is less worrisome. Lattice degeneration is present in about 8 percent of the general population and occurs in about 40 percent of eyes with retinal detachment.

CONVENTIONAL TREATMENT

Occasionally, lattice degeneration needs to be treated with freezing or laser treatments in order to prevent the possibility of retinal detachment. These treatments "spot-weld" parts of the peripheral retina to hold it into place more firmly—offering more resistance to detachment.

The above-described treatments usually are necessary only if there is a very large amount of degeneration. A second reason for these treatments is the presence of an associated hole or tear in the retina. In this circumstance, treatment is often done even if the area of degeneration is small, because the tear or hole increases the retinal-detachment risk.

If you have been diagnosed with lattice degeneration, watch for flashes of light or showers of floaters. These symptoms can indicate retinal tears or retinal detachment.

SELF-TREATMENT

Lattice degeneration is much more common in elongated (nearsighted) eyeballs. Therefore, highly nearsighted people should have a dilated eye exam on a regular (yearly) basis to ascertain that the areas of concern are healthy. Also, reducing the risk of lattice degeneration involves avoiding activities that are likely to cause trauma to the eye. Examples of such activities include boxing, hockey, football, and most contact sports.

If you have lattice degeneration, you should watch for flashes of light or a shower of many floaters in your vision. These symptoms may indicate a retinal tear or retinal detachment. And if you notice the flashes or floaters, call your eye doctor immediately for an appointment. Even without these symptoms, a diagnosis of lattice degeneration should be followed and checked on a regular basis.

NUTRITIONAL SUPPLEMENTS

SUPPLEMENT	DIRECTIONS FOR USE	COMMENTS
Vitamin A	Take 2,500 IU daily.	Good for all retinal conditions.
Vitamin C	Take 1,000–5,000 mg daily, in divided doses.	Supports all of the eye structures.

HOMEOPATHIC REMEDIES

REMEDY	DIRECTIONS FOR USE	COMMENTS
Hamamelis virginiana 6c	Place 3–4 pellets under the tongue, 3–4 times daily.	Alleviates venous congestion.
Phosphorus 6c	Place 3–4 pellets under the tongue, 3–4 times daily.	Improves the metabolism of the retinal tissue.

RECOMMENDATIONS

- If you have been diagnosed with lattice degeneration, you should avoid high-impact activities (for example, hockey, football, and wrestling).

- Request peripheral vision assessments at your yearly eye exams if you have lattice degeneration. This will help to identify affected areas of the retina.

LAZY EYE

The term "lazy eye" is commonly misunderstood by the layman. To understand what a lazy eye is, we first have to cover the conditions that exist before it. If the visual information to one eye is distorted or dissimilar in any way from the visual information to the other eye, the brain will receive two images that are very different from each other. Double vision is often the result. Since double vision is obviously an undesirable condition, the brain will "tune out" one of the two images it receives in order to see just one image again. (For a discussion of this process, see "Suppression" on page 328 and "Double Vision" on page 209.) This double vision followed by the tuning out of one eye's input can occur when strabismus causes the eyes to point at two different objects rather than at the same one (see "Strabismus" on page 320). It can also occur if the two eyes handle refraction in a dissimilar manner—for example, if one eye is nearsighted and the other is astigmatic.

Lazy eye, or amblyopia, can be treated effectively as long as it is diagnosed early in life. This is one reason why it's important to bring young children to an eye specialist for evaluation.

If the above-detailed situation exists for a long time, the eye that is not used will adapt and begin to function poorly. After some time, the best obtainable vision in that eye will not be as good as was once possible, even if the proper corrective lens is placed before the eye. This condition of having a healthy eye that cannot be fully corrected to 20/20 vision is called lazy eye, or *amblyopia* (am-blee-OH-pee-ah). The lazy eye's vision has been sacrificed to preserve the practical aspect of visual function.

Lazy eye rarely develops in adults. The misinformation between the two eyes most often begins during the first few years of life and occasionally at birth. This is another reason why it is especially important to have an eye specialist see your child as early as possible. Once the two eyes have developed their full visual capability—that is, once the two eyes have 20/20 vision—lazy eye will not likely develop. However, there are some rare instances when poisons, including tobacco and alcohol, can create an amblyopia-like condition.

CONVENTIONAL TREATMENT

Amblyopia affects about 4 million people in the United States, but there is no definitive medical treatment for it. The main conventional treatment is to try to encourage the lazy eye to see clearly by patching the good eye and making the lazy one work to its maximum potential. Amblyopia can be prevented almost 100 percent of the time if it is detected early enough (during early childhood) and if the cause is effectively treated. However, with newer techniques and technology, the age limit for treating amblyopia is no longer applicable. There have been studies that have shown improvement of vision in amblyopic adults who are in their thirties, although it takes a major commitment of time and dedication to achieve such great results.

Another common treatment mode is to use a dilating drop (atropine) instead of wearing a patch. Studies have shown that using the drop is as effective as patching. This is especially useful for children who refuse to accept the patch. This is also more cosmetically appealing. However, if the child is wearing glasses, oftentimes a piece of "frosted" tape is place over the good eye to act as a patch. Your doctor can discuss the various treatment options that might be most appropriate for your child.

Vision therapy for amblyopia involves much more than simply patching the good eye. It includes a series of techniques designed to enhance all of the visual abilities and to encourage eye teaming. Studies have shown that when combined with active visual techniques, patching for as little as two hours per day can improve the vision markedly! A behavioral optometrist who specializes in vision therapy can offer you a complete program that should be effective at resolving the amblyopia.

LUMINOPIA ONE

Luminopia One is the first FDA-approved digital therapeutic for neurovisual disorders in children, indicated to improve vision in children with amblyopia, or lazy eye. With Luminopia One, patients choose TV shows or movies to watch from a selection of 700+ hours of popular, engaging, and educational content. Patients view selected videos in real time within a virtual reality (VR) headset to promote weaker eye usage and encourage their brains to combine input from both eyes. Luminopia One has been validated through a series of clinical trials, including one that demonstrated its safety and efficacy in children aged four to seven with amblyopia. Pilot studies have also shown efficacy in older children and adolescents, where eye-patching and blurring (atropine) eye drops are largely ineffective. Ask your eyecare provider if this treatment is available in their office.

There is no surgical option for amblyopia. Since the eyes are often aligned properly and the condition exists only in one eye that is perfectly healthy, there is nothing to operate on. If the condition exists with strabismus, then the strabismus should be addressed as well. (Non-surgical techniques should be a first option).

Vision therapy can significantly improve lazy eye as long as the techniques are used on a daily basis, exactly as prescribed by your eyecare professional.

SELF-TREATMENT

Most of the vision therapy programs referred to in the section above include techniques to do at home. It is unlikely that doing therapy techniques for approximately an hour per week at a doctor's office can make a significant difference in your visual abilities. Therefore, it is critical that you maintain the effect of the therapy throughout your daily routine and practice home vision therapy. Be sure to perform the techniques on a daily basis, as prescribed. There are literally dozens of different techniques that you can perform, so vary them as needed to prevent boredom.

One other important point: if you have one good eye and one that is amblyopic, it is strongly suggested that you wear protective eyewear at all times. You never know when an object may come too close for comfort. A pair of "plano," or nonprescription, unbreakable polycarbonate lenses are the best protection you can have. Ask your optician about these lenses.

NUTRITIONAL SUPPLEMENTS

Supplement	Directions for Use	Comments
Inositol	Take 500 mg daily.	An antioxidant.
Lutein	Take 6 mg daily.	Increases macular function.
Pantothene	Take 900 mg daily.	An antioxidant.
Selenium	Take 50 mcg daily.	An antioxidant.
Vitamin A	Take 2,500 IU daily.	Good for all retinal conditions.
Vitamin-B complex	Take 75–100 mg daily.	Good for stress.
Vitamin C	Take 2,000–5,000 mg daily.	Fortifies the blood-vessel walls.
Vitamin E	Take 400 IU daily.	An antioxidant that improves retinal function.
Zinc and copper	Take 20 mg of zinc with 2 mg of copper daily.	Good for retinal health, in combination with vitamin A; also a good antioxidant. Note: The copper supplementation is necessary to balance the zinc supplementation.

HOMEOPATHIC REMEDIES

REMEDY	DIRECTIONS FOR USE	COMMENTS
Agaricus 6c	Place 3–4 pellets under the tongue, 3–4 times daily.	Good for eyelid twitching.
Aurum 6c	Place 3–4 pellets under the tongue, 3–4 times daily.	Good for lazy eye accompanied by blind spots.
Calcarea fluorica 6c	Place 3–4 pellets under the tongue, 3–4 times daily.	Supports the connective tissue.
Carboneum sulfuratum 6c	Place 3–4 pellets under the tongue, 3–4 times daily.	Good for headache.
Causticum 6c	Place 3–4 pellets under the tongue, 3–4 times daily.	Good for lazy eye accompanied by strabismus.
Conium 6c	Place 3–4 pellets under the tongue, 3–4 times daily.	Good for dizziness.
Gelsemium sempervirens 6c	Place 3–4 pellets under the tongue, 3–4 times daily.	Good for lazy eye accompanied by strabismus.
Lachesis 6c	Place 3–4 pellets under the tongue, 3–4 times daily.	Good for headache.
Lycopodium 6c	Place 3–4 pellets under the tongue, 3–4 times daily.	Good for lazy eye accompanied by blind spots.
Phosphorus 6c	Place 3–4 pellets under the tongue, 3–4 times daily.	Good for lazy eye accompanied by exhaustion.
Ruta graveolens 6c	Place 3–4 pellets under the tongue, 3–4 times daily.	Good for lazy eye resulting from over-exertion of the eyes or intense near-point work; supports the tendons and ligaments.
Sepia 6c	Place 3–4 pellets under the tongue, 3–4 times daily.	Good for lazy eye accompanied by headache.
Sulphur 6c	Place 3–4 pellets under the tongue, 3–4 times daily.	Good for lazy eye accompanied by irritation.

RECOMMENDATIONS

• If your child is six months of age or older, make an appointment for a thorough evaluation by an eye doctor, not a pediatrician. While pediatricians are excellent at reviewing general newborn health needs, vision is a specialty that deserves a specialist. There are so many optometrists and ophthalmologists who specialize in pediatrics that it should not be difficult to locate a qualified professional in your area. The examination should include a test for lazy eye. One technique uses sensors placed on the child's head. One eye is patched, and the child watches visually stimulating material on a screen while equipment monitors the activity of the unpatched eye. The procedure is then repeated for the second eye. There are several other techniques that are also effective tests of an infant's visual ability.

● The eyes develop in response to visual stimulation, so make sure that your child is surrounded with a full range of colors, lights, shapes, and sizes.

LEBER'S PRIMARY OPTIC NEUROPATHY

See Optic Atrophy, page 295.

LEGAL BLINDNESS

See Low Vision, page 271.

LENS, CLOUDED

See Cataracts, page 177.

LENS, HARDENED

See Presbyopia, page 308.

LIGHT SENSITIVITY

The eyes are designed to respond to light. However, there are a number of conditions that can make them overly sensitive to light. This light sensitivity is also known as *photophobia* (fo-toe-FO-bee-ah). Among the common causes of light sensitivity are the excessive wearing of contact lenses; poorly fitting contact lenses; eye diseases, injuries, and infections; burns to the eye; migraine headaches; meningitis; acute iritis; corneal abrasion; corneal ulcer; dilated-eye examinations; and medications and substances such as amphetamines, atropine, cocaine, cyclopentolate, idoxuridine, phenylephrine, scopolamine, trifluridine, and tropicamide (most of which dilate the pupil, causing the sensitivity to light).

There are other causes of light sensitivity, too. In fact, light sensitivity is a general and vague condition—really more a symptom than a condition. It can be caused by almost anything affecting the eyes.

CONVENTIONAL TREATMENT

The treatment for light sensitivity depends upon the cause of the problem. If the cause is an eye disorder covered in this book, see the appropriate section in Part Two for the specific conventional treatments.

SELF-TREATMENT

No matter what the specific cause of your light sensitivity is, keep your eyes shaded from excessive light by wearing optical-quality sunglasses, keeping the room lights dimmed, or simply closing your eyes. In addition, work on improving your diet. Nutrition has been shown to have a profound effect upon the eyes and visual system. A dry eye condition is often the source of the symptoms.

Sensitivity to light and glare, night blindness, and rapid tiring of the eyes are common symptoms of a vitamin-A deficiency. Excessive tearing and severe light sensitivity, along with pain and redness in the eyes, are often part of a B-complex deficiency, in particular of vitamins B_2, B_5, and B_6, as well as an omega-6/omega-3 imbalance. See the section on supplements, below, for dosage information so that you can add these important nutrients to your daily regimen.

> Light sensitivity is usually the symptom of a deeper problem. If you experience this condition, see your eye doctor and protect your eyes from excessive light by wearing sunglasses and a brimmed hat, or by dimming the lights.

NUTRITIONAL SUPPLEMENTS

SUPPLEMENT	DIRECTIONS FOR USE	COMMENTS
Vitamin A	Take 2,500 IU daily.	Good for all eye conditions.
Vitamin-B complex	Take as directed on the label.	Supports the eye tissues.
CapsiClear	Take as directed on the label.	Good for dry eyes.

HERBS AND HERBAL SUPPLEMENTS

HERB	DIRECTIONS FOR USE	COMMENTS
Eyebright	Take in supplement form as directed on the label, or use as an eyewash.	Good for external eye conditions.
Ming mu di huang wan (Brion)	Take 10 pills, 3 times daily.	Clarifies the vision.

HOMEOPATHIC REMEDIES

REMEDY	DIRECTIONS FOR USE	COMMENTS
Argentum nitricum 6c	Place 3–4 pellets under the tongue, 3–4 times daily.	Good for light sensitivity after eyestrain and for dilated pupils; maintains healthy nerves.
Arsenicum album 6c	Place 3–4 pellets under the tongue, 3–4 times daily.	Good for light sensitivity accompanied by discharge and burning.
Belladonna 6c	Place 3–4 pellets under the tongue, 3–4 times daily.	Good for dilated pupils.
Calcarea fluorica 6c	Place 3–4 pellets under the tongue, 3–4 times daily.	Good for dilated pupils.
Carboneum sulfuratum 6c	Place 3–4 pellets under the tongue, 3–4 times daily.	Good for headache.
Cinchona officinalis 6c	Place 3–4 pellets under the tongue, 3–4 times daily.	Good for dilated pupils.
Euphrasia officinalis 6c	Place 3–4 pellets under the tongue, 3–4 times daily.	Good for all eye conditions.
Graphites 6c	Place 3–4 pellets under the tongue, 3–4 times daily.	Reduces eye sensitivity.
Mercurius vivus 6c	Place 3–4 pellets under the tongue, 3–4 times daily.	Good for inflammation.
Natrum muriaticum 6c	Place 3–4 pellets under the tongue, 3–4 times daily.	Alleviates redness.
Natrum sulfuricum 6c	Place 3–4 pellets under the tongue, 3–4 times daily.	Good for inflammation; relieves mucus discharge.
Nux vomica 6c	Place 3–4 pellets under the tongue, 3–4 times daily.	Alleviates redness.
Rhus toxicodendron 6c	Place 3–4 pellets under the tongue, 3–4 times daily.	Alleviates swelling.
Silicea 6c	Place 3–4 pellets under the tongue, 3–4 times daily.	Good for chronic light sensitivity; improves nutrient absorption and metabolism; maintains healthy nerves.
Sulphur 6c	Place 3–4 pellets under the tongue, 3–4 times daily.	Good for inflammation.

RECOMMENDATIONS

• Light sensitivity is usually a symptom of a more significant condition, so appropriate diagnosis is important. Consult an eye doctor if the condition persists.

- If you wear contact lenses and experience light sensitivity with them, remove them and consult your eyecare practitioner.

- If you have allergies, light sensitivity can accompany the allergic reaction, so address that as needed.

LOW VISION

If you have been reading this book from the first page without any difficulty, your eyes must be working rather well. Congratulations! However, a great number of people cannot do this because they have a visual impairment that is not correctable, or at least not fully correctable. In fact, it is estimated that more than 10 million people in the United States are visually impaired to the degree at which they can be considered to have low vision. Low vision is defined as some type of reduction in visual acuity or the visual field that cannot be corrected. There is no clear consensus on what constitutes low vision, but individuals should be considered visually impaired. The term usually refers to those who have lost enough usable vision to make standard life tasks difficult. Their vision is not adequate for their individual needs.

> If you have impaired near vision, a simple magnifying glass may make your life easier. Look for one with an attached light so that the object is both magnified and illuminated.

Whether due to a genetic defect, a disease process, an accident, or progressive degeneration, visual impairment is a serious problem for many people. However, despite their disadvantage, these people can still be productive members of society and should be offered the opportunity to contribute. This includes those who have been termed "legally blind." The term is bandied about quite often, but it is grossly misunderstood. State and Federal laws dictate that individuals are legally blind if their best-corrected vision is 20/200 or less, or if their visual field is limited to a maximum of 20 degrees. If you're vision is extremely poor but you put on your glasses or contacts and see reasonably well, then there is no "legal" blindness to be concerned with.

CONVENTIONAL TREATMENT

The treatment for low vision depends primarily upon what visual condition is causing the problem. Most often, some kind of device is recommended to enhance the images sent to the eyes.

For impaired near vision, a simple magnifying glass is often of great help. There are some very helpful products on the market now. For example, you can purchase a magnifying glass with a light attached and a unit that is placed around the neck to allow the hands to remain free for reading, sewing, and other activities. Extremely high magnification of printed material can be obtained with closed-circuit television. The printed matter is held under the television camera, magnified, and shown on a television screen. For the truly blind, print can actually be "read" by a small camera and converted into a pattern that can be felt with the fingers. Of course, this type of equipment is expensive, but it may be worth the money if it enables you to keep earning a living or doing what you like to do. Newer technologies are continuing to be developed and, as they are, prices are likely to come down. Most computer systems have adaptability settings to help visually challenged readers.

If you have impaired distance vision, small adjustable telescopes can be attached to your eyeglasses, enabling you to see distant objects clearly within a small visual field. An eye doctor who specializes in low vision can recommend additional devices and tools to suit your condition.

For distance vision, small telescopes, which can be adjusted for focus, can be attached to your glasses. They will greatly restrict your visual field, but they may make it possible for you to see clearly within the smaller field. Pocket telescopes are also available to read such things as street signs and bus numbers. Other devices that are available include binoculars and head-mounted display units. While not necessarily allowing you to drive, at least you'll be able to navigate your way around with a bit more independence.

An optometrist who specializes in low vision, the organization titled Lighthouse for the Blind, or a low-vision center, can evaluate the appropriateness of the various devices for your particular case. For the name of a doctor or clinic in your area, contact your local branch of the Optometric Society. Moreover, surgical treatment may also be an option, depending on the specific condition that is causing your loss of vision. There have been many significant advances in eye surgery over the last several years, so consult an ophthalmologist about the options that might best serve your needs.

SELF-TREATMENT

A positive attitude and a little ingenuity can take you a long way in your efforts to adapt to low vision. Among the things you can do yourself is putting a raised dot on your oven at the 350-degree point to make setting your oven temperature easier. You can learn to punch the numbers on your telephone without having to look. You can even practice using the bottom edge of sheets of paper as a guide for signing your name on a straight line without looking. These are just a few techniques that can help you get your daily tasks done efficiently. Voice-assisted technology has helped make the life of visually challenged people much more efficient.

Quality of life is so important to maintain. Get involved in a regular exercise program, which will be good for your physical and mental health. Also, keep good music and audio-taped books on hand. Become familiar with the large-print book collection at your local library. Many communities offer support groups for people with low vision; these groups can help you with the emotional and practical aspects of your condition. Lastly, see the Resource Organizations section on page 413 for a list of groups that offer assistance to people with visual impairments.

Relatively simple modifications can make the home a friendlier place for people with low vision. Changes can include enhanced lighting, the rearrangement of furniture, or the labeling of objects with raised marks.

RECOMMENDATIONS

- Make your home as comfortable and convenient as possible. That might mean moving certain pieces of furniture into areas that are most appropriate for you—not visitors. Remind yourself that function is ultimately more important than design. Also, you can put certain raised marks or labels on items and adapt the lighting to your needs. While it may initially take a lot of energy and time to suit your surroundings to your low vision, the long-term pay-off is great and will make your life more enjoyable.

- Join a support group for your particular visual condition. It is always reassuring to know that you're not alone.

MACULAR DEGENERATION

The macula (MAC-yoo-lah) is the area of the retina that is used for direct, central vision. It is the most sensitive part of the retina. The macula begins to degenerate (deteriorate) in one out of every four people over the age of sixty-five, and in one out of every three people over the age of eighty. When macular degeneration is due to the aging process, it is simply termed age-related macular degeneration (ARMD or AMD). While both eyes usually have the disease, one may be more advanced than the other. In this circumstance, you may not notice any change taking place because the better eye will dominate your vision.

There are two types of AMD—a wet form and a dry form. The dry form of AMD constitutes 90 percent of cases and occurs when small, yellowish deposits called *drusen* (DROO-zin) start to accumulate beneath the macula. These deposits gradually break down the light-sensing cells in the macula, causing distorted vision in the eye. Vision loss from the dry form of AMD is less severe than vision loss from the wet variety. The wet form accounts for only 10 percent of cases. It occurs when tiny abnormal blood vessels begin to grow behind the retina, toward the macula. These abnormal vessels often leak blood and fluid, which damage the macula, causing rapid and severe vision loss.

There are certain risk factors that can increase your susceptibility to AMD. Age is the main one. To add to the information on age provided on the previous page, it is estimated that about 14 percent of people aged fifty-five to sixty-four years have some form of AMD. This rises to about 25 percent of persons aged sixty-five to seventy-five years, and up to 37 percent of those over seventy-five. Diet and nutrition also affect risk. The macula's fragile cells are highly susceptible to damage from the oxygen-charged molecules called free radicals. Research shows that people with a low dietary intake of antioxidants may be at risk for developing AMD. In addition, alcohol may deplete the body of antioxidants. High levels of saturated fats and cholesterol harm blood vessels and also produce free-radical reactions. If you have high blood pressure or another form of heart disease, you may also have a greater chance of getting AMD because of poor blood circulation to your eyes. So be sure to follow a diet that promotes heart health.

CATCHING IT EARLY

The cells in your eye that help you see in the dark (known as rods) are the first part of the eye affected by AMD. Because of this, the time it takes your vision to adapt from bright light to darkness can provide a very early indication of AMD. Dark adaptometry, or scotopic sensitivity, testing is helpful in measuring this transition time. Your eye doctor can use dark adaptometry to identify the presence of AMD and monitor its progression. This type of testing results in a measurement called the rod intercept time, which yields critical information to help your doctor determine your AMD status.

If you are experiencing symptoms of AMD or have multiple risk factors, you should see your eye doctor to determine your rod intercept time. Risk factors include being fifty or older; being Caucasian, a current smoker or past smoker, or overweight; and having heart disease, high blood pressure, or high cholesterol. Identifying AMD early will allow you to work with your eye doctor to take action before significant vision loss occurs. The transition from dry to wet AMD can happen rapidly. If left untreated, AMD can lead to legal blindness in as little as six months.

Exposure to certain types of light can be considered a risk factor as well. The cells of the macula are highly sensitive to sunlight. Cell damage from the sun can lead, over time, to deterioration of the macula. People with light-colored eyes may be more prone to damage from sunlight than people with dark eyes. Individuals who are exposed to high-intensity blue light for prolonged periods of time are also at higher risk for AMD. The exact reason for the blue light sensitivity is not certain, but the reduced ability of humans to produce pigment with age is being considered and reviewed in research. Thus, increasing eye pigment with age is considered a pro-active process. However, there is no conclusive research that shows that computer displays put out enough blue light to promote AMD. See the diet recommendations below.

Although age-related macular degeneration (AMD) may, in part, be inherited, there is still much you can do to avoid or slow the degeneration of the macula. One important step is to stop smoking, as tobacco more than doubles the risk of AMD.

Recent studies have shown that smoking, which reduces the level of protective antioxidants in the eye, more than doubles the risk of AMD. They found that AMD is more than twice as common in people who smoke more than one pack of cigarettes per day than in people who do not smoke. Unfortunately, the risk remains high even up to fifteen years after quitting.

A recent study has reviewed some common medications and their association with wet AMD. Here are some of those medications: Amlodipine (high blood pressure), Felodipine (high blood pressure), Bicalutamide (prostate cancer), Estradiol (hormone replacement therapy), and Atorvastatin (cholesterol). If you are taking any of these medications, inform your physician and consult with an ophthalmologist to monitor potential wet AMD complications. In addition, having diabetes is also a risk factor for wet AMD, another reason that regular retinal eye exams are critical.

While we can control some of the risk factors involved, we can't control all of them. Some studies have shown that AMD may be, in part, inherited. This means that if you have one or more immediate relatives with AMD, you may be at a higher risk for developing the condition. And gender and race factor in as well. Women over the age of seventy-five years have double the chance of developing AMD when compared with men of the same age. Low levels of estrogen in postmenopausal women may increase the risk for the condition. There is some suggestion that postmenopausal estrogen therapy may protect against AMD; more research is needed in this area. We must also take into consideration the fact that women tend to live longer than men. Regarding race, Caucasians are much more likely than African-Americans to lose vision to AMD.

Does macular degeneration ever happen to the young? There is a condition called Coat's disease, which is a form of macular degeneration that occurs in youngsters. Coats' disease is caused by a genetic defect issue—as AMD might be—but is much more uncommon.

Since the macular area is responsible for central vision only, macular degeneration does not result in total blindness, especially if only one eye is affected. However, over time, this condition can result in profound vision loss, making it difficult to read, watch television, drive, or participate in other daily activities and tasks. Therefore, if you have macular degeneration, it is important to have a comfortable rapport with your eye doctor and lots of support from friends. It is also important to do what you can to slow the progression of the disease.

CONVENTIONAL TREATMENT

Treatments for macular degeneration have changed over the past several years. At one time lasers were used in the treatment of the wet form of macular degeneration. A laser would coagulate or clot the tiny blood vessels that had grown near the macula. But more recent developments in the medical treatment of AMD, again focusing on the wet form, have taken different approaches.

Among the newer techniques, the first to be used was photo-dynamic therapy (PDT). This process employs a compound called verteporfin, which is a photosensitive drug. The drug is injected into the bloodstream, and it travels to the blood vessels in the retina. An eye doctor then shines a low-intensity laser onto the damaged area of the eye, thus activating the verteporfin. This causes a chemical reaction that destroys the abnormal blood vessels. While PDT is effective in retarding the deterioration of vision, it must be repeated several times a year.

In 2004, genetic research discovered a component of DNA that was responsible for growth of blood vessels. Researchers named it the vascular endothelial growth factor (VEGF). It was also determined that this factor was responsible for the growth of the blood vessels in the macula during AMD (and cancer tumors as well). These findings have lead to research to develop medications that inhibit this blood-vessel growth factor. As a result, we now have a category of medicines called "anti-VEGF drugs."

The first of these medications is called Macugen (pegaptanib sodium). Macugen works by blocking an essential signal that causes abnormal blood vessels to grow and leak. Macugen is not a cure, but it can help to slow further vision loss and also to help preserve what vision an individual currently has. Macugen is administered into the eye every six weeks.

A second treatment in this category is called Lucentis (ranibizumab). It also inhibits blood-vessel growth, thereby preventing scar tissue development, and protects vision. A third drug, called Avastin, is not approved for use on AMD. It is prescribed for metastatic colorectal cancer, however it has been used "off-label" in the eye and has been effective in halting the progression of AMD. A fourth option is called Eyelea (aflibercept) and has similar effects as the previous treatments but has a higher receptivity in the retina. Another entry into this category is called Beovu (brolucizumab). The injection schedule is similar to other treatments and it has been shown to be effective in increasing visual acuity. Newer drugs, such as Vabysmo, are currently being developed which require fewer injections and have a longer effectivity range.

Positive trends are being established in the treatment of AMD. However, most forms of macular degeneration cannot yet be reliably treated either medically or surgically. The best way to "treat" AMD is prevention (see below). Also, special low-vision aids can be of great help to those who suffer from AMD. These aids serve to magnify images so they are spread over a larger portion of the retina. For a description of some of these aids, see the section titled "Low Vision" on page 271.

When checking for macular degeneration, most doctors will administer a test called the Amsler Grid. For a sample grid and directions for using it, see the graphic and the associated text on page 184. This test is valuable for following the course of the disease process, but certainly does nothing to resolve the condition.

The best way to "treat" macular degeneration is through prevention:

● Practice good nutrition, including reduced fat and cholesterol intake and limited consumption of alcohol.

● Take antioxidant supplements.

● Wear sunglasses and brimmed hats to prevent damage by UV light.

● Exercise regularly.

SELF-TREATMENT

Nutrition is certainly something we have control over, and good nutrition has proven beneficial in regard to AMD. The largest study of nutritional treatment for AMD was concluded in the late 1990s. This study was called the Age-Related Eye Disease Study (AREDS). The supplement that the study participants took was a combination of beta-carotene (15 mg); vitamin C (500 mg); vitamin E (400 IU); zinc oxide (80 mg); and copper oxide (2 mg). The results showed that while there was no preventive effect or reversal of AMD, there was a slowing of the progression from stage III to stage IV (the most advanced stages). The product was supplied by Bausch & Lomb and is being marketed as Preservision.

One of the concerns I have with the study protocol was that almost two-thirds of the study's subjects were already taking a multivitamin of some form, and they were allowed to continue taking their vitamins during the study. To me, it seems that taking a vitamin while testing the effectiveness of a nutritional supplement is skewing the results, so I question the validity of this study. In addition, the amount of zinc in Preservision is way over the recommended limit of daily zinc intake, so caution should be taken with this formula. More recent research has cautioned about the amount of beta-carotene that one should take, and the AREDS study calls for an extreme amount, so be sure to review the nutritional recommendations below.

In 2007, a follow-up study called AREDS II was started to fine-tune these results and see what effect lutein, as well as zeaxanthin and omega-3 fish oils—which were added to the formula—have on AMD. My professional opinion is that the AREDS II formula is better than not doing anything, but I don't see it as the final product to help forestall the development of AMD. There are many more nutrients that can affect macular function, and I detail them in the charts below.

As previously mentioned, however, prevention is the true key to reducing the risk of AMD. While you cannot change your age, your gender, or your family tree, there are some lifestyle changes that you can adopt to help protect your eyes. First, wear sunglasses or a brimmed hat whenever you are exposed to large amounts of UV light. Moderate amounts of UV light are good for the human body, but overexposure can cause damage to some parts of the eye. Even light bulbs emit a modicum of UV light, and some people with macular degeneration have found that Chromalux full-spectrum light bulbs are easier on their eyes (see page 410 of Recommended Suppliers).

Anything that prevents clogging of your arteries may help to prevent macular degeneration (as well as the degeneration of the rest of your body). Therefore, watching your dietary fat and cholesterol, exercising regularly, not smoking, and watching your weight and blood pressure are wise moves. Limit your intake of alcohol to a maximum of six drinks per week if you are a man, and three drinks per week if you are a woman. (A discussion on the effects of red wine is in the nutrition section of Part One.)

There have been reports that a person's amount of body fat affects the amount of the antioxidant carotenoids called lutein and zeaxanthin, mentioned above, in the retina. What this means is that the higher amount of body fat you have, the less of these key nutrients is available for the retina. It seems that these nutrients are stored in fat tissue if it is available, and they are therefore not available to the eye even when needed.

Finally, most doctors recommend that their older patients take antioxidant supplements to prevent or halt the progress of macular degeneration. Recent studies indicate that a well-rounded combination of antioxidants can slow macular-degenerative changes. Several research studies on AMD are focusing on the role of carotenoids. Two of these antioxidants have already been mentioned—lutein and zeaxanthin—and they are the only dietary pigments found in the macula. In contrast, beta-carotene is virtually absent from the eye—although its cousin, vitamin A, is plentiful in the retina. Lutein and zeaxanthin can be found in almost all fruits and vegetables, but they are most likely to be present in dark green, leafy vegetables such as spinach, kale and collard greens. A study among male veterans showed that increasing the antioxidant intake can slow the progression of vision loss from dry age-related macular degeneration.

There have been a few studies on the effect of Resveratrol on macular degeneration patients. Eye researchers have been able to reduce the time it takes for older eyes to adapt to the dark with use of an oral resveratrol nutraceutical (Longevinex). Prolonged dark adaptation time is a marker of the future onset of macular degeneration.

NUTRITIONAL SUPPLEMENTS

SUPPLEMENT	DIRECTIONS FOR USE	COMMENTS
Selenium	Take 400 mcg daily.	An antioxidant.
Vitamin A	Take 2,500 IU daily.	An antioxidant. Note: Use the emulsion form for easier assimilation and greater safety.
Vitamin C with bioflavonoids	Take 1,000–2,500 mg, 4 times daily.	An antioxidant. Note: Use powdered, buffered ascorbic acid.
Vitamin E	Take 300–400 IU daily.	An antioxidant and free-radical scavenger.
Zinc and copper	Take 25–40 mg of zinc	Deficiency has been linked to eye problems. Note: Use the zinc picolinate form and be sure to include some copper; formulas that include both are available. Caution: Do not take more than 40 mg daily. It is not healthy to take excessive amounts of zinc.
Longevinex	As listed on the package	Shortens dark adaptation time, which is a measure of AMD progression.

HERBS AND HERBAL SUPPLEMENTS

Herb	Directions for Use	Comments
Bilberry	Take 160 mg daily.	Improves retinal function.
Blueberry	Drink 8–10 oz of juice daily.	Rich in flavonoids.
Ginkgo	Take as directed on the label.	The dry form stimulates blood flow in the capillaries. Do not take with wet AMD.

HOMEOPATHIC REMEDIES

Remedy	Directions for Use	Comments
Hamamelis virginiana 6c	Place 3–4 pellets under the tongue, 3–4 times daily.	Alleviates venous congestion and vascular infiltration.
Lachesis 6c	Place 3–4 pellets under the tongue, 3–4 times daily.	Good for macular degeneration with muscle fatigue.
Phosphorus 6c	Place 3–4 pellets under the tongue, 3–4 times daily.	Good for many eye conditions. Improves tissue metabolism, and reduces vascular and blood degeneration.

RECOMMENDATIONS

• While you can't stop the aging process, you can watch your diet. Eat a good-fat diet with lots of fresh vegetables and fruits, and a minimum of processed foods. Increase your consumption of legumes; yellow vegetables; flavonoid-rich berries, such as blueberries, blackberries, and cherries; and foods rich in vitamins C and E, such as raw fruits and vegetables.

• Avoid alcohol, cigarette smoke, all sugars, excessive saturated fats, and foods containing fats and oils that were subjected to heat or exposed to the air, such as fried foods, hamburgers, luncheon meats, and roasted nuts. These foods produce free radicals, which in turn contribute to poor eye health.

MEIBOMIAN CYST

See Chalazion, page 185.

MIGRAINE

See Headache, page 245.

MS, EYE PROBLEMS RELATED TO

See Multiple Sclerosis, page below.

MULTIPLE SCLEROSIS

Multiple sclerosis (MS) is an inflammatory disease of the body's central nervous system. This disease—which may, as it is now believed by many, originate with a viral infection—destroys the myelin sheaths (or coverings) of the body's nerves. Another theory is that MS is an autoimmune disease in which white blood cells attack the myelin sheaths as if they were foreign substances. The result is similar to what happens when you remove the insulation from wiring—the electrical impulses do not get to where they're going very well and escape to the wrong places.

Multiple sclerosis can affect the optic nerve itself, causing poor vision ranging from mild symptoms to changes in color vision, blind spots, and blindness. It can also affect the nerves that control the muscles of the eyes, causing double vision from strabismus, poor binocular coordination, and an uncontrollable jerking of the eye muscles. Very often, these visual problems are the first symptoms of MS.

MS is usually diagnosed between the ages of twenty-five and forty years. Women are affected nearly twice as often as men. MS is rarely diagnosed in children and in people over sixty years of age. Magnetic resonance imaging (MRI) may be used to diagnose MS. MRIs of the brain and spine can show areas of demyelination—loss of the covering of the nerve fibers. This is one marker for the disease. However, there is no single, definitive diagnostic test for MS; diagnosis must be done indirectly, by ruling out other possible causes of the symptoms.

Fortunately, most people with MS may have periods of remission during which their symptoms improve or even disappear. Many years can go by before serious visual impairment occurs, and it doesn't occur at all in some patients. Unfortunately, there is no known cure for MS, but certain dietary and supplemental approaches seem to be helpful. Long-term sufferers of MS may not benefit as much, but younger people who are just starting to exhibit symptoms may find that the correct supplements slow or even stop the progression of the disease.

Vision problems can be the first sign of multiple sclerosis. Symptoms of MS can include:

- Changes in color vision

- Blind spots

- Double vision

- Poor binocular coordination

- Uncontrollable jerking of the eye muscles

CONVENTIONAL TREATMENT

If you already have MS, you should see an eyecare professional in addition to your regular doctor. Systemic steroids and other medications are now used to improve the symptoms of multiple sclerosis, including eye problems. Such treatment options must be prescribed and monitored by a physician.

SELF-TREATMENT

A strong immune system may help to prevent the development of multiple sclerosis by assisting the body in avoiding infection, which often precedes the onset of the disease. Once you have had MS confirmed as a diagnosis, start to educate yourself and your family about the disease, and seek out sources of emotional support. Contact the National Multiple Sclerosis Society. (For the address and telephone number, see page 416 of Resource Organizations.) In addition, certain supplement and dietary recommendations, detailed below, have been known to help manage the disease. So watch your diet, take your supplements, and try to keep a positive attitude and a clean lifestyle.

NUTRITIONAL SUPPLEMENTS

SUPPLEMENT	DIRECTIONS FOR USE	COMMENTS
Choline	Take as directed on the label.	Stimulates the central nervous system and inositol protect the myelin sheaths from damage.
Coenzyme Q_{10}	Take 100 mg daily.	Boosts the circulation, improves tissue oxygenation, and strengthens the immune system.
Sulfur	Take 500 mg, 2–3 times daily.	Protects against toxic substances.
Vitamin-B complex	Take 100 mg, 3 times daily.	Aids immune function, and maintains healthy nerves. This complex should be part of your multivitamin.
Vitamin D	1,000 mg daily	Supports the immune system.

HERBS AND HERBAL SUPPLEMENTS

Herb	Directions for Use	Comments
Alfalfa	Take as directed on the label.	A good source of vitamin K.
Burdock	Take as directed on the label.	An excellent detoxifier.
Dandelion	Take as directed on the label.	An excellent detoxifier.
Echinacea	Take as directed on the label.	An excellent detoxifier.
Garlic	Take 1,000 mg, 3 times daily.	An excellent source of sulphur.
Goldenseal	Take as directed on the label.	An excellent detoxifier.
Lobelia	Take as directed on the label at bedtime.	Calms the nerves and prevents insomnia.
Red clover	Take as directed on the label.	An excellent detoxifier.
Sarsaparilla	Take as directed on the label.	An excellent detoxifier.
Skullcap	Take as directed on the label at bedtime.	Calms the nerves and prevents insomnia.
St. John's Wort	Take as directed on the label.	An excellent detoxifier.
Taheebo	Take as directed on the label.	An excellent detoxifier.
Valerian	Take as directed on the label at bedtime.	Calms the nerves and prevents insomnia.
Yarrow	Take as directed on the label.	An excellent detoxifier.

HOMEOPATHIC REMEDIES

Remedy	Directions for Use	Comments
Aurum 6c	Place 3–4 pellets under the tongue, 3–4 times daily.	Good for pain.
Gelsemium sempervirens 6c	Place 3–4 pellets under the tongue, 3–4 times daily.	Good for headaches with fever.
Hyoscyamus 6c	Place 3–4 pellets under the tongue, 3–4 times daily.	Relieves spasm.
Natrum muriaticum 6c	Place 3–4 pellets under the tongue, 3–4 times daily.	Good for pain.
Nitricum acidum 6c	Place 3–4 pellets under the tongue, 3–4 times daily.	Good for pain.

If you are young and just starting to experience the symptoms of MS, be aware that the right supplements and a healthy diet—one that is low in red meat and high in fresh fruits, vegetables, and whole grains—can slow or even stop the progression of the disease.

RECOMMENDATIONS

- The best diet for people with multiple sclerosis is one that contains no red meat. The reason is that it does not digest well—it remains in the colon for too long—and contains a lot of saturated fat.

- Eat only organically grown foods that have not been chemically treated and contain no chemical additives. Your diet should include eggs, fresh fruits, gluten-free grains, raw nuts and seeds, fresh vegetables, and cold-pressed vegetable oils.

- Eat plenty of raw sprouts and alfalfa, plus foods that contain lactic acid, such as sauerkraut and dill pickles.

- Green drinks, which contain plenty of chlorophyll, are healthy to consume, as are dark green, leafy vegetables such as spinach and kale. These are good sources of vitamin K.

- Drink at least eight 8-ounce glasses of quality water (alkaline water is suggested to reduce acidity in the body) each day to prevent toxic build-up in the muscles.

- Do not consume any alcohol, barley, chocolate, coffee, dairy products, fried foods, highly seasoned foods, red meat, oats, refined foods, rye, salt, spices, sugar, tobacco, wheat, and processed, canned, or frozen foods.

- Take a fiber supplement. Fiber is necessary for avoiding constipation. Also, periodically take warm, cleansing enemas. A clean colon is important for keeping toxic waste from interfering with muscle function.

- Avoid stress and anxiety. Attacks of MS are often precipitated by a trauma or a period of emotional distress.

MYOPIA

See Nearsightedness, below.

NEARSIGHTEDNESS

Nearsightedness, also called myopia (my-OH-pee-ah), means having good near vision but poor distance vision. For the myopic person, distant images—that is, images from objects at least 20 feet away—fall in front of the retina and look blurred. This misplacement of focus is the result of the eye being too long and therefore having a retina that is positioned farther back than normal; the cornea being too steeply curved; the eye's lens staying focused for near vision; or some combination of these and other factors. Myopia is the most common refractive error in humans, affecting over 35 percent of the population of the United States. It most often starts in childhood and continues to worsen until early adulthood, at which time, in the absence of other stress factors, it generally stabilizes.

It has been believed for a long time now that nearsightedness is inherited, and we do know that there is a heredity factor. Recent studies have shown that there is definitely a tendency for nearsightedness to develop more often in the children of nearsighted parents. However, this is probably not the whole story, because nearsightedness is much more prevalent in societies in which people do a lot of close work. Studies have found, for example, that nearsightedness is almost nonexistent in uneducated societies, and that it increases in proportion to the general level of education in the society. In other words, the more reading and near-point work a society does, the higher is its incidence of nearsightedness. Yet, there may be other environmental factors at work, which will be discussed below.

In a similar vein, studies have been conducted with Navy submariners, who are submerged for months at a time and spend their days in spaces where the maximum viewing distance is about eight feet. These studies have shown an increase in nearsightedness during these extended periods of confinement. Dr. Francis Young of Washington University has done similar research with monkeys. Dr. Young kept Rhesus monkeys in confined areas during various developmental periods of their early lives. The shorter the maximum viewing distance and the longer the confinement was, the more nearsighted the monkeys became.

So, what does this say about the way our eyes develop? The same as any biological system, our visual system adapts in response to stress. When you read, you use accomodation. Your eyes focus on a point only about 14 to 16 inches away. If you maintain a reading posture for long periods of time without taking breaks, your eyes will slowly adapt to the position in order to reduce the stress on the muscles controlling the lenses. Once adapted, the eyes can see more clearly up-close with less effort. It's as if the muscles get comfortably "stuck" in the near-focus position. To make matters worse, when the eye muscles must work constantly to accommodate for near-point work, pressure builds up in the eye. Eventually, this pressure causes the eyeball to lengthen in an effort to relieve the pressure, moving the retina

Studies have shown that nearsightedness is caused by the accommodation of the eye to near-point tasks, and tends to develop in school-aged children who are required to read constantly. Be sure that your child takes frequent breaks from near-point activities. Just looking out a window—or, better yet, getting up and going for a walk—can prevent eyes from getting "stuck" in the near-focus position.

even farther back from the lens than it was originally. Studies have shown that the sclera (the outer white coat of the eyeball) can "soften" due to a lack of nutrients or a condition called *hyperinsulinemia*, where too much insulin is produced in the body. This condition will affect genes that control growth factors, so the eyeball literally "grows too much." So, what is the result of all this? Nearsightedness. When a nearsighted eye relaxes in its attempts at accommodation and refocusing for distance vision, the images become blurred because they are too far forward of the retina. This doesn't happen just from reading steadily for a night or two. It's a gradual adaptation that your eyes make as they react to the strain of overwork.

To help prevent nearsightedness, try to keep books and other reading materials 14 to 16 inches away from your eyes. Also make sure that the room's lighting permits you to perform near-point tasks without straining.

In children, as you might expect, nearsightedness increases along with the amount of time spent focused for near-point activities. About 1.6 percent of children entering school in the United States have some degree of nearsightedness. That figure grows to 4.4 percent for seven- and eight-year-olds, 8.7 percent for nine- and ten-year-olds, 12.5 percent for eleven- and twelve-year-olds, and 14.3 percent for thirteen- and fourteen-year-olds. We used to say that the progression (worsening) of nearsightedness stabilizes at about twenty-one or twenty-two years of age. However, over the past fifteen years,

MYOPIA CONTROL

Studies show that myopic individuals are at higher risk of retinal detachment, myopic retinal degeneration, cataract, glaucoma, and other visual diseases, which is why it is so important to control the problem as best as possible. A typical program of myopia control consists of a combination of orthokeratology (see page 370), atropine eye drops, and soft multifocal contact lenses (see page 340).

Of course, it is better to avoid myopia, if possible, than to have to control it, and nutritional choices may help in this effort. Research has found that excess insulin in the bloodstream, a condition called *hyperinsulinemia*, which is generally caused by too much sugar in the diet, affects not only weight gain but

also a weakening and thinning of the sclera. With a combination of a weakened sclera and excessive near-point viewing, the eye tends to become elongated, creating a "long" eyeball, which is exactly the cause of myopia. Unfortunately, once the sclera has been elongated, it cannot be returned to its normal shape. Therefore, reversal of myopia is not possible simply by changes in diet.

It is imperative that parents be aware of their children's insulin levels, especially if either parent is myopic. Limiting your child's near-point viewing and making sure your child spends at least two hours outdoors every day can help to prevent the development of myopia.

eye doctors have seen more nearsightedness progressing well into the late twenties and even thirties. The reason? We're not quite sure, but computers are almost certainly one of the culprits. They require constant near-point focus, and an increasing number of children and adults are spending more of their time in front of computer displays and cell phones.

CONVENTIONAL TREATMENT

There is probably no escape from activities that require near-point focus. Consider all of the things we do with our eyes at the near point—reading, writing, drawing, computing, painting, sewing, crocheting, and even cooking and eating, to name just a few. And then there are those intermediate-distance tasks, such as playing the piano (reading music), shopping, working at computers, card playing, watching television, and enjoying a variety of hobbies. During the grade-school years, children read the equivalent of about 700 books. When this reading time is added to play time and computer time, it's not hard to see why so many people develop nearsightedness. Have you ever seen a lawyer, for example, who doesn't wear glasses? (If you have, that individual is probably wearing contacts!)

So, what can be done about all of this? Well, you could stay away from near-point activities, but that's not too practical. It is better to first make an appointment for a complete vision examination with an optometrist who performs near-vision tests. Many doctors omit the more thorough tests because they take an extended time to perform and evaluate than the simple tests for distance vision.

If glasses are prescribed, they won't "cure" you, but they certainly will improve your distance vision. However, you might be advised to remove your glasses for reading and other near-point activities, since wearing them for those activities will only force your eyes to accommodate more and may hasten the progression of your nearsightedness. Or, you might be given bifocals, with each eyeglass lens including a prescription section for distance vision and a section of lesser power for near vision. With these kinds of bifocals, you don't have to keep taking your glasses off for near-point activities. (No-line bifocals can work fine here too.) However, it has been confirmed that this technique to slow the progression of myopia is not very effective.

Although it is easier to prevent nearsightedness than it is to reverse it, vision therapy can diminish the condition. However, you must seriously dedicate yourself to your vision therapy program.

For many centuries, the only treatment for nearsightedness was eyeglasses. The eyeglass lenses were, and still are, designed to weaken the focusing strength of the light entering the eye so that it falls farther back toward the retina. Then, in the mid-1950s, contact lenses became a possible vision-correction device. Since then, many individuals have corrected their myopic vision by wearing contacts. The idea of using lenses that are in direct contact with the eye was actually conceived by Leonardo da Vinci. However, his idea didn't take off. Fast-forward a number of centuries, and we find that today there are many types of lenses available in several materials. For a description of the different types of contact lenses currently available, see page 338.

However, there are several drawbacks to using eyeglasses or contact lenses to correct nearsightedness. Glasses have a limited ability to correct peripheral vision. In addition, the thickness of the lenses can be extreme and can cause perceptual distortions. Contact lenses can overcome these difficulties, but they have problems of their own. Since they are in direct contact with the eye tissue, they can accumulate debris and proteins from the tears and harbor bacteria, which can lead to infections. The eye can react to the lens material or to the debris on the lens, both of which can decrease your ability to wear the lenses successfully.

More recently, a third alternative has emerged. It is called refractive surgery, and the term is an umbrella term for a number of procedures. But, in general, all of the procedures under that label attempt to move the point of focus of the light that is entering the eye more closely to the retina by surgically altering the shape of the cornea. Each of the surgical procedures has positive and negative aspects. For a discussion of the different types of refractive surgery being performed today, see page 371.

SELF-TREATMENT

At home, make sure that you have enough light for your near-point activities, and do not perform near-point work at a table or desk facing a wall. You want to be able to look up and focus for distance from time to time. Remember to follow the "20-20-20" rule: Every 20 minutes, take 20 seconds and look 20 feet away. Reading distance should be kept at 14 to 16 inches—no closer! (If you are not able to read at this distance, something is wrong and a full examination is indicated.) In short, give your eyes a chance to relax when doing a lot of close work, and schedule routine eye examinations to be sure everything is working properly.

Vision therapy is another alternative for nearsightedness. However, it is more difficult to reverse nearsightedness than it is to prevent it. If you are attempting to diminish your nearsightedness, you must seriously dedicate yourself to your vision therapy program, doing all of the required techniques on a regular basis. Changing the way you see is a monumental task, but you may be able to do it if you commit to the process and follow through completely. Usually, people with more severe nearsightedness can improve their myopia to a small degree with vision therapy, not enough to avoid the need for glasses or contacts lenses.

NUTRITIONAL SUPPLEMENTS

SUPPLEMENT	DIRECTIONS FOR USE	COMMENTS
Calcium	Take 800 mg daily.	Important in collagen formation.
Chromium	Take 80–100 mg daily.	Deficiencies have been found in persons with nearsightedness.
Copper	Take 2 mg daily.	Important in collagen formation.
Vitamin A	Take 2,500 IU daily.	Good for all eye conditions.
Vitamin C	Take 2,500 mg daily.	Strengthens the collagen for stronger eyes.

HERBS AND HERBAL SUPPLEMENTS

HERB	DIRECTIONS FOR USE	COMMENTS
Eyebright	Take as directed on the label.	Good for the eye tissues.
Ming mu shang qing pian (Brion)	Take 4 pills, 2 times daily.	Clarifies the vision. Caution: Do not use during pregnancy.

Because night blindness is usually caused by a vitamin-A deficiency, it is a rare condition in the United States. If you are having difficulty seeing at night, a full eye examination is recommended because this may be a symptom of a more serious eye disorder.

RECOMMENDATIONS

• Have your eyes checked regularly. This is especially important for school-aged children. Make sure that your near vision is tested.

• When doing a near-point activity, follow the "20-20-20" rule to give your eyes a rest.

• Increase your intake of protein and fiber, and reduce your intake of simple carbohydrates (sugar). Avoid most processed foods. High sugar content alters the structure of the lens inside the eye and can cause it to swell, creating a myopic condition.

• If you are sick with a fever, avoid near-point activities. High temperatures weaken and soften the collagen, which can easily become stretched with increased eye pressure.

NIGHT BLINDNESS

True night blindness is a relatively rare condition in the United States. The main symptom of this disorder is a decrease in visual acuity under nighttime viewing conditions. Most often, night blindness is caused by a nutritional deficiency—specifically, a vitamin-A deficiency—and is common in under-developed countries. Vitamin A is necessary for the formation of "visual purple," the pigment required by the retina to convert light energy to nerve energy. Other causes of night blindness are fatigue, emotional disturbances, and hereditary factors.

It is very common for persons who are just beginning to become near-sighted to complain of difficulty seeing clearly at night. This is different from true night blindness. The retina has a dual sensitivity; it is sharp in one area for daytime vision and in another for nighttime vision. The eyes generally become more nearsighted at night. In addition, our eyes are usually more fatigued after being used all day in stressful situations, thus leading to a poorer focusing ability by late in the day. Finally, when the light is dim, the pupil dilates, causing the visual image to be somewhat distorted. In addition, those who start developing cataracts will also notice difficulty seeing at night, typically due to the scattering of light associated with cataract formation.

There are, however, some very serious eye conditions in which the main symptom is night blindness. Most notable is retinitis pigmentosa, which is described in more detail beginning on page 318. Night driving is one of the most difficult tasks we do with our eyes. So, if you notice that you are having difficulty reading those street signs at night, a complete eye examination is in order.

CONVENTIONAL TREATMENT

The treatment for night blindness depends on the cause of the problem. For the simple problem of nearsightedness, glasses are normally prescribed, often just for nighttime driving. Contact lenses may also be recommended, but most likely for full-time wear rather than just nighttime viewing. If your eyes are not permanently nearsighted but merely overstressed, you may be advised to use reading glasses for your daily near-viewing activities. These will allow the eyes to relax more during close work and therefore keep them from being stressed for nighttime viewing.

For the serious causes, such as retinitis pigmentosa, there are no con-ventional treatments available. However, new research is showing that nutritional supplementation with vitamin A might have a slowing effect on the progression of the disease. However, this should be done under the supervision of a medical professional and is not something to be attempted on your own.

SELF-TREATMENT

In general, supplementing your diet with vitamin A will help to protect your eyes against night blindness. Also, vitamins B_1, B_2, and B_3, as well as zinc, have been reported to relieve night blindness when vitamin A does not produce a response. See the nutritional supplement chart below for dosage information.

However, the best thing that you can do if you notice a problem with your nighttime distance vision is to make an appointment for a full eye examination. It is important to confirm that there are no other underlying problems. Ask your doctor what alternatives are available for your specific condition.

NUTRITIONAL SUPPLEMENTS

SUPPLEMENT	DIRECTIONS FOR USE	COMMENTS
Vitamin A	Take 2,500 IU daily.	Supports the retina.
Vitamin-B complex	Take 75–100 mg daily.	Good for nerve function.
Zinc and copper	Take 25 mg of zinc and 2 mg of copper daily.	Good in combination with vitamin A. Note: The copper supplementation balances the zinc supplementation.

HERBS AND HERBAL SUPPLEMENTS

HERB	DIRECTIONS FOR USE	COMMENTS
Eyebright	Take as directed on the label.	Good for all eye conditions.
Qi ju di huang wan (Brion)	Take 8 pills, 3 times daily, or drink as a tea.	Aids liver function.

RECOMMENDATIONS

• Have a complete eye examination once a year. Regular examinations can catch night blindness before it becomes disabling.

- Remember, large doses of vitamin A can be harmful on a long-term basis, so if starting on a program to take this for a long period, please do so under your eye doctor's supervision.

NIGHT VISION, DECREASED

See Night Blindness, page 290.

NYSTAGMUS

Nystagmus (nis-TAG-mus) is characterized by involuntary movement—or "jerkiness"—of the eyes, which often seriously reduces vision. About 1 in every 1,000 people have this disorder, which is usually present at birth. Nystagmus often affects the nerves around the eye rather than the eye itself. Sufferers of nystagmus are not simply nearsighted. Many can and do register as "partially sighted" or even "legally blind." Their vision often varies throughout the day and is likely to be influenced by emotional and physical factors such as stress, fatigue, nervousness, and lack of familiarity with surroundings.

Most people with nystagmus encounter difficulties, both practical and social, in their everyday lives. For example, few can drive a car. Some even lose out on education and employment opportunities. Because depth perception is reduced by nystagmus, clumsiness and a proclivity for tripping result. People who have this disorder are generally coordinated enough to accomplish basic tasks but not activities that require good hand-eye coordination, such as sports.

Nystagmus may be inherited or it may be the result of a sensory problem. In fact, it can be one of the first signs of multiple sclerosis. (For a discussion of multiple sclerosis, see page 281.) It is also a common occurrence in albinism (see page 156). In a small number of cases, nystagmus occurs for no known reason. It can also develop later in life, sometimes as a result of an accident or illness, especially if the motor-muscle system has been affected.

If you are concerned that you or a member of your family has nystagmus, consult an eye doctor. Nystagmus affects different people in different ways. While there are general patterns, good advice for one person may be inappropriate or even bad for another, especially if additional eye problems are present.

Eyeglasses cannot correct nystagmus, but some simple changes can help you cope with this condition:

- When reading, find the angle of vision at which the print seems clear.

- Whenever possible, use large-print books.

- When working at a computer, make simple modifications to suit your needs. Adjust the position of the screen, increase or decrease brightness, and customize the size of the characters.

CONVENTIONAL TREATMENT

Since nystagmus most commonly begins at birth, the main goal of treatment is to minimize the visual disturbances caused by the condition. Nystagmus cannot be corrected with eyeglasses. However, contact lenses, especially the gas permeable type, occasionally are useful in reducing the magnitude of the jerkiness. We're not exactly sure why this happens, but many think that the "feel" of the lenses gives some feedback to the brain and the eye movements slow down as a result. Others think that the contact lens provides a more stable image to the eye, so it slows down the movement.

In some cases, vision therapy (see page 385) may help to reduce the symptoms somewhat and give the person some control of her eye muscles. But there is no real treatment specifically for nystagmus. Keep in mind; it can simply be a symptom of a more severe condition.

SELF-TREATMENT

For people with nystagmus, the angle of vision is important. Most sufferers have something called a "null point," an angle where eye movement is reduced and vision is improved. Those with a null point often adopt an awkward head posture that makes the best use of their vision.

As far as classroom or office work is concerned, sitting to one side of the computer monitor or blackboard often helps. Many can read very small print if they get close enough or use a visual aid. However, the option of using large-print material should be available, and all written matter should be clear. It is very hard for a person with nystagmus to share a book with someone else because the book will probably be too far away or at the wrong angle. In addition, reading speed might be reduced because of the extra time needed to scan. But this should not be taken as a sign of poor reading ability.

Good lighting is essential to the person with nystagmus. If necessary, find a lighting specialist who can make sure that all tasks are well illuminated.

Computers are used by many people with nystagmus who find it helpful to be able to position the screen, adjust the brightness, customize the character sizes, and so on, to suit their own needs. However, that being said, some people find it difficult to read traditional computer screens. So, each separate case of nystagmus must be managed according to the individual's specific needs.

Depending on the cause of the nystagmus, color therapy may also be appropriate. Color therapy serves to stimulate the eyes to maximize the vision. For a complete discussion of color therapy, see "Syntonics" on page 383. See the "Recommendations" area of this discussion for further pointers on dealing with nystagmus.

Since nystagmus causes the eyes to jerk involuntarily, it's common to lose your place while reading. A dark card that marks the line being read can make the task far easier.

NUTRITIONAL SUPPLEMENTS

SUPPLEMENT	DIRECTIONS FOR USE	COMMENTS
Vitamin-B complex	Take at least 100 mg daily.	Good for nerve function.

HOMEOPATHIC REMEDIES

REMEDY	DIRECTIONS FOR USE	COMMENTS
Calacarea carbonica 6c	Place 3–4 pellets under the tongue, 3–4 times daily.	Improves mineral absorption and utilization.
Magnesia phosphorica 6c	Place 3–4 pellets under the tongue, 3–4 times daily.	Relieves muscle spasm.

RECOMMENDATIONS

• Good lighting is important, especially since some persons with nystagmus are also light sensitive. If necessary, hire a lighting specialist to make your home a more comfortable place in which to live.

• Ask your doctor about having an MRI. A brain scan will help to rule out disorders that may be contributing to the nystagmus, or even causing it.

• If you are a parent or teacher of an individual who has nystagmus, encourage the student to explain her visual needs to classmates and other teachers. However, avoid continual and undue attention to those needs. The remaining tips are also for the parent and/or teacher of a person with nystagmus:

■ Allow the individual to hold books and other objects close to the eyes, to tilt the head, and to adopt any other body posture that enhances vision.

■ Provide her with personal books and worksheets, as sharing is impractical.

■ Enlarging the text of printed materials often helps, although good contrast may suffice.

■ Use strong color contrast between letters, figures, lines, and the background. Make sure to use good spacing.

■ Place wall displays for reference at eye level (not above a filing cabinet or table, for example) and where the person with nystagmus can stand close to it.

- Allow the student to choose where she sits. Often, that will be in front of and near to the board, but it may also be off to one side. In addition, allow the student to sit closely to demonstrations during activities.

- Store visual aids so that the individual with nystagmus can easily reach them when needed.

- Allow the student to use prescribed tinted glasses, a cap, a hat, or eye-shades to reduce the effects of glare.

- Read aloud when you write on the board, and describe any diagrams you draw.

- Allow the student sufficient time to complete tasks and to examine materials and objects.

- Good (although not necessarily bright) lighting is essential. The light should be behind the student and directed onto the object being viewed. Matte surfaces on walls, boards, and paper prevent light reflection and glare.

- To help the child with nystagmus keep track of her place while reading, encourage the use of a dark card or a finger. Keep on hand exercise books with matte paper, different colors, and ruled lines.

OPTIC ATROPHY

Optic atrophy (AT-troh-fee) was first described by the German eye specialist Theodore Leber in 1871, so it is often known as "Leber's hereditary optic neuropathy" (noor-OP-ath-ee), or LHON. It consists of a slow decaying, or dying, of the optic nerve. The illness usually occurs in males, although some females are affected. There is no warning of the onset of the condition.

Once a member of a family is diagnosed as having optic atrophy, other members of the family become potential sufferers or carriers. Only females can pass the problem on to their children; males are not known to transmit the disease. Fortunately, not every at-risk individual will become a sufferer. Unfortunately, there is no way of predicting who will develop the symptoms. If the symptoms do develop, both eyes are normally involved, even if to varying degrees. Some of the early changes that occur in the eyes of sufferers, such as an increase in the number of minute blood vessels at the back of the eye and the loss of color vision prior to vision loss, may also be found in subjects at risk. But, as indicated above, this does not help to predict which people will lose their sight. The eyesight can deteriorate over a period of hours or months. Very rarely, the eyesight may partially or completely improve again. Early eye exams are essential.

In 1988 researchers discovered that LHON is one of a group of mitochondrial genetic diseases that are inherited only through the mother. As we have reviewed, the mitochondria are the cell bodies where energy needed for the activities of the cell is produced from oxygen. There are now some twenty different genes known to take part in the development of LHON. Three particular mutations account for 85 to 90 percent of the cases of LHON. However, the mitochondrial mutation is clearly not the only genetic factor involved in the disease, as not every carrier is affected and men are at higher risk than women.

Most sufferers of optic atrophy are registered as legally blind, although many retain enough usable eyesight to remain navigational—that is, they can move around fairly well in familiar surroundings, but cannot drive and cannot read without massive magnification. Typically, sufferers cannot recognize people in the street, although they may be able to discern moving shapes as those people approach. There is often no way of recognizing a sufferer in public because the defect is in the optic nerve. The eyes appear normal to the casual onlooker.

There is no proven cause of or cure for the disease. As mentioned, genetic defects have been identified in some sufferers, but they do not yet help to predict future sufferers, as many people carry the defects but do not lose their vision. Research has shown a deficiency of an enzyme called rhodanese in those who suffer from optic atrophy, but the significance of this finding is also unknown. However, since one of the functions of rhodanese is to detoxify cyanide, doctors recommend that subjects at risk of developing optic neuropathy do not smoke.

Because there is no way to halt or treat this disorder, the only applicable advice to offer is that if you are diagnosed with optic atrophy, make sure you surround yourself with a solid support team. Also, maintain your health as much as possible so that you have the energy, motivation, and insights to develop a lifestyle that allows you to accomplish what you desire.

If you have been diagnosed with optic atrophy, avoid smoking, smoke-filled rooms, and alcohol. This may help slow the progression of the disease.

CONVENTIONAL TREATMENT

Glasses and contact lenses are of no practical help for those who struggle with optic atrophy. Unfortunately, doctors cannot offer conventional therapeutic aid. They do recommend a cessation of physical exercise during the acute phase of sight loss, however.

SELF-TREATMENT

As detailed above, optic atrophy is a severe condition that is not considered treatable. Some limited benefits may be derived from syntonics (see page 383), a type of color therapy that can serve to stimulate and balance the nerves in the proper way. Other than that, maintaining a healthy lifestyle can help those with optic atrophy to keep the body and mind functioning as optimally as possible, therefore allowing an overall sense of well-being.

NUTRITIONAL SUPPLEMENTS

SUPPLEMENT	DIRECTIONS FOR USE	COMMENTS
Vitamin A	Take 2,500 IU daily.	Good for all eye conditions.
Vitamin-B complex	Take 75–100 mg daily.	Maintains healthy nerves.

HOMEOPATHIC REMEDIES

REMEDY	DIRECTIONS FOR USE	COMMENTS
Nux vomica 6c	Place 3–4 pellets under the tongue, 3–4 times daily.	Reduces nerve and vascular irritability.
Phosphorus 6c	Place 3–4 pellets under the tongue, 3–4 times daily.	Improves tissue metabolism and supports nerve and vascular integrity.

Symptoms of optic neuritis—inflammation of the optic nerve—include eye pain, disturbed color vision, and loss of vision. Fortunately, the majority of patients recover their vision within a few months.

RECOMMENDATIONS

• Avoid smoking and smoke-filled rooms. (See the section on "Conventional Treatments" on page 296 for an explanation.)

• Eliminate alcohol consumption, especially if you are in the process of losing your sight. There is a disorder called alcohol amblyopia that is a secondary blindness caused by alcohol intoxication. Clearly, someone who is already ocularly disadvantaged would not want to exacerbate occurring vision problems.

OPTIC NERVE, DECAY OF

See Optic Atrophy, page 295.

OPTIC NERVE, INFLAMMATION OF

See Optic Neuritis, below.

OPTIC NEURITIS

Optic neuritis (nur-EYE-tis) is an inflammation of the optic nerve. It is also known as retrobulbar neuritis, since the nerve is behind (retro) the globe of the eye. Optic neuritis is generally experienced as an acute blurring, graying, or loss of vision. This disorder usually occurs in one eye, although occasionally in both eyes (see below). The visual deficit tends to reach its maximum within a few days and then improve within eight to twelve weeks.

Optic neuritis typically presents with a triad of symptoms—loss of vision, disturbed color vision, and eye pain (often with eye movement). The initial attack is in just one eye in 70 percent of adult patients and in both eyes in 30 percent. The mean age-range of onset of the disorder is the twenties, but it can develop anytime from birth through the sixties. The annual incidence of optic neuritis ranges from 1.4 to 6.4 new cases per 100,000 people. Associated visual symptoms include reduced perception of light intensity and loss of vision induced by exercise or increased body temperature.

The visual loss accompanying optic neuritis can be subtle or profound. In some cases, the vision may be 20/20 with blurring upon exertion as the only symptom. The rate of visual decline varies; it can occur over a period of hours (rarely) to days (most commonly). The peak visual loss most often is about one week after the onset of the disorder.

The prognosis for visual recovery usually is good. The majority of patients—that is, 65 to 80 percent—recover a visual acuity of 20/30 or better. Most patients recover their visual acuity within a few months, although they often report some residual visual defects. These residual defects have included decreased contrast sensitivity, disturbed color vision, visual field constriction, and light sensitivity.

Optic neuritis is sometimes caused by a vitamin-B deficiency. In this case, vitamin-B supplementation usually results in recovery within three to four days.

Sometimes optic neuritis is associated with a vitamin-B deficiency, but most of the time it is caused by another disease process. In a young, otherwise healthy person, multiple sclerosis (MS) is the most likely cause. It has been estimated that about 55 percent of patients with multiple sclerosis have an episode of optic neuritis. Frequently, optic neuritis is the first symptom of MS. While estimates of the subsequent development of MS in a person who presents with optic neuritis vary, studies that include up to ten years of follow-up have demonstrated that approximately 50 to 60 percent of patients with isolated optic neuritis go on to develop MS. A more recent study reported that persons with optic neuritis who also had abnormalities in their spinal fluid were more likely to develop MS. Other studies have demonstrated that a majority of patients with optic neuritis have evidence of demyelination (wearing away of the nerve sheath) in the brain, as evidenced on MRI scanning. For a more comprehensive discussion of MS, see page 281.

CONVENTIONAL TREATMENT

There are no optical corrections that will help with the loss of vision caused by optic neuritis. Recent studies suggest that a short course of intravenous steroids, followed by a tapered course of oral steroids, may be useful in helping to reverse and restore vision damaged by optic neuritis. However, there is no definitive evidence that treatment with steroids affects a more complete recovery than no treatment at all. Also, long-term steroid use is discouraged due to the long list of complications from such therapy. MRIs are standard protocol for this condition.

SELF-TREATMENT

When a B-complex or vitamin-B_1 deficiency is responsible for the optic neuritis, supplementing with these vitamins will result in recovery within three to four days. The B vitamins must be taken in adequate amounts even when a deficiency doesn't exist. They are needed for the general health of nerve tissue.

A well-balanced diet is important for the maintenance and repair of the muscles and nerves. Whenever you have an infection, you should boost your protein, calorie, and fluid intakes. Flare-ups of optic neuritis should be managed similarly. Take care to eat well, rest well, and avoid unnecessary stress.

NUTRITIONAL SUPPLEMENTS

SUPPLEMENT	DIRECTIONS FOR USE	COMMENTS
Essential fatty acids	Take 1,000 mg EPA/DHA daily.	Repair and rebuild the nerves.
Glutathione	Take 500–1,000 mg daily.	Supports the nerve and brain tissues.
Lecithin	Take 2 tbsp, 2 times daily.	Protects and repairs the nerves. Note: Use the granular form.
Magnesium	Take 400 mg daily.	Helps the body to utilize the B-complex vitamins.

SUPPLEMENT	DIRECTIONS FOR USE	COMMENTS
Protein	Take .5 gm for every 1 lb of body weight daily.	Important for the repair of body tissues.
Vitamin-B complex	Take at least 100 mg daily.	Good for nerve function.

HERBS AND HERBAL SUPPLEMENTS

HERB	DIRECTIONS FOR USE	COMMENTS
Bilberry	Take 60 mg daily.	An antioxidant.
Oats	Take as directed on the label.	Calms the nerves and soothes the mucous membranes.
Skullcap	Take as directed on the label.	Calms the nerves and relieves spasm.
St. John's wort	Take as directed on the label.	An anti-inflammatory that repairs and rebuilds the nerves, as well as increases blood flow.
Valerian	Take as directed on the label.	Calms the nerves and relieves spasm.

HOMEOPATHIC REMEDIES

REMEDY	DIRECTIONS FOR USE	COMMENTS
Aconite 6c	Place 3–4 pellets under the tongue, 3–4 times daily.	Good for optic neuritis in the early stages, as well as for pain and inflammation.
Apis mellifica 6c	Place 3–4 pellets under the tongue, 3–4 times daily.	Good for inflammation.
Hypericum perforatum 6c	Place 3–4 pellets under the tongue, 3–4 times daily.	Reduces nerve irritability.
Phosphorus 6c	Place 3–4 pellets under the tongue, 3–4 times daily.	Good for many eye conditions.
Spigelia 6c	Place 3–4 pellets under the tongue, 3–4 times daily.	Good for pain and nerve sensitivity.

RECOMMENDATIONS

• Relaxation is a key component of the healing process. Reduce the stress level in all of the areas of your life.

• Avoid stimulants such as coffee, carbonated beverages, and cigarettes, which can irritate the nervous system and, thus, the optic nerve.

- Increase your fluid intake, as that helps to wash away irritants and toxins, as well as maintain good fluid balance.

- Eat a diet of fresh fruits and vegetables, raw nuts and seeds, and whole grains. Good dietary decisions will help your body to recover more quickly.

OVERCONVERGENCE OF THE EYES

See Convergence Excess, page 193.

PHOTOPHOBIA

See Light Sensitivity, page 268.

PIGMENT DEFICIENCY

See Albinism, page 156.

PIMPLE ON THE EYELID

See Stye, page 324.

PINGUECULA

The word *pinguecula* (pin-GWEK-yoo-lah) comes from the Latin word for "fatty." A pinguecula is a yellowish patch that forms in the white part of the eye, often at the three-o'clock or nine-o'clock position in relation to the cornea. See the illustration provided by Figure 2.6. There may be more than one pinguecula present in each eye. Pingueculae are completely different from jaundice, which causes a generalized yellowing of the entire sclera. They are believed to be caused by exposure to excessive UV light, dust, or wind, and are common in farmers, gardeners, lifeguards, surfers, and construction workers—if these individuals work outdoors and don't wear good protective sunglasses.

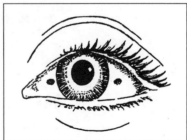

FIGURE 2.6
An Eye Affected by Pingueculae.

Pingueculae do not need to be removed since they do not affect the vision of the patient. These patches do tend to swell when irritated, but they return to a stable condition once the irritant has been removed.

CONVENTIONAL TREATMENT

Currently, there is no medical treatment for pingueculae because they are not sight-threatening. They are more cosmetically unappealing than dangerous. However, the presence of pingueculae does indicate that the eye is under environmental stress, and that some action needs to be taken. In general, the conventional treatment for pingueculae is to reduce the irritation to the eye. Many doctors simply recommend over-the-counter eye lubricants.

SELF-TREATMENT

A soothing eyewash is the best remedy to quiet a pinguecula that is irritated. Use the herbal remedies recommended below as eyewashes. Do not use eye drops that are intended to whiten the eye. However, as mentioned above, the new eye drop called Lumify (Baush+Lomb) does effectively whiten the eye with no "rebound" effect.

Moreover, stay out of irritating environments such as dusty or heavily polluted areas. That way, the swelling can be reduced or avoided. And wear sunglasses when outdoors for extended periods of time. If your eyes also feel dry, follow the suggestions in the section on dry eye disease (see page 215).

NUTRITIONAL SUPPLEMENTS

SUPPLEMENT	DIRECTIONS FOR USE	COMMENTS
CapsiClear	Take 1 gelcap, 2 times daily.	Maintains proper tear film.
Vitamin A	Take 2,500 IU daily.	Good for all eye conditions.
Vitamin C	Take 1,000–3,000 mg daily, in divided doses.	Protects the eye and aids tissue healing.
Zinc and copper	Take 25 mg of zinc and 2 mg of copper daily.	Enhances the immune response.

HERBS AND HERBAL SUPPLEMENTS

HERB	DIRECTIONS FOR USE	COMMENTS
Chamomile	Apply as a hot compress, or use as an eyewash.	Soothing for the eye tissues.
Eyebright and fennel	Apply as a hot compress, or use as a cool eyewash.	Good for inflammation.

HOMEOPATHIC REMEDIES

REMEDY	DIRECTIONS FOR USE	COMMENTS
Apis mellifica 6c	Place 3–4 pellets under the tongue, 3–4 times daily.	Relieves swelling around the eyes.
Pulsatilla 6c	Place 3–4 pellets under the tongue, 3–4 times daily.	Good for eyelids that are stuck together, although this does not typically happen with pinguecula—only if the eyelids are inflamed.
Ruta graveolens 6c	Place 3–4 pellets under the tongue, 3–4 times daily.	Good for hot, red, inflamed eyes.
Sulphur 6c	Place 3–4 pellets under the tongue, 3–4 times daily.	Good for red, inflamed eyelids.

RECOMMENDATIONS

• If you believe that you may have a pinguecula, see your eye doctor. A routine examination should confirm your self-diagnosis and allay any fears that your condition is more serious.

• Watch your cholesterol level. Some experts feel that a pinguecula might indicate a high blood-cholesterol level. However, no research has been conducted as of yet to explore this connection.

PINKEYE

Pinkeye, more properly known as *conjunctivitis* (con-junk-tiv-EYE-tis), refers to an inflammation of the conjunctiva. That is the mucous membrane that lines the eyelids and also covers the exposed surface of the sclera. Pinkeye can be caused by a bacterial, viral, or fungal infection; by an allergy; or by anything that has irritated the conjunctiva.

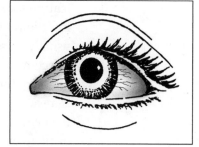

Bacterial conjunctivitis can be recognized by a discharge that contains pus and sticky, crusty eyelids that may have to be pried open in the morning. The mucous tissue under the eyelids is beefy red, and the eyes feel sore. The white part of the eyes looks red, with large, twisted blood vessels. See Figure 2.7, "An Eye Affected by Pinkeye." Bacterial conjunctivitis can strike people of all ages, but it's especially common in children, whose hand-washing

FIGURE 2.7
An Eye Affected by Pinkeye.

and other hygienic practices tend to be less than adequate. In fact, children should be encouraged not to rub their eyes with dirty fingers because it is easy to develop bacterial conjunctivitis when they do so. This type of conjunctivitis is usually self-limiting and generally responds to hot compresses. However, if it doesn't resolve within a few days, you should see an eye doctor.

Viral conjunctivitis looks a little different from the bacterial type. The viral type is somewhat more common in adults rather than in children, although children also get it. This kind of infection may start in the eyes, or it may be a part of a systemic virus that is also causing a cold or sore throat. When this happens, it just means that the virus has gotten into the conjunctiva along with other parts of the body. The discharge from the eyes is usually more watery and less sticky than that associated with a bacterial infection. The conjunctiva inside the eyelid is red and sometimes has raised spots that look like little cobblestones. The eyes hurt and look red. Antibiotics don't help viral conjunctivitis, but the infection usually clears up within a few days without any treatment.

Fungal infections of the conjunctiva can also occur, especially in people whose immune systems are not functioning properly, such as cancer and AIDS patients and people taking medications that suppress the immune system. The latter might include, for example, someone who has had an organ transplant. Fungal infections can be dangerous, and so they require prompt treatment with special anti-fungal medications. It's hard to diagnose fungal conjunctivitis by yourself, but if you develop any kind of conjunctival infection while on medications that suppress your immunity or while being treated for AIDS or cancer, see your doctor immediately. Fungal infections can also occur with poor hygiene and contact lens wearing.

Allergic conjunctivitis is pinkeye caused by an allergy. An important feature that distinguishes allergic from infectious conjunctivitis is itching. Infections of the conjunctiva hurt; allergic reactions itch. Also, the eyelashes usually do not become matted with allergic conjunctivitis as they do with an infection, especially a bacterial one. The conjunctiva is usually swollen, and although the sclera may be red, the undersides of the eyelids are pale. There is a watery discharge that weeps from the eye. Allergic reactions involving the eyes also frequently involve sneezing, wheezing, and other symptoms of allergies to animals or plants. These reactions can be treated with antihistamines by mouth or with eye drops that block allergic reactions.

In general, pinkeye can be a very trivial or a potentially serious problem. See your eye doctor if your pinkeye doesn't clear up within a couple of days.

FIRST AID FOR PINKEYE

- Call your eye doctor as soon as possible after noticing the first symptoms.

- Avoid touching your eyes, especially with unclean hands.

- Apply a warm, wet washcloth to the affected eye several times per day.

When pinkeye is caused by an infection, it is highly contagious. It can be spread by sharing a towel, handkerchief, or makeup brush. Therefore, if you have contracted pinkeye, you should not share personal items and should wash your hands frequently.

CONVENTIONAL TREATMENT

The conventional treatment for pinkeye generally depends on the cause of the condition. Bacterial conjunctivitis is usually treated with antibiotics. The treatments are most often topical.

Viral conjunctivitis can be treated with antiviral medications, but often it is left untreated because it may clear up as a result of the treatments already being used for the systemic viral condition. In other words, since the conjunctivitis is part of a virus' path, the usual treatment addresses the general virus situation, not the eye specifically. Some doctors recommend the use of steroid ointments or eye drops to alleviate the inflammation in viral conjunctivitis, but this may be dangerous if misdiagnosed. And if the infection happens to be caused by a herpes virus, the steroids can make it much worse. Sometimes it's best to just leave well enough alone.

Fungal forms of conjunctivitis are treated with topical antifungals. Allergic conjunctivitis is usually treated symptomatically—that is, by reducing the itching and inflammation of the eye tissue along with treating the rest of the allergy symptoms. Topical antihistamines are generally the medications of choice for that type of conjunctivitis. To avoid allergic conjunctivitis, it is very helpful to flush your eyes with an eyewash if you've been around something to which you're allergic.

If your conjunctivitis symptoms include itching, the condition is probably caused by an allergy and can be relieved with topical antihistamines. Once the eye recovers, try periodically flushing it with eyewash to remove pollen and other allergens.

SELF-TREATMENT

You can try to treat your pinkeye with a hot compress—that is, very warm water on a clean washcloth—two or three times per day. Use this treatment specifically if your lids are sticking together in the morning. However, if the pinkeye doesn't resolve within a few days, see your doctor. Importantly, if you suspect allergic conjunctivitis, use a *cold* compress to reduce the itching.

In addition, be sure to clean your hands and face often, and splash your eyes with cold water. Do not use any over-the-counter preparations that promise to remove redness from the eyes. However, there are several herbal and homeopathic eye treatments that may help. See the following page.

NUTRITIONAL SUPPLEMENTS

SUPPLEMENT	DIRECTIONS FOR USE	COMMENTS
Vitamin A	Take 2,500 IU daily.	Good for all eye conditions.
Vitamin C	Take 1,000–3,000 mg daily, in divided doses.	Protects the eye, and aids tissue healing.
Zinc and copper	Take 25 mg of zinc and 2 mg of copper daily.	Enhances the immune response.

HERBS AND HERBAL SUPPLEMENTS

HERB	DIRECTIONS FOR USE	COMMENTS
An mian pian (Brion)	Take 4 pills, 3 times daily.	Purges "heat" from the liver.
Chamomile	Apply as a hot compress, or use as an eyewash.	Soothing for the eye tissues.
Eyebright and fennel	Apply as a hot compress, or use as an eyewash.	Boost the circulation.
Long dan xie gan wan (Brion)	Take 6 pills, 2 times daily.	Purges "heat" from the liver and gallbladder.
Ming mu di huang wan (Brion)	Take 10 pills, 3 times daily.	Good for red or itchy eyes.
Ming mu shang qing pian (Brion)	Take 4 pills, 2 times daily.	Good for red, itchy, or burning eyes. Caution: Do not use during pregnancy.
Nei zhang ming yan wan (Brion)	Take 8 pills, 3 times daily.	Good for itchy, painful eyes. Caution: Contains aluminum, so limit its use.
Shi hu ye guang wan (Brion)	Take 1 pill, 2 times daily.	Good for red or itchy eyes.
Xiao yao wan (Brion)	Take 8 pills, 3 times daily.	Invigorates a congested liver.

The eyes' focusing ability peaks at about ten years of age. As an individual gets older, the eyes' lenses become thicker and stiffer, eventually leading to presbyopia, or the inability to focus on near-point objects.

HOMEOPATHIC REMEDIES

REMEDY	DIRECTIONS FOR USE	COMMENTS
Aconite 6c	Place 3–4 pellets under the tongue, 3–4 times daily.	Good for inflammation.
Allium cepa 6c	Place 3–4 pellets under the tongue.	Good for inflammation.
Anacardium 6c	Place 3–4 pellets under the tongue.	Alleviates swelling.

REMEDY	DIRECTIONS FOR USE	COMMENTS
Apis mellifica 6c	Place 3–4 pellets under the tongue.	Good for pinkeye with swollen eyelids; alleviates edema and inflammation.
Arnica montana 6c	Place 3–4 pellets under the tongue.	Good for inflammation.
Arsenicum album 6c	Place 3–4 pellets under the tongue.	Good for inflammation.
Belladonna 6c	Place 3–4 pellets under the tongue.	Good for inflammation.
Calcarea fluorica 6c	Place 3–4 pellets under the tongue, 3–4 times daily.	Good for inflammation; relieves discharge.
Calcarea sulfurica 6c	Place 3–4 pellets under the tongue, 3–4 times daily.	Good for inflammation; relieves discharge.
Causticum 6c	Place 3–4 pellets under the tongue.	Relieves discharge.
Euphrasia officinalis 6c	Place 3–4 pellets under the tongue, 3–4 times daily.	Good for inflammation.
Graphites 9c	Place 3–4 pellets under the tongue, 3–4 times daily.	Good for inflamed eyelids.
Mercurius corrosivus 6c	Place 3–4 pellets under the tongue, 3–4 times daily.	An infection fighter; good for pinkeye with mucus discharge.
Mercurius vivus 6c	Place 3–4 pellets under the tongue, 3–4 times daily.	Good for inflammation; relieves discharge.
Natrum muriaticum 6c	Place 3–4 pellets under the tongue, 3–4 times daily.	Good for inflammation.
Pulsatilla 6c	Place 3–4 pellets under the tongue, 3–4 times daily.	Good for inflammation and for allergic conjunctivitis; relieves discharge.
Rhus toxicodendron 6c	Place 3–4 pellets under the tongue, 3–4 times daily.	Good for inflammation; alleviates swelling.
Ruta graveolens 6c	Place 3–4 pellets under the tongue, 3–4 times daily.	Good for inflammation.
Sepia 6c	Place 3–4 pellets under the tongue, 3–4 times daily.	Good for inflammation; alleviates swelling.
Silicea 6c	Place 3–4 pellets under the tongue, 3–4 times daily.	Good for inflammation.
Sulphur 6c	Place 3–4 pellets under the tongue, 3–4 times daily.	Good for inflammation and for allergic conjunctivitis.

RECOMMENDATIONS

● Pinkeye is one of the most contagious diseases currently known. Children seem to be more susceptible to it, probably due to their lack of proper hygiene. Teach your child to wash her hands properly and to keep the hands away from the eyes.

● You should identify what type of pinkeye you have so that treatments are effective. If you are unsure of the type, see an eye doctor for proper diagnosis.

PINKEYE, CONTACT LENS-RELATED

See Giant Papillary Conjunctivitis, page 230.

PRESBYOPIA

During our first thirty to forty years of life, our eyes work busily to see everything they can, especially when we read and perform other near-point tasks. When our eyes are relaxed, they are, theoretically, in focus for distance vision. As we move closer to an object, we must actively increase the focal power of the lenses inside our eyes to keep the object clear. This is very easy to do when our eyes, and our bodies, are young. In fact, our focusing ability is at its maximum when we are about ten years old. As we grow older, however, our eyes' lenses become thicker and stiffer, and our maximum focusing ability—actually, the ability of our lenses to become rounded, as they must to do near-point work—diminishes. Eventually, we notice a blur at close range.

Although this process of the lenses becoming hardened is continuous throughout life, it isn't given a name until we are unable to focus on the near image (16 inches away or less) comfortably. The condition is then called presbyopia (prez-bee-OH-pee-ah). The word comes from the Greek word *presbys*, which means "old," and *opia*, which refers to "vision."

Looking at this problem in perspective should help to give you a better idea of why it happens. Consider prehistoric man. In those early caveman days, the life expectancy was only about twenty-five to thirty years. The only near-point activities were cooking and making weapons, neither of which was extremely detailed work. Most of the visual requirements at that

Drugstore reading glasses are inexpensive and easy to obtain, but are really not the best option for people with presbyopia. In fact, these "cheater" glasses can actually increase eyestrain. Instead, get prescription glasses, which are of better optical quality and will provide you with the exact prescription you need.

time were distance tasks, such as spotting that night's dinner and keeping from becoming someone else's dinner. So, really, the eyes were originally designed to focus adequately for an entire lifetime. Now, though, people live a lot longer than thirty years!

CONVENTIONAL TREATMENT

One way to compensate for the deficiency in near vision is to use a prescription lens that helps the eye to focus. If you already wear glasses to see clearly at a distance, you'll need two different lens prescriptions—one for distance vision and one for near vision. One way to handle this double prescription is with bifocals or progressive addition lenses. The top half of the lens is for distance vision, and the lower half is for near vision.

Do not use the kind of reading glasses that can be bought without a prescription. They are not likely to be the exact prescription you need, and the lenses will be of poor optical quality. Many people use these "cheater" reading glasses for extensive near work such as computer use. But this can cause more strain on the eyes.

Recently, eye drops have been marketed to allow those with presbyopia to read without glasses. The Vuity (Abbie) medication is a reformulated glaucoma medication (pilocarpine) that constricts (makes smaller) the pupil. This effectively increases the focal "depth of field," allowing clearer near vision. It's not for everyone, and they claim that it works most effectively on those between the ages of forty and fifty-five (early presbyopia). As with all medications, there are some side effects but there will be some who appreciate putting off reading glasses for a few years. Ask your doctor for advice.

SELF-TREATMENT

There is a school of thought that says presbyopia is not an inevitable consequence of aging, but instead is the result of years of improper nutrition, stress, inadequate exercise, and faulty oxygenation of the body. Even if you do everything right, you cannot prevent the development of presbyopia entirely, but you may be able to postpone it or slow it down with good nutrition, aerobic exercise, and generally healthful living. Like any part of the body, the lens will stay younger longer with the aid of good overall health.

In addition to general exercise and good nutrition, before you approach the "bifocal age," you should do the following simple technique several times each day. The technique consists of focusing from near to far (at least 20 feet away) and back to near again. This keeps the muscle that controls the lens in good working order and the lens as flexible as possible. For more techniques that may help, see "Vision Therapy" on page 385.

NUTRITIONAL SUPPLEMENTS

SUPPLEMENT	DIRECTIONS FOR USE	COMMENTS
Glutathione	Take as directed on the label.	Maintains the clarity of the lens.
Vitamin B$_2$	Take 50 mg daily.	Alleviates eye fatigue.
Vitamin C	Take 2,000–3,000 mg daily in divided doses.	Maintains the flexibility of the lens.
Vitamin E	Take 400 IU daily.	Alleviates eyestrain.

HOMEOPATHIC REMEDIES

REMEDY	DIRECTIONS FOR USE	COMMENTS
Calcarea fluorica 6c	Place 3–4 pellets under the tongue, 3–4 times daily.	Supports the connective tissue.

RECOMMENDATIONS

● Presbyopia is a gradual process, though you may wake up one day and discover that reading is suddenly difficult. Maintaining your focusing ability is much easier than trying to regain a lost ability. So, watch what you eat, get enough exercise, and try to keep your stress level down.

● Sometimes a medication can cause a fairly rapid loss of focusing ability if it affects muscle function. If you are taking medications and notice a loss of focusing ability, be sure to check with your doctor and tell him about your symptoms.

● As you approach your fortieth birthday, practice the focusing technique described under "Self-Treatment," on previous page.

PTERYGIUM

A *pterygium* (ter-IDJ-ee-um) has some similarity to a pinguecula, but it is shaped differently, is located in a different spot in the eye, and has more blood vessels. A pinguecula is a yellowish patch on the white part of the eye. (For a complete discussion of pingueculae, see page 301.) A pterygium is a triangular-shaped white area containing a lot of blood vessels. In fact, the word "pterygium" comes from the Greek word for "wing." (See Figure 2.8 at right.) While a pinguecula does not interfere with vision and therefore does not need to be removed, a pterygium grows onto the cornea, where it can obscure vision. Before it reaches that point, it has to be removed.

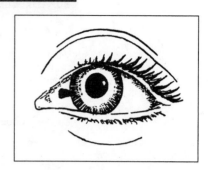

FIGURE 2.8
An Eye Affected by a Pterygium.

To determine if what you have is a pinguecula or a pterygium, look in the mirror. If the patch is starting to cover a part of your iris, you have a pterygium. There is usually only one pterygium in the eye, and it is most often located on the nasal side of the eye— that is, nearer to the nose instead of the ear. No exact cause for pterygia is known, but the condition does occur more frequently in hot, dusty climates, and it is often seen among surfers, who spend hours in the windy ocean spray and sun, and in farmers, whose eyes are frequently exposed to hot, sunny, and debris-laden conditions.

CONVENTIONAL TREATMENT

Most eye doctors prefer to leave pterygia alone until they begin to encroach on the line of sight, where they can interfere with vision. Previously, pterygia tended to grow back after being removed. However, the newer procedures are more effective at removing them, and re-growth is now rare. Sometimes a graft of tissue from underneath the inside of the upper eyelid is used to cover the area where tissue was removed. While this is still a complicated procedure, it can be very effective in allowing you to look and feel good afterward.

SELF-TREATMENT

Once a pterygium has started to grow, the best thing you can do is to reduce the environmental assault on it. Stay out of windy, dusty, sunny, and smoky environments. In addition, keep your eyes lubricated and moist. Wear high-quality sunglasses that block out 100 percent of UV radiation.

If you have a pterygium, try to avoid windy, dusty, sunny, and smoky environments, all of which can aggravate the condition. High-quality sunglasses that block all UV radiation are a must.

NUTRITIONAL SUPPLEMENTS

Supplement	Directions for Use	Comments
CapsiClear	Take 2 gelcaps, 2 times daily.	Supports the tear film.
Vitamin A	Take 2,500 IU daily.	Good for all eye conditions.
Vitamin C	Take 1,000–3,000 mg daily, in divided doses.	Protects the eye and aids tissue healing.
Zinc and copper	Take 25 mg of zinc and 2 mg of copper daily.	Enhances the immune response. Note: The copper supplementation is needed to balance the zinc supplementation.

HERBS AND HERBAL SUPPLEMENTS

Herb	Directions for Use	Comments
Chamomile	Apply as a hot compress, or use as an eyewash.	Soothing for the eye tissues.
Eyebright and fennel	Apply as a hot compress, or use as an eyewash.	Boost the circulation.

HOMEOPATHIC REMEDIES

Remedy	Directions for Use	Comments
Acidium Sulfuricum	Place 4 pellets under the tongue, 3–4 times daily.	Resolves pH imbalances.
Apis mellifica 6c	Place 3–4 pellets under the tongue, 3–4 times daily.	Relieves swelling around the eyes.
Bellis perrenis	Place 3–4 pellets under the tongue, 3–4 times daily.	Helps with healing and treating capillary weakness.
Cantharis	Place 3–4 pellets under the tongue, 3–4 times daily.	Increases kidney excretion of toxins.
Lachesis	Place 3–4 pellets under the tongue, 3–4 times daily.	Reduces inflammation.
Ruta graveolens 6c	Place 3–4 pellets under the tongue, 3–4 times daily.	Good for hot, red, inflamed eyes.
Sulphur 6c	Place 3–4 pellets under the tongue, 3–4 times daily.	Good for red, inflamed eyelids.

RECOMMENDATIONS

- Always wear good quality sunglasses when spending excessive time in the sun; be sure they have 100 percent UV absorption and good optical quality.

- Keep your eyes moist and lubricated at all times.

PTOSIS

See Drooping Eyelids, page 212.

PUPILS, DIFFERENT-SIZED

See Anisocoria, page 159.

RECURRENT CORNEAL EROSION

Recurrent corneal erosion is a condition in which the outermost cells of the cornea fail to adhere to their basement membrane. It usually follows a corneal abrasion, and most often happens in dry eye conditions.

The outermost cells of the cornea are about five rows deep and are anchored to the membrane located behind them. When you scratch your cornea, these cells are scraped away, exposing sensitive nerves, which result in pain. Normally, the cells grow back rapidly, usually within twenty-four hours. However, if the scrape is unusually deep, you may have lost all five layers of cells and exposed the bare membrane. In this situation, it will take longer for the cells to grow back because of the extent of the damage.

In addition, while your eye heals, you may try to function normally but in doing so may irritate the area and stall the healing process. The new cells might be brushed off before they have had a chance to adhere firmly to the basement membrane. This can happen if you scratch your eye or have a dry eye condition, both of which make it more difficult for the cells to grow back properly. Even opening your eyes first thing in the morning (or rubbing them when you do) can rub away those cells and re-injure the area. So instead of going on with chores as usual, allow your eye some special treatment.

Recurrent corneal erosion needs time to heal. If you have been diagnosed with this condition, take time off from daily chores; avoid rubbing your eyes; stay away from wind, dust, smoke, sun, and other drying environments; and follow your doctor's treatment program until your eye has fully recovered.

CONVENTIONAL TREATMENT

The mildest approach to treating this disorder is to use either artificial tears or a temporary antibiotic in order to keep the eyes moist and free of bacteria. This is often accompanied by the use of a lubricating ointment at bedtime to prevent the eyelids from sticking to the loose corneal cells. If this approach is not successful, a bandage contact lens may be used to protect the cornea from physical contact with the eyelids. This bandage contact lens will likely be in the form of a disposable soft contact. If the scratch is deep, a pressure bandage may be required.

If these mild treatments are not effective, a more radical approach will be necessary. This radical approach is called anterior stromal puncture (ASP), in which about forty to sixty micropunctures are made into the front part of the cornea. The eye is numbed and a needle is used. The micropunctures allow the cells to adhere better to the basement membrane. Though somewhat painful, ASP is effective in severe cases of recurrent corneal erosion.

SELF-TREATMENT

If your doctor diagnoses recurrent corneal erosion, prepare yourself for a long healing process. It will take anywhere from a week to a month or more, and will depend mostly on your environment. Use the lubricants prescribed by your doctor as often as necessary. Even more important are the ointments prescribed for application at bedtime.

In the morning, use warm compresses to relax your eyes before you open them. Obviously, you will need help preparing them. Suggestions for compresses are found in the chart on herbal treatments, below. Finally, stay out of dry or smoky environments, as such atmospheres can irritate your eyes and delay healing.

NUTRITIONAL SUPPLEMENTS

Supplement	Directions for Use	Comments
Vitamin A	Take 2,500 IU per day.	Supports the corneal tissue as it heals.
Vitamin C	Take 500 mg, 2 times daily, for 2 days.	Builds collagen tissue.
CapsiClear	Take 1 gelcaps, 2 times daily.	Supports the tear film.

HERBS AND HERBAL SUPPLEMENTS

HERB	DIRECTIONS FOR USE	COMMENTS
Bayberry, eyebright, and goldenseal	Use as an eyewash, 2 times daily.	Good for all eye conditions. Caution: Do not take goldenseal internally for more than 1 week, and do not use goldenseal during pregnancy.
Comfrey	Use as an eyewash.	Promotes healing.
White willow bark	Take 400 mg, as needed.	Good for pain.

HOMEOPATHIC REMEDIES

REMEDY	DIRECTIONS FOR USE	COMMENTS
Aconite 6c	Place 3–4 pellets under the tongue, every 3–4 hours, or put 2 drops in 1 cup of water and use as an eyewash.	Good for pain and for inflammation.
Hypericum perforatum 6c	Place 3–4 pellets under the tongue, every 3–4 hours, or put 2 drops in 1 cup of water and use as an eyewash.	Reduces the effects of a nerve injury.

RECOMMENDATIONS

• Keep your eyes well-lubricated at all times. Even during sleep, the lids may creep apart, allowing the eyes to dry out to some degree. If necessary, use surgical tape to keep the lids closed while sleeping.

• Avoid sunny, windy, dusty, and other drying environments so that your eyes can heal properly and as quickly as possible.

RED EYES

See Bloodshot Eyes, page 174.

REFRACTIVE ERRORS, DIFFERING

See Anisometropia, page 161.

RETINA, PEELING

See Retinal Detachment, below.

RETINAL BLEEDING

See Diabetic Retinopathy, page 205.

RETINAL DETACHMENT

SYMPTOMS OF RETINAL DETACHMENT

- Flashes of light that look like sparks or flickers

- A large number of floaters

- A shadow or curtain that spreads from the edge of the visual field to the central vision

- A shimmering effect

A retinal detachment is the peeling away of the retina from the back of the eye, the way you might imagine wallpaper peeling away from a wall. A healthy retina is securely attached to the choroid layer of the eye. In retinal detachment, a hole or tear in the retina allows fluid to collect between the retina and the choroid, leading to separation.

Retinal detachment can occur for many reasons, not all of them injuries, although a blunt or penetrating injury to the eye is a common cause of the condition. Extremely nearsighted eyes and protruding eyes are more prone to retinal detachment than farsighted eyes and normal eyes, probably because the retinas are more tautly stretched. Recent cataract surgery is another risk factor.

You should know the symptoms of retinal detachment because failure to seek treatment in time can result in blindness in the affected eye. A developing retinal detachment is heralded by flashes of light that look like sparks or flickers, a large number of floaters in the field of vision, and a shadow or curtain that spreads from the edge of the visual field to the central vision. You may also notice a shimmering effect, such as what you see when you look through gelatin. However, you will not feel pain from the retina, since the retina does not contain pain receptors. You may, of course, feel pain from elsewhere in the eye if an injury caused the detachment.

CONVENTIONAL TREATMENT

A detached retina can be reattached by an ophthalmologist if it is caught in time. If there is only a small hole, a laser may be used to seal it. If there is a large tear and the retina is actually peeling away from the eye, a freezing probe will be used to make the retina adhere to the choroid again. Many times, a strap called a scleral buckle is permanently attached around the eyeball to compress it slightly and allow the retina to contact the choroid once again.

In extreme cases, an air or oil bubble is injected into the vitreous portion of the eye. Air bubbles always rise, so the patient is put on a tilted table and rotated to the position that will allow the rising bubble to push the retina back into place. Patients may be placed in this position for several hours to several weeks!

SELF-TREATMENT

There isn't much that you can do for yourself to reattach a detached retina. Getting prompt attention is your first priority—seconds count! The only thing to do is to lie down very quietly and stay in that position until help is available. This occasionally allows the retina to fall back into place. Do not make any sudden moves, either with your head or your eyes, and stay quiet and relaxed until you can see an ophthalmologist.

NUTRITIONAL SUPPLEMENTS

SUPPLEMENT	DIRECTIONS FOR USE	COMMENTS
Vitamin A	Take 2,500 IU daily.	Supports the retina.
Vitamin-B complex	Take at least 100 mg daily.	Good for nerve function.

RECOMMENDATIONS

• Time is of the essence when it comes to treating a retinal detachment. Be sure to review the symptoms and also share them with family members and children.

• From time to time, a retinal detachment is caused by extreme physical exercise such as heavy weight lifting. However, this is not a common cause of the disorder.

RETINAL HOLES OR TEARS

See Lattice Degeneration, page 262.

FIRST AID FOR RETINAL DETACHMENT

• Stabilize your eye—lie down and keep your eyes very still, preferably closed.

• Have someone take you to an eye doctor or emergency room quickly, but carefully.

RETINITIS PIGMENTOSA

Retinitis pigmentosa (ret-in-EYE-tis pig-ment-OH-sah) is an inherited disease that affects approximately 1 out of every 3,700 people. It causes deterioration of the retina, with progressive loss of sight starting at about the age of ten. The first symptoms of retinitis pigmentosa (RP) are increasing night blindness and difficulty seeing in dim light. Then, the peripheral vision gradually decreases, until you feel as if you are looking through a tunnel (tunnel vision), with only a small "island" of central vision. Fortunately, this island may last until you are well along in years. However, the loss of peripheral vision will eventually make it impossible for you to drive or do many mobile tasks.

CONVENTIONAL TREATMENT

If you have been diagnosed with retinitis pigmentosa, consult a low-vision specialist who can recommend aids that are suited to your needs.

Generally, the medical community has no treatment for RP. Medical practitioners recommend getting in touch with a low-vision clinic. The staff at the clinic can teach you how to obtain and use the best low-vision aids that are available.

However, a recent breakthrough in tackling retinitis pigmentosa was made by a team of molecular geneticists in New Zealand. The researchers found defects in two genes in the retinal epithelium, a layer of cells at the back of the eye. They discovered that a number of retinal diseases are caused by genetic mutations in the epithelium. The two defective genes give instructions to two proteins that play a vital role in transporting vitamin A to the eyes' light-detecting cells, which need a continuous supply of the nutrient to function. These researchers believe certain RP cases can be cured by supplementation with raised levels of vitamin A, something that has been suspected for many years but could not be proved. The mineral zinc most often accomplishes the transport of vitamin A. Thus, increased zinc is being considered as a treatment as well. The drawback of excessive zinc must be overcome, however, because zinc can be toxic at high levels.

One of the New Zealand researchers conducted much of his practical research in India and said that it might take generations to prove vitamin A is a preventive cure. But for some known sufferers, vitamin A treatment could be as dramatic as insulin treatment is for diabetics. Interestingly, the ancient Egyptians treated blindness with ground-up roasted ox liver. We have come to realize that liver is a high source of vitamin A.

For people with RP who do not respond to vitamin A, another treatment possibility is transplantation of the epithelial layer. This technology, which is already within grasp, may offer a cure to up to one-third of RP sufferers. There are numerous research studies being conducted, but none have proven to be the final answer as of yet.

SELF-TREATMENT

Once your doctor has developed a protocol with you for supplementation of vitamin A, you can obviously administer the vitamin to yourself. *Do not attempt to design a high-dose vitamin-A supplementation plan on your own.* Vitamin A can be toxic in extremely high levels. Thus, your program must be overseen by your eyecare professional.

Although research indicates that vitamin A may be a preventive cure for retinitis pigmentosa, you should not implement a vitamin-A regimen on your own. Because high doses of this supplement can be toxic, therapy must be overseen by your physician.

NUTRITIONAL SUPPLEMENTS

SUPPLEMENT	DIRECTIONS FOR USE	COMMENTS
Vitamin A	Take 2,500 IU daily.	Good for all retinal conditions. Note: Use the emulsion form for easier assimilation and greater safety. Also, use under supervision of a doctor.
Zinc and copper	Take up to 40 mg of zinc and 2 mg of copper daily.	Aids in the transport of vitamin A. Note: The copper supplementation is needed to balance the zinc supplementation.
Lutein	Take 12 mg daily.	Supports retinal function.

HOMEOPATHIC REMEDIES

REMEDY	DIRECTIONS FOR USE	COMMENTS
Nux vomica 6c	Place 3–4 pellets under the tongue, 3–4 times daily.	Good for nerve inflammation.
Phosphorus 6c	Place 3–4 pellets under the tongue, 3–4 times daily.	Supports nerve and vascular integrity.

RECOMMENDATIONS

• For more information on RP, contact the Retinitis Pigmentosa Foundation. For the address and other contact information, see page 414 of the Resource Organizations section.

• If you have any family history of retinitis pigmentosa, have a routine dilated-eye exam yearly to assure that your vision is intact.

RETROBULBAR NEURITIS

See Optic Neuritis, page 298.

SCRATCHED CORNEA

See Corneal Abrasion, page 197.

SPOTS BEFORE THE EYES

See Floaters, page 228.

STRABISMUS

Strabismus (stra-BIZ-muss) is the technical term for crossed eyes. Actually, "crossed" is somewhat of a misnomer, because in strabismus, an eye can be turned upward, downward, inward, or outward. When an eye is turned toward the nose—that is, turned nasally—the individual is commonly labeled as "cross-eyed." When an eye is turned toward the ear—or turned temporally—the individual is usually referred to as "wall-eyed." See Figures 2.9 and 2.10 for helpful illustrations.

FIGURE 2.9
An Eye Affected by Strabismus, Turned Nasally.

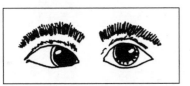

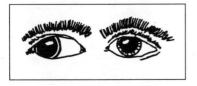

FIGURE 2.10
An Eye Affected by Strabismus, Turned Temporally.

About half of the people who have strabismus were born with it. Somewhere along the line, the eye-brain hookup became incorrectly "wired." In children, strabismus usually involves an eye that is turned nasally. Some authorities believe that strabismus is hereditary. It may be, since it often occurs in the same family.

What are other causes of strabismus? Believe it or not, we don't really know for sure what the root problem is in many cases. Strabismus may be induced by a poor visual environment—for example, by isolating an infant in a dark room or by keeping an infant positioned with the same eye closer to the mattress. The eyes are intended to receive light; they function best in light. The more they are used during our growing stage, the better they develop. The more visual stimulation a child is given, the more visual experience the child has, and the better is her visual development. If a child's visual stimulation is deficient or limited to one side, the child's visual system will not develop symmetrically.

The eyes are directly connected to the brain and are controlled from there. So are the six sets of eye muscles attached to the eyeballs. For an illustration of the eye muscles, see Figure 2.11, "The Muscles That Control the Eye." These muscles control where the eyes are aimed. Years ago, doctors thought that the incorrect turning of an eye was a purely mechanical error, caused by an eye muscle that was too long or too short. They believed that all they had to do to straighten out the eye was to surgically shorten or move a muscle. Sound logical? Well, maybe. But consider this: An eye muscle is more than a hundred times stronger than it needs to be to turn an eyeball. Why, then, can't it just pull the eye in the correct direction without the benefit of surgery?

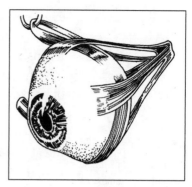

FIGURE 2.11
The Muscles That Control the Eye.

The answer turns out to be that strabismus is usually a problem of eye-brain coordination, not just of muscles being weak, too short, or too long. When the eye muscles of a child with strabismus are tested, they are usually found to be in perfect working order—even though the child can't aim both of the eyes in the same direction at the same time.

CONVENTIONAL TREATMENT

Some ophthalmologists still routinely recommend eye surgery to correct strabismus. However, I usually advise against such surgery as a first option, although it does help in some extreme cases. Most of the time, I find that surgery doesn't really correct the problem; it only makes the eyes appear to be aimed at the same point. The brain may still not "fuse" the images together, and therefore suppression (see page 328) will simply occur. Also, it is very easy to believe that the eyes are aimed properly but, in truth, they could be slightly off. If you have been given a recommendation to have this type of surgery, consult an ophthalmologist who specializes in the procedure, as well as an optometrist who uses non-surgical therapeutic techniques to teach the eyes to work together. (For a discussion of non-surgical therapeutic techniques, see "Vision Therapy" on page 385.)

Surgical procedures can be helpful for extreme cases of strabismus, but other forms of treatment, such as vision therapy, should be tried first. For some individuals, prescription eyeglasses may provide an effective nonsurgical solution to the problem.

Surgical treatment for strabismus is beneficial in some cases. For children, pediatric ophthalmologists sometimes choose to operate on the muscles of both eyes, even though only one eye may be turned. These doctors move the muscles on both eyes farther back, thus loosening the tension on the muscles. Both eyes are operated on because it has been found that when only one eye is operated on, the other eye may end up "following" the first eye. For example, if a nasally-turned eye is operated on and pulled temporally, the other eye may turn nasally. Both eyes will tend toward the right, for instance. Therefore, the operation that is often performed to straighten a nasally-turned eye will weaken the power of the muscles on the nasal side of both eyes.

Another surgical procedure for strabismus involves the turned eye only. If the eye is turned nasally, the muscle on the nasal side is moved back, as in the above-described operation, to reduce the tension on that side. In addition, the muscle on the temporal side is shortened to increase the tension on *that* side, thus pulling the eye toward the temporal side. Likewise, to turn an eye toward the nasal side, the muscle on the temporal side is moved back, with the muscle on the nasal side shortened.

A number of simple at-home games can provide the stimulation a child's eyes need to develop and focus correctly.

It is common in the arena of eye muscle surgery that there may need to be more than one procedure performed. My impression of this process is that we can never be exactly sure how the person will react to the procedure; the realignment of the eye muscles is an inexact science. Thus, I believe that all efforts short of surgery should be explored first. Once the eye muscles have been relocated, it changes the eye muscle-brain connection and makes binocular vision more difficult to achieve.

There are several ways to treat strabismus without surgery. One way is to "force" the child to use the turned eye by covering the good eye for prescribed periods of time. This is called *occluding* the vision in the good eye. The more functional eye can be covered with a patch or with a translucent lens in a pair of eyeglasses. The vision in the good eye can also be occluded with the use of eye drops that cause blurring. However, you have to be careful not to obscure the vision in the good eye for too many hours of the day or you may risk losing the good vision it has. Furthermore, because strabismus is a binocular problem, using one eye is not the final answer. It is simply a first step in assuring that each eye works to its maximum ability. Your developmental optometrist should be able to guide you to the best non-surgical therapy.

Another way to treat strabismus without surgery is to use eyeglasses. Sometimes, childhood strabismus is caused by farsightedness. The child tries to compensate for the farsightedness by over-converging the eyes— that is, making both of the eyes turn inward too much. This kind of strabismus should be treated with glasses or contact lenses that correct the farsightedness.

SELF-TREATMENT

There are a number of at-home techniques and activities that can be done to prevent or treat strabismus in an infant or child. For starters, place your infant on her back. Standing directly in front of the child, gently grasp both of the child's wrists and slowly lift her up into sitting position. Repeat this technique a few times as if it were a game, being careful not to tire the child. This technique will help the child's neck muscles to develop properly. Good control of the neck muscles aids in the development of binocular vision.

Hold your infant in the air and attract her attention to your face. Gradually bring the child closer to you, causing the child's eyes to converge. Bring the child all the way to your face, make a funny sound when your noses touch, and then lift the child away again. Repeat this technique a few times as if it were a game, being careful not to tire the child. This technique will develop the child's ability to converge the eyes effectively.

Drape a piece of material with bold black and white stripes over the edge of your child's crib. The stripes will stimulate the child's visual development. Alternate the material so that the stripes align both horizontally and vertically, in order to balance out the visual development. Of course, be sure the material in not within reach of the child, as that would create a hazard.

Place your child in an infant seat or high chair, and line up four or five squeaky toys just out of her reach. Sitting across from your child, squeeze the farthest toy on your left. As soon as your child looks at that toy and attempts to grasp it, squeeze the farthest toy on your right. When your child reaches for this second toy, squeeze a toy on your left again. Continue squeezing different toys only as long as the child feels it's a game; stop if the child becomes frustrated or irritable. This technique will stimulate the child's eyes to move in both directions. (It's also a nice little hearing test.)

Have your older child look through a stereoscopic viewer, such as a View-Master, at three-dimensional reels. These reels are available with cartoon characters and other images that kids enjoy. Ask the child whether the character or animal looks as if it's "sticking out" or "jumping out." The child will see a three-dimensional image only if she uses binocular vision.

If your child is under twelve years of age, ask your pediatrician for the proper dosage of the following nutrients.

NUTRITIONAL SUPPLEMENTS

SUPPLEMENT	DIRECTIONS FOR USE	COMMENTS
Manganese	Take 4 mg daily.	Stimulates the nerve-muscle connection.
Vitamin A	Take 2,500 IU daily.	Good for all eye conditions.
Vitamin-B complex	Take 100 mg daily.	Good for proper nerve growth.

HOMEOPATHIC REMEDIES

REMEDY	DIRECTIONS FOR USE	COMMENTS
Aluminum 6c	Place 3–4 pellets under the tongue, 3–4 times daily.	Good for strabismus affecting the right eye; improves coordination.
Calcarea carbonica 6c	Place 3–4 pellets under the tongue, 3–4 times daily.	Good for strabismus affecting the left eye; relieves spasm.
Phosphorus 6c	Place 3–4 pellets under the tongue, 3–4 times daily.	Good for many eye conditions.

RECOMMENDATIONS

• Always get a second opinion if your doctor recommends surgery for strabismus. Once the muscles are cut from the eyeball, their signals to move the eye are never the same.

• Therapists very often recommend gross-motor techniques, such as ball bouncing, hopping, jumping, and crawling, to help the body acclimate to bilateral stimulation. Trampolines are an excellent option but exercise caution due to potential injuries. Play games with your child that incorporate these movements, such as basketball, hopscotch, and jumping rope.

• Under the "Self-Treatment" heading in this section, there are a number of exercises recommended for the prevention of and treatment for strabismus in infants. For older children, try the techniques recommended for coordination on page 45.

STYE

A stye, technically called a *hordeolum* (hord-ee-OH-lum), is a common problem caused by a bacterial infection in one of the small glands on the edges of the eyelids or just under the eyelids. A stye looks and feels like a pimple on the eyelid—because that's exactly what it is. See Figure 2.12 for an illustration. It is often somewhat painful. Children frequently get styes from rubbing their eyes with dirty hands. But adults also get them from time to time, and sometimes it's hard to say how the infection got started.

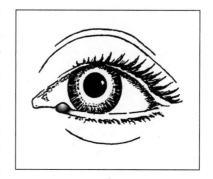

FIGURE 2.12
An Eye Affected by a Stye.

You can differentiate a stye from a chalazion, a similar infection, by tugging slightly at the eyelid skin. If the pimple or swollen area moves with the skin, it's probably a stye. If the skin slides over the mass, it's most likely a chalazion. Also, unlike styes, chalazia are usually painless. (For a complete discussion of chalazia, see page 185.) Most styes go away within a week or so.

CONVENTIONAL TREATMENT

Medical attention is rarely needed for styes. However, a stubborn stye can be incised and drained by a doctor—after numbing, of course. Topical antibiotics are also sometimes used.

SELF-TREATMENT

A stye can be brought to a head by steam bathing. One way to do this is to simply boil some water and pour it into a cup. Then, just close the eye and lean over the cup so that the steam rises toward the stye. You can also use a washcloth soaked in warm water or one of the herbs listed on page 326. I usually suggest not breaking the stye once it does come to a "head." There are some pretty nasty bugs in the fluid inside the stye, and the area is pretty close to the eye. So just let the stye's material get absorbed naturally by the body.

Moist heat from warm compresses can relieve the discomfort of a stye and promote faster healing. Steam from a bowl of boiled water can also be effective.

There are some over-the-counter remedies for styes that contain a compound called mercuric oxide. These remedies may work, but the mercury in these preparations can be very irritating to the eye. Mercury causes itching, stinging, and redness in many people. For these reasons, I don't recommend these products.

NUTRITIONAL SUPPLEMENTS

SUPPLEMENT	DIRECTIONS FOR USE	COMMENTS
Vitamin A	Take 2,500 IU daily.	Good for all eye conditions; especially beneficial if styes are a frequent problem.

HERBS AND HERBAL SUPPLEMENTS

HERB	DIRECTIONS FOR USE	COMMENTS
Eyebright	Apply as a compress or use as an eyewash.	Good for all eye conditions.
Raspberry	Apply as a compress or use as an eyewash.	Alleviates redness and irritation.

HOMEOPATHIC REMEDIES

REMEDY	DIRECTIONS FOR USE	COMMENTS
Apis mellifica 6c	Place 3–4 pellets under the tongue, 3–4 times daily.	Alleviates swelling.
Graphites 6c	Place 3–4 pellets under the tongue, 3–4 times daily.	Good for styes accompanied by severe discharge.
Lycopodium 6c	Place 3–4 pellets under the tongue, 3–4 times daily.	Good for styes accompanied by severe discharge.
Pulsatilla 6c	Place 3–4 pellets under the tongue, 3–4 times daily.	Good for styes accompanied by mucus discharge; especially good for styes in the upper eyelids of children and for inflammation.
Sepia 6c	Place 3–4 pellets under the tongue, 3–4 times daily.	Good for styes accompanied by watery discharge.
Staphysagria 6c	Place 3–4 pellets under the tongue, 3–4 times daily.	Good for lumps in the eyelids, especially for recurrent styes, and for inflammation; supports the connective tissue.
Sulphur 6c	Place 3–4 pellets under the tongue, 3–4 times daily.	Good for recurrent styes and good for inflammation.

RECOMMENDATIONS

• Do not attempt to drain the head of a mature stye. Doing this can lead to more serious problems. Instead, contact your doctor for proper treatment if the swelling does not go away on its own within a reasonable amount of time.

• Taking omega-3 oils or fish oils internally might help not only to fight the infection but also to keep the eyelid oils cleaner and less likely to plug up.

SUBCONJUNCTIVAL HEMORRHAGE

A subconjunctival (SUB-con-junk-TIE-val) hemorrhage is bleeding from broken blood vessels under the conjunctiva of the eye. More specifically, the bleeding occurs between the conjunctiva and the sclera. It is a problem that usually looks much more serious than it is. The area where the bleeding occurs appears as a bright red patch on the white sclera. There is no pain, and vision is not affected. See Figure 2.13 for a helpful illustration.

A subconjunctival hemorrhage can result from a jarring injury, such as a blow to the head, or from anything that increases the pressure in the delicate blood vessels of the conjunctiva, such as intense coughing, sneezing, vomiting, or pushing during childbirth. Of course, if you're having any additional symptoms that concern you, such as pain or visual disturbances, see your eye doctor.

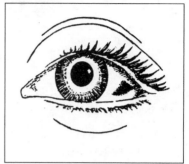

FIGURE 2.13

An Eye Affected by a Subconjunctival Hemorrhage.

CONVENTIONAL TREATMENT

Since the blood will be absorbed and the eye will return to normal within one to three weeks, a subconjunctival hemorrhage does not need to be treated. In fact, no real treatment exists for this particular problem. However, in cases in which subconjunctival hemorrhages are caused by trauma to the eye, it is important to have a professional evaluation performed to assure that all of the structures of the eye are intact and functioning normally.

SELF-TREATMENT

If you notice a subconjunctival hemorrhage and know when you received it, apply cold (or crushed ice) compresses to your closed eyelid for the first day or two. This will slow any bleeding. For the next day or two, do nothing. Then begin to apply warm compresses. This treatment will help the pooled blood to break down more quickly and the condition to resolve. In any case, a subconjunctival hemorrhage will usually disappear on its own within a short time.

NUTRITIONAL SUPPLEMENTS

SUPPLEMENT	DIRECTIONS FOR USE	COMMENTS
Calcium and magnesium	Take 1,000–1,500 mg of a combination supplement daily.	Essential for blood clotting.

**FIRST AID FOR A
SUBCONJUNCTIVAL
HEMORRHAGE**

• Apply a cold,
wet washcloth as
a compress to the
affected eye when you
first notice a subcon-
junctival hemorrhage.

• Repeat the cold
compress several
times during the first
twenty-four hours. No
additional treatment is
necessary during the
next forty-eight hours.

• On the fourth day,
begin applying warm
compresses to the
affected eye. This will
hasten the breakdown
of the visible blood.

SUPPLEMENT	DIRECTIONS FOR USE	COMMENTS
Vitamin A	Take 2,500 IU daily.	Good for all eye conditions.
Vitamin C	Take 3,000 mg daily.	Important for blood clotting.

HERBS AND HERBAL SUPPLEMENTS

HERB	DIRECTIONS FOR USE	COMMENTS
Alfalfa	Take as directed on the label.	A good source of vitamin K.

HOMEOPATHIC REMEDIES

REMEDY	DIRECTIONS FOR USE	COMMENTS
Arnica montana 6c	Place 3–4 pellets under the tongue, 3–4 times daily.	Reduces hemorrhaging and venous congestion; good for subconjunctival hemorrhage caused by injury.
Sanguinaria 6c	Place 3–4 pellets under the tongue, 3–4 times daily.	Improves vasomotor activity and reduces congestion.

RECOMMENDATIONS

• If you experience subconjunctival hemorrhages frequently, especially without apparent causes, you should consult your medical doctor.

• Make sure you're not over-dosing on some common nutrients, like vitamin E or fish oils, as high doses may make you more susceptible to bleeding.

SUPPRESSION

Your two eyes receive images that must be fused together in the brain to form one picture. If this fusion isn't accomplished with efficiency, you will experience two images. In other words, you will see "double." Since double vision is a most unwanted condition, the brain will probably turn off one of the two images it perceives. This is called suppression.

Fortunately for your brain and visual system, you can experience double vision without ever being aware of it. Unfortunately, there may be no clues that let you know you need to seek professional help. The suppression of images can go on for many years with no indication of a problem, especially when the disorder begins early in life. This problem often results in loss of stereo vision and could lead to a permanent loss of best vision in the eye that's being suppressed.

Studies have found that children who are efficient at suppression are actually good readers and learners. This may sound contradictory, but it really isn't. If there is a severe conflict between the two eyes and the brain has a very difficult time fusing the two images, it makes it very easy for the brain to suppress one image and see fine with the one eye that it chooses to use. However, if there is a very subtle difference between the two eyes and the brain occasionally suppresses one image, or if the two eyes constantly battle for fusion, there will be a conflict and the symptoms of poor reading and decreased learning will become apparent.

CONVENTIONAL TREATMENT

The treatment for suppression depends, unfortunately, on the doctor you see for your eye examination. Since suppression in some people is subtle and occasional, it takes a special in-depth type of examination of the visual system to be detected. If your doctor is more interested in just making sure that your eyes are healthy and seeing 20/20, your suppression problem may be missed.

Since suppression problems affect children and their learning abilities the most, it is critical that an examination for this condition be included in all of their vision exams. An optometrist who specializes in functional, or behavioral, vision will give the most appropriate evaluation. If found early, suppression can be treated with a program of vision therapy. (For a discussion of vision therapy, see page 385.)

Suppression can be missed in a general eye examination. Because it can affect children and their learning abilities the most, all children's vision exams should include a test for this disorder.

SELF-TREATMENT

Since the visual system follows the path of least resistance to seeing, there may not be much that you can do to force your brain not to suppress the images coming from one of your eyes. However, a good vision-therapy program will include techniques that you can perform at home on a regular basis. These techniques should allow you to use both eyes efficiently and effectively. Check with your doctor to see what kind of vision therapy would be best for your particular condition. Also, consult the vision therapy section of this book, page 385.

RECOMMENDATIONS

- Vision therapy is not a quick-fix, so be patient (no pun intended). However, you also need to be aggressive in taking control of your vision.

- Have your eye doctor evaluate you—and your children, if applicable—for more than just 20/20 vision. Checking for suppression should be part of your exam. An annual eye exam will assure that any visual deficiencies are caught early and therefore will be easier to treat.

THYROID EYE DISEASE

See Graves' Disease, page 240.

TUNNEL VISION

See Retinitis Pigmentosa, page 318.

UNDERCONVERGENCE OF THE EYES

See Convergence Insufficiency, page 195.

VISION, DISTORTED

See Astigmatism, page 164.

VISION SUPPRESSED IN ONE EYE

See Suppression, page 328.

WALL EYES

See Strabismus, page 320.

WHITE PATCH ON THE CORNEA

See Pterygium, page 311.

YELLOW PATCH ON THE SCLERA

See Pinguecula, page 301.

PART THREE

Therapies, Procedures, and Eyewear for Eye Care

There are several therapies, procedures, and eye "appliances" offered by eyecare specialists to serve visual needs. In Part Three, we will review those techniques and treatments concerned with preserving and improving vision. There is a good deal to cover in this section, which is arranged alphabetically by topic.

In this last part of the book, we will examine what may be considered lesser-known methods for eye care, namely acupuncture and acupressure, orthokeratology, and color therapy, also called syntonics. Of course, we will also cover more common corrective methods, such as eyeglasses and contact lenses. And as promised throughout Part Two, we will delve

more deeply into surgical procedures for the eyes, including cataract surgery, corneal transplant, and refractive surgery. Finally, we will also spend a good deal of time on vision therapy.

Hopefully, you will gain enough of an understanding of each of these therapies and procedures to enable you to discuss them with your eye doctor if you ever need to decide upon the most appropriate method for resolving your particular condition. Remember, good vision involves more than periodic eye exams and a healthy lifestyle. It also requires that you educate yourself on ways to optimize your vision. Part Three provides the latest information so that you can make that possible.

ACUPUNCTURE AND ACUPRESSURE

Acupuncture is the basis of traditional Chinese medicine. This method of treatment has been practiced for about 5,000 years, and textbooks on the subject go back about 2,000 years. It is a technique for treating certain conditions, relieving particular symptoms, and even producing the same effects as anesthesia, all of which are accomplished by passing long thin needles through the skin and into specific points that affect the nerve-transmission signals. The practice of acupressure uses those same points but simply involves the application of pressure rather than penetration with needles. Let's learn a little more about these two therapeutic techniques and how they apply to eye care.

BASIC BACKGROUND

As described above, acupuncture is an ancient healing modality. It relies on a system of meridians, or pathways, in the body. Generally, subscribers to the methodology of acupuncture and acupressure believe that energy should flow easily along these pathways, supplying vitality and, when necessary, healing. But due to various factors—for example, stress or injury—the energy can become blocked and result in pain, illness, and dysfunction. To fix the problem, practitioners of acupuncture and acupressure locate an area where there is a blockage, or an area that serves to reach a blockage via a meridian, and apply treatment to restore energy flow. The meridians allow them to treat certain parts of the body by applying needles or pressure to other areas along a given pathway. For example, they

can relieve tension in the head by massaging certain areas of the hands because a meridian connects those areas.

As mentioned previously, acupuncture can also be applied to numb an area so that further treatment can be administered. It has been used in place of conventional anesthesia, although this should be done only by highly trained practitioners. In fact, acupuncture was largely introduced to the West in 1971, after James Reston, an American journalist who was working for *The New York Times*, needed an emergency appendectomy while on location in China. He was amazed at the effects when acupuncture was administered to relieve his severe post-surgical pain. As his American audience began to read about Reston's experience, they began to consider acupuncture and acupressure as viable therapies.

Acupuncture evolved alongside—not in conjunction with—modern scientific medicine, but the acupuncture mechanism has been positively evaluated. Acupuncture stimuli activate the tissues and cells to promote effective cellular activities, especially triggering the mitochondrial citric cycles (or Krebs cycle) by which the particular cells rejuvenate and remodel themselves, therefore creating a healing and/or health-enhancing effect on the tissues involved. The American Medical Association has formally acknowledged acupuncture as a legitimate healing modality. However, today it still remains in the domain of "alternative" treatment in the West.

As I have suggested above, the technique known as acupressure is a modification of acupuncture. By massaging the same points that acupuncture penetrates with needles, relaxation and the inducing of healthy tissue changes, such as increased blood flow, can be achieved. Acupressure is a safe, simple, and inexpensive treatment. It is considered a milder therapy than acupuncture, and it therefore is less effective than stimulation with needles.

ACUPRESSURE MASSAGES FOR EYE HEALTH

Although acupressure and acupuncture have been promoted as pain-reducing procedures, they can also increase energy to particular points in the body and achieve a number of specialized results. Some of the points used in both acupuncture and acupressure are shown in the illustrations included in this section. Certain points on the face and hands are used by Chinese acupuncturists to treat conditions such as nearsightedness and other refractive errors, excessive tearing, eyelid twitching, sinusitis, and strabismus. You can use these points to give your eyes and head area a healthful, relaxing massage. A more complete program to improve visual functions must be administered by a licensed acupuncturist.

To give yourself an acupressure massage, refer to the illustrations as you read the following instructions. Also, keep in mind that to massage an acupressure point, apply threshold pressure to the point with your finger or thumb. Threshold pressure is firm pressure— pressure on the "threshold" of becoming painful. The idea behind acupressure is to stimulate the point, but not cause the muscles to tighten from pain. The pressure should be firm but gentle. Apply threshold pressure to a point for ten seconds, then release for ten seconds. Repeat the pressure-release cycle eight times. Another method is to apply continuous pressure for one to five minutes.

First, see Figure 3.1, below. Locate the point on your hand called *hoku*. To do this, on the hand that you wish to massage, move the thumb up next to the forefinger. Notice the hump that results in the muscle within the "V" formed by the bones of the thumb and forefinger. The peak of that hump is the hoku point. Press the point while relaxing the other muscles in that hand. Repeat on the remaining hand. Massaging the hoku point is believed to increase circulation and nerve energy to the head.

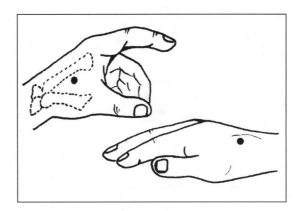

FIGURE 3.1 **The Hoku Point.**

Next, using the thumb and forefinger of one hand, massage the two points on either side of the bridge of your nose at the level of your eyes. These points are called *jing ming*, and are illustrated in Figure 3.2. Massaging them is believed to fight eye disease and facial paralysis.

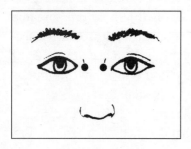

FIGURE 3.2
The Jing Ming Points.

Press the forefingers and middle fingers of each hand together. Then place the pairs of fingers on your cheeks next to your nose near the nostrils. Anchor your thumbs under your lower jawbone, then remove your middle fingers and massage your cheeks with your forefingers. These points on your cheeks, which are illustrated in Figure 3.3, are called *si bai*. Massaging them is believed to combat various eye disorders, headache, and eyelid twitching.

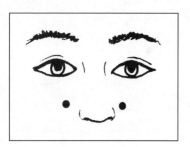

FIGURE 3.3
The Si Bai Points.

Using the outsides of your forefingers, rub along the bony ridges above and below your eyes. See Figure 3.4. Keep your other fingers curled under, and anchor your thumbs on each side of your forehead. By rubbing along the bony ridges, you will massage four points around each eye—*zan zhu* (point 1 in the illustration), located above the inside corner of the eye; *yang bai* (point 2 in the illustration),

located over the eye; *tong zi liao* (point 3 in the illustration), located at the outside corner of the eye; and *cheng qi* (point 4 in the illustration), located below the eye. Massaging the zan zhu point is believed to fight headaches. Massaging the yang bai point is believed to help night blindness and glaucoma. Massaging the tong zi liao point is believed to combat the headaches accompanying eye diseases. And massaging the cheng qi point is believed to help alleviate conjunctivitis, nearsightedness, and optic atrophy.

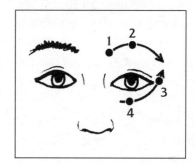

FIGURE 3.4
The Zan Zhu (Point 1), Yang Bai (Point 2), Tong Zi Liao (Point 3), and Cheng Gi (Point 4) Acupressure Points.

CONCLUSION

While it is beyond the scope of *Smart Medicine for Your Eyes* to delve into the entire theory of acupuncture, it is important to be aware that this ancient discipline is finally being accepted by the Western medical community. As of 2002, the American Medical Association acknowledged the effectiveness of acupuncture for several conditions and for pain control. More is continually being learned about the theories, procedures, and uses of acupuncture. Look for this practice to gain continued acceptance as time goes on.

CATARACT SURGERY

A cataract is a clouding of the lens within the eye. As discussed in "Cataracts" on page 177, the clouding can be partial or complete. Therefore, the interference to vision that cataracts cause runs the gamut from slight to severe. Moreover, a cataract that causes a slight problem today may develop into a disabling condition in the future. This is because the type of cataract that occurs with advancing age is generally progressive. Luckily, not all cataracts reach the point at which they obscure vision. Those that are considerably disabling, though, generally require surgery. This section will provide some helpful information on cataract surgery and what can be expected to follow it.

TYPES OF CATARACT SURGERY

Most eye doctors will ask you how well you feel you are functioning in your daily life with your cataract. Your answer will be a determining factor in the decision on whether or not to operate. When your cataract does interfere significantly with your vision and your lifestyle, your doctor will most likely recommend surgery. Consider that cataract surgery is the most common surgical procedure done in the United States today, with about 4 million operations performed annually. A few different surgical techniques are currently in common use, and you and your surgeon can decide which one is best for you. Most often, cataract surgery can be done as an outpatient procedure.

There are two types of surgery most commonly used for cataracts. The first is called *extracapsular cataract extraction*. The lens of the eye is surrounded by a capsule that helps to keep it in place. In extracapsular cataract extraction, a bit of this capsule is removed and the cloudy lens is taken out. The main advantage of this procedure is that most of the capsule is left intact to continue performing its function of dividing the front and back parts of the eye. In addition, that remaining capsule can support an artificial lens implanted in your eye as a replacement for the extracted lens. (For a further discussion of this, see "Sight After Lens Removal," in the next section.) Extracapsular cataract extraction is now used in about 95 percent of cataract operations.

A technique that can be used during an extracapsular extraction is *phacoemulsification* (fake-oh-ee-MUL-si-fi-KAY-shun). With this technique, the cataract is emulsified (broken up) using ultrasonic energy. Once emulsified, it is aspirated (sucked out). Phacoemulsification has the advantages of a smaller incision and faster post-surgical wound healing when compared with other methods of extraction. This method has also led to the use of a foldable intraocular replacement lens (IOL). The lens is made of a rubbery material so that it can be folded and inserted into the eye through a small slit. Once inside the eye, it expands and is wedged into place by the surgeon. Almost all lenses used these days are capable of being inserted in the folded position.

Another way to remove a cataract is to remove the cloudy lens while it is in its capsule—that is, both the lens and lens capsule are removed. This procedure is called intracapsular cataract extraction. These days, the lens and capsule usually are frozen first to make extraction easier and to minimize bleeding. The main advantage of this method is that every bit of lens and capsule tissue is removed so that no secondary cataract or cloudiness of the capsule can form in the future. When the capsule is left in the eye (as it is in the extracapsular technique), it may itself become opaque, or remnants of the old lens may grow over it and make it cloudy. These problems are known as secondary cataracts, or "after-cataracts." The disadvantage of intracapsular cataract extraction is that, once the lens capsule has been removed, the vitreous humor no longer has a dam to prevent it from oozing into the front part of the eye, where it doesn't belong and can cause trouble. Another problem is that the capsule is not present to support an artificial lens implant.

Contrary to what many people believe, lasers are not normally used in cataract surgery. Lasers burn holes in tissue, and a lens with a hole isn't any better than a lens with a cataract. However, lasers are often used to cut the front of the capsule, thus making a clean surface to remove the lens, as well as to resolve secondary cataracts (a clouding of the capsule) by burning a small hole in the remaining capsule so that you can see through it.

New and better procedures are now being developed to remove cataracts. The new procedures involve smaller incisions and have fewer complications. Most often, cataract surgery takes less than one hour to complete.

SIGHT AFTER LENS REMOVAL

By now, you may be wondering, "But if my lens is removed, how well will I see afterward?" Without a lens, you will have very poor visual acuity. Fortunately, there are ways to get around this problem. You may have heard of cataract glasses or may have even seen people wearing them. Years ago, these heavy, thick glasses had to be worn after cataract surgery. They were not only unsightly, but they also left something to be desired in terms of optical correction. Nowadays, people who have a lens removed have it replaced with a plastic lens inserted into the eye right where the original lens used to be. The latter type of lens, called an *intraocular lens*, or IOL, is put into place immediately, during the cataract surgery. Today, almost 100 percent of persons who have a cataract extracted have an intraocular lens implanted within the eye.

Traditional IOLs are monofocal, meaning they offer vision at one distance only, and that's usually distance vision. Therefore, you would have to wear eyeglasses or contacts in order to read, use a computer, or view objects in the middle distance. But there are now newer IOLs that incorporate a "multifocal" technology and even some that accommodate like your original lens! Let's review the current models and see what might be the best option for your needs.

Diffractive Technology Lenses

Multifocal intraocular lens (IOL) designs provide correction for both near and distance vision, and both near and far objects can be in focus at the same time. Your brain must learn to select the visual information it needs to form an image of either near or distant objects, so multifocal IOLs may require some adjustment. A person may adjust better to multifocal IOLs if they are placed in both eyes. This type of lens is not an option for some people.

The first multifocal intraocular lenses we'll discuss are the ReSTOR lens made by Alcon, Inc. and the Tecnis Multifocal IOL made by Abbott Medical Optics. These designs use diffractive technology, which is composed of a series of small concentric circles of differing powers that change from the center of the lens to the periphery. This allows light to be focused on two different planes—distance and near.

Studies have shown that more than 80 percent of the patients who use ReSTOR do not require glasses for near or distant vision, and that Tecnis results in excellent vision with superior depth of focus. However, there is one main drawback with ReSTOR—a tendency toward glare and halos at night. Plus, vision at an intermediate or arm's-length distance, such as that required for computer use, is often not sharp. Both these lenses have upgraded technology over the past few years.

Five-Zone Lenses

Another lens option is the ReZoom Multifocal Lens by Abbott Medical Optics. This acrylic lens distributes light over five optical zones to provide near, intermediate, and distance vision. Surveys have shown that 93 percent of ReZoom recipients report never or only occasionally needing glasses. However, while distance and intermediate vision are often clear, near vision can be problematic.

Accommodative Lenses

Then there are the lenses that accommodate, or focus, like your original lens—well, almost. Several designs are currently approved and many more are in clinical trials. The first one to be approved is called the Crystalens, by Bausch & Lomb. This lens is a hinged-plate silicone IOL that attaches to the capsule of the old lens. The contraction of your eye's ciliary muscle, used to accommodate (see page 153), causes pressure to move the hinged IOL forward, thereby changing the effective power of the eye. This lens allows fair near vision in 16 percent of patients. However, it provides excellent intermediate vision at 24 inches in 94 percent of patients. The drawbacks are related to lens positioning—if it becomes dislodged, the optics become distorted and vision is poor.

Extended Depth of Field Lenses

Another lens that uses a different technology is called the Technis Symfony IOL. Rather than splitting light into distinct focal points, the TECNIS Symfony IOL elongates focus, resulting in an increased depth of field. This empowers the patient to experience a full range of continuous vision while maintaining high image contrast. Unlike other IOLs, TECNIS material is not associated with glistenings. Glistenings cause light scatter, which can be distracting, especially with night driving.

With all of these lens implants, the visual outcome varies and some "re-learning" is required. Thus, it may take four to six weeks before your vision is completely stabilized. Be sure to discuss all of the pros and cons of the various lenses with your doctor before you agree to surgery. The newer multifocal lenses are more costly and may not provide the best vision in some cases.

The goal of using multifocal IOLs is to be independent of glasses. A recent analysis of studies revealed evidence of high levels of patient's satisfaction in general. The spectacle independence was 80 percent or more in 91.6 percent for distance vision, 100 percent for intermediate vision, and 70 percent for near vision in the different groups studied. The binocular uncorrected vision of 20/20 was achieved in 100 percent for distance visual acuity, 96 percent for intermediate visual acuity, and 97.3 percent for near visual acuity of the patients included in the study.

One thing that all of these IOLs have in common is that they absorb UV light. The crystalline lens (your real one) is the main absorber of UV light in the eye. Without that ability, UV radiation would reach the retina and cause significant damage.

The greatest drawback of all of these lenses is that great surgical expertise is required for precise placement in the eye, especially if the lenses are also going to correct for astigmatism. For this reason, it is vital that you seek out a surgeon who has had extensive experience with the implantation of multifocal lenses. As long as the lenses are appropriately chosen and positioned, the quality of vision is better than that with less sophisticated lenses and certainly better than it would be with thick glasses. Most likely, reading glasses will be required for special needs, but that's a small price to pay for overall clear vision.

CONCLUSION

Cataract surgery has come a long way, and it continues to improve. It is important to emphasize that there is no optimal surgery or lens protocol; the best choice truly depends on your particular eye structure and eye condition. Be sure to discuss all of the options with your cataract surgeon or your co-managing optometrist so that you are well aware of what to expect before, during, and after the procedure.

CONTACT LENSES

Contact lenses are an optical device made to fit over the cornea of the eye to change its refractive characteristics and improve vision. The idea of using lenses that are in direct contact with the eye was actually conceived centuries ago by Leonardo da Vinci. But such lenses did not become practical, everyday items until the mid-1950s. Today, there are many types of lenses available and a great number of people who use them. This section will explore the different kinds of contacts available. It will also offer instructions on how to wear them and care for them.

A GENERAL PERSPECTIVE ON CONTACT LENSES

Many people ask me how I, as an optometrist, feel about contact lenses. I feel perfectly fine about contacts. I have fit several thousand patients with contact lenses, and while experiences with contact lenses are highly individualized, most of the patients with whom I have worked are very happy with their lenses. They are able to find a type of lens that is compatible with their eyes, and they are thrilled to be able to see more clearly without glasses.

About 45 million Americans now wear contact lenses, and many additional people give them a trial run every year. Given the convenience and cosmetic benefits of contact lenses, why would some choose not to use them? Well, a good number of people think that the idea of "sticking something in your eye" is too uncomfortable. If you are among such thinkers, consider that the contact lens is designed to be worn *on* the eye—not *in* it. Then maybe you can look at this with a more positive perspective.

Perhaps the most obvious motivation to use contacts is that the majority of people prefer the way they look without glasses. Moreover, contacts have become accessories of sorts. You can go one step beyond just removing your glasses—you can actually change your eye color through the use of tinted contacts.

However, appearance is not the only reason to wear contact lenses. If you're very nearsighted, for example, your eyeglass lenses will be concave in shape (see "Types of Eyeglass Lenses" on page 355). When you look straight ahead through the centers of the lenses, you will find that your prescriptions are exactly what you need, but as you get away from the centers and move out toward the peripheries of the lenses, you will experience a lot of distortion. The lenses of the glasses are, out of necessity, thicker around the peripheries, so they don't correct your vision very well when you look through that part. Nor do you have any correction beyond the edges of the frame. With contacts, the lenses stay right on the corneas and move with your eyes, so you are always looking through their optical centers, where there is virtually no visual distortion.

TYPES OF CONTACT LENSES

Very early contact lenses, or those used prior to the 1950s, covered the entire front of the eye, not just the cornea as they do now. The cornea needs to take in oxygen and get rid of carbon dioxide, and it must stay wet. The early contacts didn't permit oxygen and carbon dioxide to permeate, thus causing the cornea to swell. The wearing time on these lenses was very limited.

"Modern" contact lenses have been around since the 1950s (the first patent on one was in 1955), but they've come a long way since then in terms of the materials from which they're made, their comfort and "wearability," and the kinds of conditions that they can correct. Contact lenses were originally made of hard, impermeable materials—glass until the late 1940s, and a hard plastic until the 1970s. Then, in the 1970s, new materials became available, and lenses that were gas permeable (transmitted oxygen through the lens) and hydrophilic (water-loving) were developed. And the science of contact lenses has continued to progress over the years. Today, lenses are available in soft, rigid, and combination materials to suit a variety of needs.

Despite the fact that, in general, today's contacts are much more comfortable than those of the past, not everyone who requires corrective lenses can wear them. Among those who have difficulty with contact lenses are people with chronically dry eyes because of a medical condition or medication (for example, antihistamines can dry the eyes out); people who have allergies that make their eyes itch and swell; and people who have extremely sensitive eyes and, therefore, cannot tolerate lenses resting on their eyeballs. But with the variety of materials and designs that are available today, most people are able to find something that fits their individual needs.

Let's review what has been available over the years, and what is currently available and recommended.

The Original Hard Contacts

The earliest contact lenses were developed in Germany in 1927. They were made of glass and covered the entire visible sclera. In 1937, an early type of plastic was developed for use in contact lenses, but the lenses still covered the whole visible sclera. These newer lenses were introduced in the United States in 1938. In 1940, a plastic called polymethylmethacrylate (PMMA) came into use for contacts, which were still made to cover the whole front of the eyeball.

It wasn't until 1955 that the first patent was granted for lenses made of PMMA that covered only the cornea. These smaller plastic lenses were routinely fitted during the 1950s. They were somewhat flexible, but they still earned the name "hard lenses." The plastic could be molded inexpensively, polished to a smooth optical surface, and modified with relative ease. A minor prescription change was an in-office procedure. The lenses maintained a good optical transparency that did not fade with time. Moreover, they didn't crack too easily, they didn't sustain bacterial growth (which could cause infection), and they could be tinted slightly to make them easier to find if dropped.

These lenses also had a downside. The material had no ability to transmit oxygen or carbon dioxide, which made them unhealthy for the cornea. In addition, solutions had to be used to help water or tears adhere to the surface. It took some determination to wear these lenses because they were so uncomfortable. However, a certain number of brave souls were able to tolerate them, and the lenses were a definite improvement for those with very high prescriptions. The lenses, if not lost, could sometimes last for as long as ten or fifteen years! Please note, though, that no contact lens should be used for that long.

Today, those original PMMA hard contact lenses are obsolete. The newer materials have all but displaced them from optometrists' inventories. Newer lenses are comfortable and healthier for your eyes.

Soft Contacts for Daily Wear

In the early 1960s, a Czechoslovakian chemist named Dr. Otto Wichterle developed a new type of plastic that he originally thought could be utilized to make artificial blood vessels and organs. He then used a child's "lab" set to experiment with using the plastic for contact lenses. Called hydroxyethylmethacrylate, or HEMA, this material changed the world of eye care forever. "Soft contacts" had arrived on the scene.

These soft contacts—now referred to as "daily-wear soft lenses"—were introduced to the public in 1971 by the Bausch & Lomb Company of Rochester, New York. They marked the beginning of a whole new era in contact lens technology. The material was 38 percent water and was called hydrophilic, or "water-loving," because it also absorbed water. The lenses were more permeable to oxygen and carbon dioxide than hard lenses, and their comfort level was incredible compared to that of the hard lenses.

However, the vision through the soft lenses was not quite as sharp as that through the hard lenses, and these early lenses could not correct for astigmatism. Also, in addition to absorbing water, these lenses had an affinity for infection-causing bacteria. The care of the lenses was therefore complicated, often calling for disinfection by heat unit every night. (Those of us in the field called them "boiler units.") Despite the disinfection techniques, the incidence of eye infections in soft-lens wearers remained higher than that in hard-lens wearers. The soft lenses also tended to yellow with age, could rip rather easily, and lasted for only a year or two in spite of their substantial price. But for persons who were nearsighted, did not have astigmatism, and were reliable enough to disinfect the lenses every night and replace them every year or two, these lenses were wonderful.

In 1976, soft contact lenses became available for people with astigmatism too. These lenses, called "toric lenses" (*torus* is Latin for "bulge"), were manufactured using a computerized lathe that could cut different curves into different areas of a lens in much the same way that eyeglass lenses are made. These contact lenses were unable to correct for large amounts of astigmatism, but they worked very well for many people.

There were other limitations though. The first astigmatism lenses were slightly uncomfortable because they had a bulge on the lower edge to keep them positioned properly over the cornea. This thickness was noticeable, but the lenses were still more comfortable than the

original hard lenses. They were made of the same material as other daily-wear soft contacts, so their care was the same, but so were the other problems mentioned above.

Today, soft contacts for daily wear are still available and can be chemically disinfected instead of needing to be sterilized with heat. Thus, maintenance of the lenses is much easier. Also, the current astigmatism lenses have thinner edges, so they are much more comfortable and are also available in several other types of plastic material.

Rigid Gas Permeable Contacts for Daily Wear

Patented in 1974 and introduced to the public in 1978, rigid gas permeable lenses were the next advancement in technology for hard lenses. They looked and acted like hard lenses, but they could absorb small amounts of fluid and were able to transmit oxygen and carbon dioxide to and from the eye. This was due to the addition of silicone to the plastic material. The silicone made the lenses more comfortable and adaptable than the original hard lenses. Because these new lenses were not as hard as the original lenses but they still held their shape on the eye, they were called "rigid" rather than "hard."

Many people who wore the old hard lenses but had some discomfort were now able to upgrade to the newer material with almost no change in their vision or care regimen. The only drawback to the updated plastic material was that, although the silicone aided in gas transmission, it made the surface more difficult to wet, similar to the original hard lens. Therefore, some people experienced a drying of the eyes toward the end of a day of wearing these lenses. Luckily, this was more of a discomfort than a danger.

Today, there is a newer generation of gas permeable lenses that can be comfortably worn all day by most people. They have increased oxygen transmission and fluid-attraction ability. These lenses are a good alternative for those patients who can't get good visual correction with soft lenses or who don't want the risk of infection that soft lenses pose.

Soft Contacts for Extended Wear

Probably the biggest explosion in the contact lens field was the advent of contact lenses that could actually be worn overnight for days at a time. The only problem seemed to be that the original soft extended-wear lenses were extremely fragile—they used lots of water to increase oxygen transmission. That drawback has been significantly improved since those early days.

In 1981, the FDA approved extended-wear soft contacts designed to be worn for thirty days at a time without cleaning or disinfecting. Unfortunately, this proved to be too long of a wearing period and earned the lenses some bad press that was not entirely undeserved. In September of 1989, the *New England Journal of Medicine* published an article based on a study sponsored by the Contact Lens Institute, a group of contact lens manufacturers. The study noted that the risk of corneal ulcers, which can occur with infections of the cornea, was five times greater in extended-wear lens users than in daily-wear lens users, although the problem still occurred in only 0.2 percent (2 out of every 1,000) of all extended-wear lens

users. All of a sudden, everyone was afraid to sleep with contact lenses in their eyes. Many medical practitioners called for no overnight wear of lenses, even though the study did note that the risk of infection increased proportionally with the wearing time.

Until recently, daily wear was the only wearing schedule eye doctors considered safe enough for soft lenses. However, with the introduction of Silicone Hydrogel materials, things have changed. I'll cover those in a separate section below.

Rigid Gas Permeable Contacts for Extended Wear

In early 1987, the FDA approved rigid gas permeable contact lenses that could be worn overnight for up to seven days. These lenses were made of a material specifically designed for extended wear. They had the optical and handling advantages of hard lenses combined with a wearability closer to that of soft lenses. The key difference was the addition of fluorine to the silicone material during the manufacturing process. This allowed the best combination of gas transmission and moisture maintenance of any lenses yet developed.

Rigid gas permeable lenses for extended wear have been available for some time now, with several manufacturers elaborating on the basic concept. The lenses offer many advantages in the areas of lens life and visual clarity. The material allows for a flexible wearing schedule similar to that of extended-wear soft lenses. It is durable enough to be handled daily, yet apparently is safe enough to be left in the eye for several days. The 1989 Contact Lens Institute study on extended-wear problems did not include any rigid gas permeable lenses. But these lenses are now being used with a special orthokeratology program (see "Orthokeratology" on page 370).

Disposable Soft Contacts

In 1987, Johnson & Johnson's contact lens subsidiary, Vistakon, released the first disposable contact lenses. They were called Acuvue. These lenses were similar to daily-wear soft lenses, but they were made in an entirely new way. In fact, the new process enabled the lenses to be produced and sold so cheaply that they could be discarded after being worn on a daily-wear basis (not overnight) for just one or two weeks.

I often recommend that disposables worn on a daily basis be used for up to two weeks. And I tell my patients who wear the disposables to use a disinfecting solution on the lenses every night. Most contact lens companies make disposables, and almost all eye doctors fit them. If you choose to wear disposable contacts, just be sure that you complete the follow-up care. Wearers of disposable lenses should visit their optometrists for a vision examination every year, and more often if any problems occur. Simply ordering lenses through the mail or Internet, without an exam and current prescription, is asking for trouble and is now illegal.

Most contact lens companies have kept pace with the changes in contact lenses by introducing "daily-disposable" lenses. These are lenses that are put on in the morning and thrown away at night. They are a bit more expensive than the other types of lenses, especially since you need 720 lenses per year, but they do have some unique applications, and no care solutions are needed. They are a problem-solver for many patients who want to wear contact lenses without the burden of cleaning and caring for their lenses. And they are also useful for patients who have allergies or who build up deposits on their regular lenses.

New features continue to develop. For example, you can also get disposable contacts that are clear but block up to 90 percent of UV light. These contacts do not qualify as a substitute for a good pair of UV-blocking sunglasses, but people concerned about UV exposure to the eye may find them very useful. Also, Vistakon has released lenses that change with the UV light, just like photochromic glass lenses (see page 361).

Bifocal Contacts

Even back in the 1970s, bifocal contacts were available. However, the original bifocal contacts were hard lenses, had all of the drawbacks of hard lenses, and weren't tolerated very well by a large number of patients. Nowadays, bifocal contacts are available in rigid gas permeable and soft materials. The rigid types have a success rate for vision correction of about 70 percent, and people who are already comfortable with that material seem to have little trouble adapting to the bifocal version.

The first bifocal *soft* contact lenses became available in 1985. The theory of how they should work was well developed, yet in practice the lenses did not perform as expected. Since then, there have been several different forms of multifocal soft contacts, each using a different technique to achieve clarity for near as well as distance vision. Unfortunately, no one design has proven to be perfect for the majority of those who try soft bifocal contacts.

Current success rates for vision correction through bifocal contact lenses are running at about 70 to 80 percent. But presbyopes—that is, those of you who require bifocals—take heart! Since most contact lens wearers are baby boomers who are now reaching their early sixties, many contact lens manufacturers are putting big money and effort into the research and development of a successful and comfortable bifocal contact lens. New designs are being developed constantly, so it should be only a short time before the next generation of lenses hits the market. Currently, there are even bifocal disposable and bifocal astigmatism lenses available.

Because bifocal contact lenses don't work for all of the population, many doctors are using a technique called *monovision* for bifocal patients who want contacts. In the monovision technique, one eye is fitted with a near-vision prescription lens, and the other eye is fitted with a distance-vision prescription lens. Then, because of our ability to suppress a blurred image (see "Suppression" on page 328), the brain shuts off the image from the distance lens when you look at something close up, and alternately shuts off the image from the near lens when you focus for distance. You don't develop lazy eye because each eye is used some of the time. This way of seeing usually takes the brain a few weeks to learn, but it works surprisingly well (although not perfectly). If you don't want to wear glasses but need bifocals, and if the current bifocal lenses don't suit you, you might want to give monovision a try.

Tinted Contacts

For many years, hard and rigid gas permeable contact lenses have been available with a slight tint called a *handling tint*. It is not really visible on the eye, but it is just dark enough to allow the lenses to be found if accidentally dropped. Manufacturers haven't, and probably won't, try to make these lenses capable of changing a person's eye color because both these types of lenses are slightly smaller than soft lenses and don't quite cover the entire iris. If you have brown eyes and wore a pair of these lenses tinted blue, for example, you'd see a blue lens ringed by a brown iris, which might look interesting at Halloween but isn't likely to become popular.

Beginning in about 1984, however, a process of tinting lenses enough to change eye color was developed for soft lenses. These tinted soft lenses caught on and gave lens wearers an additional choice. The first tinted lenses were capable only of changing the color of light blue or green eyes. Then, in 1986, Wesley-Jessen, Inc., of Chicago introduced lenses with an opaque tint that would actually make a brown eye appear blue, green, or aquamarine. The interest in contact lenses boomed again. About a third of the new tinted soft lenses that were sold had no prescription; they were purchased for cosmetic purposes only. Today, these lenses are available in colors with names such as baby blue, sapphire, and misty gray, and many optometrists offer free trials to see what difference they can make in your appearance. Theoretically, there's nothing wrong with wearing contact lenses to change your eye color, but it's important to remember that these lenses are made of the same material as prescription daily-wear and extended-wear soft lenses, so they need to be given the same care. They are still medical devices, not makeup.

Since I mentioned Halloween, you'll likely see ads for "Wild Eyes" or other tinted contact lenses with very unusual configurations—8-balls, flames, cat's eyes, sparkles, just to name a few. Again, these contacts are still considered medical devices and must be fit by a certified professional and not just purchased at a beauty shop or swap meet. Severe eye infections have occurred with lenses being bought without the proper care instructions. A spooky night out is not worth risking your eyesight!

Silicone Hydrogel Soft Lenses

In 2001, a new material was introduced. This material has incorporated the best of the traditional soft HEMA material with a blend of silicone to create a material that allows an enormous amount of oxygen through the lens. There is so much oxygen passing through the lens that even with the eyes closed—that is, during sleep—the cornea receives enough oxygen to maintain its clarity and health. Thus, this lens material is now FDA-approved for extended wear. As of this writing, there are five different lenses that fit into this category and all have their advantages over traditional soft lenses.

Now, it is important to know that, although the lenses are approved for extended wear (anywhere from one week to one month), they can be worn just on a daily basis as well. Thus, silicone hydrogels are most likely the future of soft contact lenses, and more designs and options—for example, bifocals and astigmatism lenses—are now available. Whether or not you decide to sleep in this lens, the

material is excellent for general wear and allows more oxygen through it than any other lens available. Ask your optometrist about silicone hydrogel as an option if you are getting fitted for contacts.

Hybrid Contact Lenses

In the mid-1980s, a new development in contact lenses combined the two types of lenses—rigid gas permeable and soft. These hybrid lenses had a central section that was made of a gas permeable material, and then a surrounding "skirt" of soft lens material. There were some technological problems with fitting and comfort, and the lenses tore easily, but through continued development there is now a new generation of this lens called Synergeyes of Carlsbad, CA.

The Synergeyes lens maintains the same design—a rigid center with a soft skirt— but uses materials that allow for great oxygen transmission through the lens. Fitting of the lens is easy and the success rate is high. Most doctors use this as a "niche lens"—something they can prescribe if no other lens is appropriate for the correction of a patient's vision. If you are not completely satisfied with your current contact lenses, ask your eye doctor if he works with this lens.

Daily Disposable

Today we have lenses that are put on in the morning and thrown away at the end of the day. This is by far the most convenient (no solutions or case is needed) and healthiest option for wearing contact lenses. You typically purchase a six- or twelve-month supply of lenses and use them on a daily basis. These are perfect for swimmers/surfers or anyone who needs to travel and not carry solutions with them. These lenses are now available in multifocal and astigmatism corrections, so they are quickly becoming the state-of-the-art choice of the contact lens-wearing public. Ask your doctor if these lenses are available for your optical needs.

Scleral Contact Lenses

The very early contact lenses didn't just fit over the cornea but covered much of the sclera (white) of the eye. While it may seem like a throwback to early days, there are new versions of these lenses that are now very popular. They are termed scleral lenses and have some advantages for special cases. Some doctors fit them only for dry eye patients, but there are many other conditions where a scleral lens might be the best option. Conditions such as keratoconus, corneal degeneration, trauma, corneal transplant (see page 353), chemical burns, and more.

The scleral lens/prosthetic device is clear and can vary in size. It can be anywhere from the size of a nickel to a quarter, or even a little larger. It is made from a gas-permeable plastic that allows oxygen to reach the eye's surface. This device will rest on the conjunctiva, the clear tissue over the sclera (the white part of the eye). This part of the eye is much less sensitive than the cornea. By resting on the conjunctiva/sclera only, this lens will vault over the distorted/damaged part of the cornea. This creates a new, smooth optical surface that protects the eye from the environment and any mechanical trauma that can be caused by

blinking action. Review the Resource Organizations on page 413 for practitioners who specialize in this type of contact lens fitting.

If you are considering contact lenses, hopefully this section has helped you identify the correct questions to ask your eye doctor. And if you are a wearer of contact lenses, you might now have an "eye" on a new type of lens. Why not find out if a newer, more versatile lens works for you?

We have certainly journeyed through quite a world of contact lenses. Now you know a good deal of the history, applicability, and even possible future of each type of lens. For summarized comparisons of the types of lenses, especially on key qualities that might help you select a particular lens, see the table below entitled "Characteristics of Various Types of Contact Lenses."

HOW TO WEAR AND CARE FOR YOUR LENSES

Once you decide to use contact lenses to correct your vision, you will have to add some new habits and precautions to your lifestyle. That being said, most wearers of contacts find that the brief time it takes to care for their lenses is well worth it. As a new wearer, you will need to adapt to the lenses. Once the eyes are used to the lenses, however, it will simply be maintenance as usual. Here is some practical advice on wearing and caring for your lenses.

The Process of Adapting to Contact Lenses

The contact lens experience is a very individual one. However, there are a few common

CHARACTERISTICS OF VARIOUS TYPES OF CONTACT LENSES

CHARACTERISTIC	SOFT LENSES	RIGID GAS PERMEABLE LENSES	DISPOSABLE LENSES	SILICONE HYDROGEL DISPOSABLE LENSES	SCLERAL LENSES
Visual acuity	Good	Excellent	Good	Good	Excellent
Resistance to deposits	Poor	Good	Poor Fair (lipids)	Excellent (proteins);	Good
Comfort during first 1–2 weeks	Excellent	Fair	Excellent	Excellent	Good
Comfort after first 1–2 weeks	Excellent	Good	Excellent	Excellent	Good
Gas permeability	Good	Good to excellent*	Good	Excellent	Good
Durability	Fair	Good	Poor	Fair	Excellent
Ability to retain moisture	Fair	Good to excellent	Good	Excellent	Good
Ease of care	Fair	*Excellent*	*Excellent*	Excellent	Excellent
Ease of customizing fit	Fair	Excellent	Fair	Fair	Good
Flexibility in wearing time	Good	Good to excellent	Fair	Excellent	Good
Tintability	Excellent	Good	Good	N/A	Good

* Rigid gas permeable lenses vary in their exact formulation depending on the manufacturer, so it is more difficult to generalize about their characteristics than it is to generalize about the characteristics of other types of lenses.

experiences, as well as symptoms of problems, of which you should be aware. So, let's summarize some initial issues you might experience when you start wearing contacts, as well as a few warning signs to look out for regarding possible complications.

When you first start wearing contact lenses, your eyes will go through a period of physiological adaptation; they will actually "learn" to ignore the contact lenses. This is not asking something unreasonable from your eyes. In fact, you could adapt to and ignore an eyelash stuck in your eye if it were present long enough! Adaptation to rigid lenses can take up

to a week or two, but soft lenses might take only up to a few hours to get used to. Contacts (unlike eyelashes) are designed to be on your eyes, and most people will eventually adapt to them. By the way, to dispel an old wives' tale, calluses do not build up on the insides of the eyelids when you wear contacts, as some people believe.

When you first get your lenses, your eye doctor will put you on a wearing schedule. Be sure to stick to the wearing times, even if the lenses feel great. Sometimes a problem may exist that you can't feel until the lens is removed. An average wearing schedule for adapting to soft lenses and rigid gas permeables is as follows: four to five hours on the first day, five to six hours on the second day, and so on, adding progressively more hours every day until you can wear your lenses for the duration of all your waking hours by the seventh day. Follow your doctor's advice about adapting to your lenses, and know that your wearing schedule might vary from this sample one.

Some of the sensations you may notice with rigid gas permeable lenses include an increased sensitivity to the sun and wind, awareness of the lenses, frequent blinking, fluctuating tear flow, and transient blurred vision. If any of these symptoms persist for more than seven days, tell your doctor when you return for your follow-up exam, which is usually in one week.

Soft lens adaptation is much more subtle. The lens sensation usually disappears within the first thirty to ninety minutes of wearing time. Although soft lenses are very comfortable, your vision may occasionally blur, and you may experience some drying of the lenses and of your eyes. Again, let your doctor know what you experience.

The Maintenance of Your Contact Lenses

Rigid gas permeable and soft contacts require slightly different kinds of care. We can apply some of the same rules for maintaining their effectiveness, but then there are specialized instructions as well. First, I will share with you what I tell my patients about the wearing of and caring for their contact lenses in general. Then I'll follow that up with specific recommendations for the two types of lenses under discussion, and even a little bit of advice on such topics as swimming with your contacts and spending time outdoors with your contacts. Your doctor might have other "dos and don'ts" to add to my suggestions, so be sure to have a full discussion with him as well.

ORDERING CONTACT LENSES

These days there are numerous brands and types of contact lenses available for purchase, and many places from which to purchase them. While it may seem like all contact lenses are essentially the same, they are still FDA-controlled prosthetic devices that require a prescription to acquire. Eye doctors know their patients' eyes and will recommend specific lenses that will be safe and effective for them. If you decide to buy your contacts online, you are likely to find cheaper but similar options being offered in addition to the kind your doctor has prescribed. These lenses, however, may feature old lens technology (sometimes from the 1990s) and may not be the best choices when it comes to the health of your eyes. If you would like to order contact lenses that are different from those listed on your prescription, talk to your eye doctor, whose primary interest is maintaining your eye health.

Preparing to Insert Your Contacts

There are some very important steps to take as you go through the process of inserting your contact lenses. First, wash your hands with a *non-creamy, non-oily* soap before handling your lenses. Most pump soaps contain creams. Both Ivory and a clear soap such as Neutrogena are good examples of soaps that are appropriate to wash with prior to inserting your contacts.

Also, keep your fingernails manicured and short. This allows for easier hygiene and reduces the chance that you will scratch your eye in the process of inserting a lens. Plus, short, manicured nails allow you to maneuver the lens more effectively as you are placing it in your eye.

Never insert lenses if your eyes are red or irritated. Wait a few hours to see if the redness and/or irritation pass. If the symptoms persist, call your doctor. Of course, if there is any severe pain, call the doctor immediately.

Close the drain when you insert or remove your lenses over a sink. Finally, check your lenses often for nicks and other damage. It is easy to do this just prior to inserting them, as you already have them in your hand and they are clean. If a lens has a defect, you can still wear it if it's comfortable, but be especially careful about how you handle it. Order a replacement lens as soon as possible.

Moistening Your Contacts

Contact lenses can become dry due to environmental conditions or simply your eyes' natural tendencies. *Never use saliva to wet your contact lenses.* Saliva is full of bacteria. It's not the same as tears, which are free of bacteria unless you have an eye infection. You can cause a very serious infection by inserting saliva-coated lenses into your eyes.

Please note that it's better to put rigid gas permeable lenses on dry than to wet them with saliva. If necessary, you can wet rigid lenses with bottled, distilled, or filtered tap water. As for moistening soft lenses, use only a designated wetting solution, such as saline solution or a store-bought soft-contact lens rinse—never plain water. In particular, soft-lens wearers should always have a wetting solution on hand to use in an emergency.

Regarding the wetting of either type of lens, *do not use water from the faucet.* Unfiltered tap water is not clean enough. Any kind of water, including bottled and distilled, will be absorbed by the lenses and may cause variation in the lens material.

Conducting Your Cosmetic Routine

Many of your morning habits involving sprays and makeups might have to be adjusted now that you are concerned with maintaining the integrity of your lenses. First, do not insert your lenses until after you have used hair spray. The spray can quickly ruin a lens. However, you should put your lenses in *before* doing your makeup. There's more to say on the subject of cosmetics.

The accumulation of makeup oils and face creams can cause a film to build up on the lenses. The use of cream, instead of powdered, eye shadow and water-soluble makeup reduces the chances that your lenses will become compromised. You can also find makeup products that are specifically designed for contact wearers. They tend to wash away more easily and be less irritating to the eyes.

MAKEUP AND CONTACT LENSES

You can certainly use makeup if you wear contacts, but you should be a little more careful about your makeup routine. Here are a few tips to help you to protect your eyes and your contact lenses.

- Look for oil-free makeup. Makeup with oil could spread around your face, get in your eyes, and blur your lenses.

- Use liquid eyeliner. It is tricky but much safer. Be especially careful if you decide to use a pencil eyeliner. Putting pressure on your eye with a sharp object is risky in any situation, but even worse if you're wearing contacts.

- Choose the right mascara. There are countless types of mascara to choose from, so look for one that doesn't clump or flake. Those that do can irritate your eyes and cause problems with your lenses.

- Use creams or pressed powder. Loose powder makeup can easily get in your eyes, which can cause irritation, damage to your lenses, and even infections. In most cases, creams are best, but a good alternative is a pressed powder, which is less likely than loose powder to get in your eyes.

- Put your contact lenses in *before* you start applying your makeup. Putting the lenses in after you've applied makeup makes it easier for your lenses to get dirty and damaged, and for makeup to get trapped in your eye.

- Never put eyeliner inside your eyelids. Putting liner on the water line makes it very easy for makeup to spread to your eye and get trapped by your lenses, causing irritation or infection.

- Never go to bed with your makeup on. Removing your makeup before going to bed is important because it keeps your face clean and prevents makeup from getting in your eyes and causing infections.

- Remember to remove your contact lenses *before* removing your makeup.

- It may be wise to use a wipe designed specifically for removing eye makeup, since eye makeup can be difficult to remove. Instead of scrubbing your face and irritating your eyes, use a wipe to remove the makeup gently.

Removing and Cleaning Your Lenses

It is smart to establish a routine of always removing the lens from the same eye first, to avoid accidentally interchanging your lenses. In other words, you might want to start habitually with your right eye, removing the lens, cleaning it and placing it in the proper case chamber, before moving on to the left lens.

Clean your lenses, rinse them thoroughly, and disinfect them daily as directed. And don't be afraid of rubbing a soft lens—they are very sturdy (despite their soft feel) and should be rubbed *firmly* in a straight back-and-forth motion to clean them completely. The only caution involves your fingernails; be sure they do not cut the edge of the lens. In addition, change the storing solution daily.

How well you clean your contact lenses

has a profound effect on how long your lenses will last. Be sure to use the cleaning and storing solutions that your eye doctor recommends. There are hundreds of different solutions on the market today, and you have to be careful about what you buy if you switch brands. Do not switch solutions without your doctor's approval.

Moreover, clean your lens case periodically by boiling a pot of water, removing it from the heat, and soaking your empty case for at least twenty minutes. A dirty case can contaminate clean lenses. Of course, so can dirty fingernails.

Taking Extra Precautions

There are some general precautions to take if you wear contacts. First, do not rub your eyes intensely while the lenses are in place. You could tear the lens, irritate your eye, or even cause the lens to get stuck temporarily above your eyelid. Also, avoid anything that may cause dry eyes, such as smoke, wind, and dust. When outdoors, wear sunglasses to help reduce any light sensitivity caused by your lenses.

Remove a lens immediately if a foreign body becomes lodged in your eye. Rinse your eye and the lens thoroughly before reinserting the contact. Do not wear the lens if the discomfort continues.

Do not wear lenses when using eye medications or when you have an eye infection. Call your doctor if you have a question about wearing your lenses while using a systemic medication. If your eyes are red but you have contacts in, don't use eye-whitening drops.

Do not sleep with your lenses without your doctor's approval. In addition, keep a backup pair of glasses on hand, even if you wear your lenses all the time. There may be a

time when you are unable to wear your contacts because of either an infection or a lost lens. Lastly, have your ocular health, visual acuity, and lens performance evaluated at least once each year.

Swimming With Contact Lenses

In general, do not swim with your lenses inserted unless you wear goggles. Wait at least one hour after swimming in chlorinated water to reinsert the lenses. If you are a soft lens wearer and like water activities, there are some additional questions you might have regarding the safety and effectiveness of using soft contact lenses for these activities. Here is some useful information.

When engaging in water sports, you basically have three options. First, you can avoid swimming with contacts. Second, you can remove and dispose of the lenses should they be accidentally exposed to water. And third, you can wear watertight goggles. These options are likely not to please you but they are the safest ways to maintain eye health and the full lifespan of your contacts.

Properly maintained swimming pools are treated with chlorine and other chemicals. Soft lenses may absorb these chemicals, which can irritate the cornea, conjunctiva, and eyelids. If you do wear your contacts into a pool—let's assume you are taking precaution and wearing goggles, but water gets into them—you'll likely have symptoms of redness, discomfort, and light sensitivity. Generally, this reaction is short-lived and doesn't result in permanent damage to the tissues. But to avoid the symptoms as much as possible, remove your lenses as soon as possible and wash your eyes out with artificial tears.

Swimming in the ocean is different. While there are no chemicals to consider, the high concentration of salt in the water will cause the lenses to tighten on the eye. While this is handy to keep the lenses from floating away, it can also cause fitting problems. To resolve this problem, use plenty of lubrication after swimming with the lenses on. And, of course, never swim or surf in polluted water; it can contain microorganisms, which can create infectious conditions for the eye. If you like to swim in lakes or rivers, again be cautious because they can harbor more microorganisms than the ocean. Wearing disposable lenses is the best option here just to make sure that you can replace any possibly contaminated lens immediately. Of course, it is worth repeating that you should not go underwater when wearing contact lenses unless you have goggles in place.

If you are a diver or like to snorkel, a good mask or pair of goggles is essential. There might be some swelling of the cornea during ascension from a dive; thus, your vision will be hazy or cloudy. Wearing the right type of lens—that is, one with high oxygen transmission—will help, but also using lubricating solution immediately after surfacing will help reduce this effect. In addition, it is advisable to wait five minutes before attempting to remove your lenses, just in case they are stuck on your eyes.

For gas permeable lens wearers, the main problem is that the lenses can float off the eye while you are underwater. But a rigid gas permeable or silicone hydrogel lens is the best type for diving, so just be sure to wear a mask and have it properly sealed.

Learning a Little More About Soft Contacts

There are a few extra points to be made about soft lenses in particular. Handle your soft lenses as little as possible, and then only with your fingertips. Never handle your lenses with your fingernails. And be careful not to crease your lenses, which is easier to do if they are very dry.

It is important to check your lenses before inserting them to make sure they are not inside out. If a lens is inside out, it may pop out of your eye when you blink or cause irritation, discomfort, or blurred vision. And once your lenses are removed from your eyes, keep them wet. Should a lens dry out, carefully place it in your storing solution or saline for at least four hours. If it is intact, feels comfortable in your eye, and does not negatively affect your vision, it can be safely worn. However, once a lens has dried, it is weakened and may tear more easily.

Properly cleaning your soft lenses is key to getting them to last their full lifespan. Use only the disinfecting method prescribed by your doctor. Do not change methods without getting your doctor's approval. Generic store-brand contact-cleaning solutions may not be appropriate for newer materials. In addition, ask your doctor about ultrasonic cleaning, which is highly effective in slowing down the build-up on lenses when performed regularly but is not usually necessary for disposable lenses. Lastly, be aware that, unlike rigid lenses, soft lenses cannot be polished.

We have completed the ABCs of wearing and caring for contact lenses. When you first start wearing contact lenses, all of the necessities and precautions might seem a little intimidating. But rest assured that these safety practices all become habit after a while, and very soon, you won't even have to think about most of these steps. A few lifestyle adjustments initially will have to be made, but when the newness wears off, you'll forget what it's like *not* to have contacts and you will become very confident as you wear and care for your lenses.

CONCLUSION

Most vision problems today can be at least partially corrected with contact lenses. Much of the success of contacts, however, still depends on the motivation to maintain them properly and the selection of the proper type of lens. In my practice, I prefer to start a patient with soft lenses because of the comfort factor, and then to move to rigid lenses if the soft lenses aren't satisfactory. That being said, some optometrists like to start with rigid gas permeable lenses, then go to soft lenses if the rigid ones don't work out. They are really apples and oranges, and thus difficult to compare.

All in all, the decision of what type of lens is best must be made on an individual basis, and only after a thorough discussion between you and your eyecare practitioner. The circumstances of some individuals call for a gas permeable fit right away. If you've been wearing hard lenses without much discomfort for the past several years, then you should probably go to rigid gas permeable rather than soft lenses. Why? First of all, the visual acuity is somewhat better when rigid lenses are worn. Second, the required care and handling of the lenses will be closer to what you're used to. As is evident, there are many factors to consider before you make a final decision. So, if you're interested in wearing contacts or in trying a different type, you should ask your eye doctor for the latest information on the lenses that are appropriate for your particular eye problem.

CORNEAL TRANSPLANT

There may come a time when the cornea becomes deformed or defective. One of the more common causes of this is *keratoconus*. (For a complete discussion of keratoconus, see page 259.) Whatever the cause of the corneal deformity or defect, there is a procedure in which the damaged cornea can be removed and replaced with a donor cornea. This section briefly discusses the corneal transplant process.

THE TRANSPLANT

Eye banks in major cities collect healthy corneas from recently deceased individuals who had indicated they wished to donate their organs. Interestingly, the corneas are the only usable parts of donated eyes. The eye banks then fulfill requests from eye surgeons for these corneas. The system of banking and distributing corneas is highly organized and sophisticated.

Corneal transplant surgery involves the use of a *trephine* (TREH-feen), which is used like a cookie cutter, first to remove your distorted cornea and then to cut a similar "button" from the donor cornea. This process is sometimes performed with lasers. The donor cornea button is placed in the round hole of your cornea and stitched in place. The suture (thread) that is used is much finer than a human hair and is easily overlooked by the naked eye.

Not only is corneal transplant surgery the most successful of all the transplant procedures, and very common too, but also the techniques are being improved constantly. Either general or local anesthesia can be used in this surgery, and you may need to spend a night or two in the hospital, but that's usually the maximum stay. You will need someone to drive you home, and once there, you will have to rest and relax for several days.

While corneal transplantation, technically called *penetrating keratoplasty* (PKP), has a 95 percent rate of success, this procedure involves potentially serious risks, as do all operations. In cases in which the first transplant is not successful, a second can be undertaken with success. However, permanent loss of vision, though extremely rare, can also occur. Corneal transplantation is considered only in those cases in which contact lenses cannot be worn or provide inadequate vision correction. It is also the surgery of choice when the cornea becomes clouded or scarred beyond medical treatment.

AFTER THE SURGERY

Most people experience surprisingly little pain and discomfort following a corneal transplant. The time taken off from work varies with the individual and the kind of work the individual does. Generally, if you have a sedentary job, you will be back to work in a week or two. Your bandages may likely be removed in one to two weeks after the surgery, but you will not be able to see clearly yet. It will probably be several months before your vision stabilizes, but your doctor may prescribe eyeglasses or contact lenses to assist you along the process. Individual cases vary, so the time frames mentioned should be considered very general.

The probability that a receiver of a donated cornea will reject the cornea is less than that for any other transplanted organ, simply because the cornea has no blood supply. The rejection of other organs is usually due to incompatibility between the donor and the recipient and is mediated by blood cells.

While the surgical transplantation of a new cornea resolves the basic problem of corneal surface irregularity, eyeglasses or contact lenses are usually still needed for vision correction. In many cases, rigid gas permeable or scleral contact lenses are required to correct the large amount of visual distortion that is associated with transplants. This type of contact lens in discussed in depth on page 346.

CONCLUSION

I feel it is important to repeat that the technology involved in corneal transplants continues to progress. Therefore, it would not be productive to provide very detailed descriptions of the equipment used and steps taken during this process. However, the summary provided in previous pages should give you a good idea of how a corneal transplant is generally approached and accomplished. I hope this summary has also been encouraging to you, as I have stressed how very successful this operation is for the vast majority of patients.

EYEGLASSES

Many people who regularly wear eyeglasses do not think about them very often. The glasses have become a normal part of their life and are easy to take for granted. But the fact is that millions of us wouldn't be able to function without our eyeglasses. It's worth taking a look at how eyeglasses work, how they're made, and how you can choose a pair that's attractive, functional, and durable.

TYPES OF EYEGLASS LENSES

There are two basic types of eyeglass lenses prescribed for vision correction—lenses for nearsightedness and lenses for farsightedness. Both can include astigmatism correction. These two basic types of lenses can also be combined into one lens that corrects for both near and distance problems, as well as one lens that corrects for near, distance, and intermediate problems. Furthermore, such combination lenses can be crafted to meet the specific requirements of a certain work situation or hobby. In this section, we will discuss the two basic types of lenses and the variations that are in popular use today.

Minus Lenses and Plus Lenses

The two basic types of lenses prescribed for vision correction are referred to as minus lenses and plus lenses. The minus lens corrects for nearsightedness. It is concave in shape and thinner in the center than at the edges. Because of this shape, the minus lens weakens the focusing power of light before it enters the eye, so that the image of the object that the eye

is observing falls farther back, on the retina. See Figure 3.5. The minus lens is needed for the nearsighted eye to see clearly at a distance.

The plus lens corrects for farsightedness. It is convex in shape, much like the shape of the crystalline lens in the eye. It is thicker in the center than at the edges, and increases the focusing power of light before it enters the eye. Because of this, images fall farther forward in relation to the retina (see Figure 3.6). This increase in focusing power is needed for the farsighted eye to see clearly.

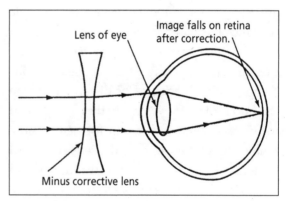

FIGURE 3.5 **How a Minus Lens Works.**

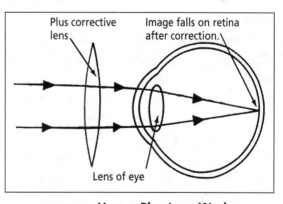

FIGURE 3.6 **How a Plus Lens Works.**

A plus lens is also used to correct presbyopia. In presbyopia, which is a normal part of aging, the eyes' own lenses have hardened and can no longer accommodate to see things up-close. (For a complete discussion of presbyopia, see page 308.) A lens that moves images farther forward to fall on the retina—in other words, a lens that corrects for farsightedness—can compensate for an eye that cannot accommodate for near vision.

The lens used for astigmatism is usually a combination of plus and minus lenses to fit the particular curvatures of the astigmatic eye. This type of lens does not look like either a minus or a plus lens because of the way lenses are now manufactured. However, the principle on which it is based is the same.

Your eye doctor will prescribe exactly the lens power you need to see clearly. Your doctor also will measure the distance between the pupils of your eyes when they are aligned for distance, and then again for near vision. Finally, he will make sure the lenses' optical centers—the parts you look through when you look straight ahead—correspond to those distances.

If you need glasses, it is important to work with an eyecare professional. Beware of "over-the-counter" reading glasses available at pharmacies and discount stores. These glasses are not of high optical quality, and, needless to say, they were not made with your exact prescription in mind. The optical centers of pharmacy glasses will probably be different from those of your eyes, which can cause a lot of eyestrain. Also, such lenses never compensate for astigmatism.

Bifocals

Let's say you need your distance prescription to see the television when you're sitting and the road when you're driving, but you also need some correction for very close work such as reading. In other words, you now have a problem with both near and distance vision, and you have only a narrow range in-between at which you can see without correction. You could keep wearing your distance glasses for getting around in the world and also get a pair of reading glasses for near work. Some people do this. Or, you could enter the world of bifocals.

Bifocals, as their name implies, are lenses that have two focal corrections—one for near-point work and one for distance. If your eye examination reveals that you need bifocals, take heart, for you aren't the first, and you certainly won't be the last person who needs them. Let's explore the world of bifocals to see where they came from and where they're going. You might be surprised.

The first bifocal was developed by Benjamin Franklin in the late 1700s—yes, he was quite the inventor! He took his distance glasses and cut them in half, took his reading glasses and cut them in half, and then glued the two halves together so that the distance lens was on top of the near lens. This primitive but functional solution kept Franklin from having to switch back and forth between two pairs of glasses.

In 1908, John Borsch, Jr., created the first "fused" bifocal. He cut a segment out of the lower portion of a distance lens, inserted a portion of a near lens in the hole, and then heated the two sections to melt them together. The lines between the two lens pieces were not as obvious as those in the Franklin bifocal, but the optics were not as sharp either.

The first truly effective "one-piece" bifocal came along in 1910, when technology had advanced enough to allow the production of a single glass lens with two different curves—one curve for each focal point. The reading segment of this bifocal was large, which sounds appealing to those who need help focusing on near-point work, but the line between the segments was obvious and the glass lenses were heavy. However, this is the same type of lens as today's "executive bifocal," which has a line going all the way across the lens. The executive bifocal is available in either glass or plastic. Its major drawbacks are the prominent line between the segments and the "jump" in image as the eye passes from the distance segment to the near segment. Given the state of technology these days, this type of bifocal is rarely prescribed.

After the first effective one-piece bifocal came the flat-top bifocal, which has been the most popular type of bifocal in recent times. The flat-top is similar to the fused lens invented by Borsch, but the top portion of the reading segment is made of the same material as the distance lens so that, when the lenses are fused, the line between the two sections "disappears" and leaves a crescent-shaped reading segment. This lens has some significant optical advantages, as well as a very thin, hardly noticeable line. Many of today's bifocals are made this way.

Finally, in 1946, a bifocal was developed that was similar, again, to the Borsch lens, but the distance and near segments were blended together at their junction to reveal no noticeable line at all. This was cosmetically appealing because the lens did not look like a bifocal. However, when the wearer changed focus, his vision blurred significantly in the transition zone between the two segments. This was unacceptable to most wearers, so the flat-top remains the bifocal of choice today.

Trifocals and Progressive Addition Lenses (PALs)

Bifocals are adequate for the majority of people with a need for both distance- and near-vision corrections. Most people's eyes can focus for intermediate activities—such as computer work, card playing, music reading, seeing prices on grocery shelves, and working at a large desk—by using either the distance-lens or near-lens segment of their glasses. But there are some people whose eyes need a special lens for this intermediate, arm's-length distance. The answer for these people is—you guessed it—trifocals. Trifocals correct vision at three different focal distances.

The first trifocals were developed in the 1940s and were similar in design to the flat-top bifocals. The only difference was that the trifocals had a third lens segment for intermediate vision, inserted between the near and distance segments. However, the fitting of these lenses was extremely difficult. The intermediate segment needed to be low enough so that the wearer could look comfortably through the distance segment while driving, but it also needed to be high enough so the wearer could look comfortably through the reading segment at, for example, groceries on a supermarket shelf while keeping the head in a normal position. It was no surprise that few people adapted well to the first trifocals.

The next stage of evolution in trifocals occurred in France in the early 1950s. Bernard Maitenaz developed a single lens that incorporated the distance, intermediate, and near prescriptions without any visible lines. This lens was called a progressive addition lens (PAL) because the power change from distance to near was gradual and uninterrupted, similar to the power change normally accomplished by the eye itself. Many people today mistakenly call this lens a "no-line bifocal," but it is more accurately termed a "multifocal" lens. Unfortunately, Maitenaz's first-generation design caused severe distortions at the edges of the lens, which created a swimming effect when walking.

These days, technological advances in optics have not only overcome most of the problems in Maitenaz's lens, but also have improved the lens enough so that it is now the correction of choice in many situations. Currently, more than twenty companies make over three hundred variations of PALs, and the latest versions seem to be easy to adapt to and comfortable to wear. The topmost part of the lens corrects for distance viewing; the central part corrects for intermediate viewing; and the bottom part corrects for near viewing. The head positions required, although still a consideration, are not nearly as much of a complicating factor because of the gradual transition in lens power.

Occupational Progressive Lenses (OPALs)

As they perform their jobs, many people find that conventional lenses don't allow clear or comfortable vision. This can be due to unusual working distances or angles. For example, computer users must be able to clearly see their monitors, which are often positioned straight ahead at an intermediate distance. In addition, they need to see the keyboard very clearly, as well as papers on their desk. Thus, one pair of glasses may not serve all situations. Occupational progressive lenses, or OPALs, are specifically designed to solve challenging on-the-job situations. Occupational lenses come in many forms, but the most current technology allows multiple viewing distances without incorporating any lines in the lenses.

Since your job may have a variety of visual requirements, discuss your needs with your eye doctor to see if there is a lens that is appropriate for you. There are a number of lenses available that are designed with computer use in mind, as well as other types of unusual designs for different working conditions. It is important to have accurate measurements of all your working distances and angles so that your doctor can make the proper recommendations.

For those who don't wear glasses, the world of eyeglasses might seem rather simple and straightforward. But people who must correct vision problems know that obtaining the best eyeglasses for their specific needs and environmental conditions can be a technical and complicated matter. Many factors go into creating effective corrective eyeglass lenses. However, now that online options are promoted for eyeglasses ("we'll send you five pairs to try on"), it still does not replace the interpersonal aspect of eyeglass fitting. You must realize that the technology and training to fit a pair of glasses with a complicated lens correctly requires on-site evaluations and determinations. Now that we have reviewed the general types available, let's learn more about the materials used in lenses.

EYEGLASS LENS MATERIALS

Up until the late 1950s, all eyeglass lenses were made of glass—which is why they weren't called "eyeplastics." Since then, however, the advent of an optical plastic called CR-39 has revolutionized lenses. This material was originally developed during World War II, but over time it was refined to improve its optical properties. CR-39 plastic is now used in over 90 percent of American lens prescriptions. However, there are still options, and we should look at all of them.

Various Plastics

As already mentioned, CR-39 is currently the most widely used material for lenses placed into frames. The main advantage of CR-39 over glass is that it is light in weight—about 50 percent of the weight of a glass lens per diopter of power. (As discussed later in this chapter, the diopter is the unit of measurement for the strength of a prescription.) This makes it much more comfortable to wear, especially for people with a higher prescription, either for nearsightedness or farsightedness.

Plastic also offers much more protection to the eyes. A plastic lens can still break, but it takes a much greater force to break plastic than it does to break glass. In addition, plastic does not splinter into tiny slivers the way glass does. And if you like rimless frames, plastic is the lens material you should choose because it won't chip at the exposed edge nearly as easily as glass does.

Plastic lenses can easily be tinted different colors, and the color can be changed if desired. Glass cannot be so easily tinted, although it can be done. To add to the

positives, plastic lenses can be treated to block out ultraviolet light, which makes it as good a material for sunglasses as glass. Incidentally, glass lenses block most UV light without being treated.

In 1985, a new kind of plastic lens, called *polycarbonate,* entered the market, and it has some advantages over the CR-39 lens. The bending ability of this plastic allows it to be formed into lenses that are much thinner than the lenses made of CR-39 plastic and yet achieve equal optical power. Polycarbonate lenses are also 50 percent lighter than conventional plastic lenses, have inherent UV protection, and can be treated to be scratch-resistant.

One of the most impressive properties of polycarbonate plastic is that it is practically unbreakable. A twelve-gauge shotgun fired at a polycarbonate lens at close range will only dent it! This is obviously the ideal material to use for protective eyewear. The only significant drawback is that the usable optical zone—the part through which you see—of polycarbonate lenses is slightly narrower than that of conventional plastic lenses, so distortions can occur in the peripheral vision, which bothers some people with a higher prescription. A further consideration is that polycarbonate lenses are not tinted as darkly as the other plastics.

Adding to the choices now is a higher-density plastic, called "high-index" plastic. This plastic is similar to CR-39 plastic, except it is denser, allowing lenses to be thinner and lighter, even lighter than polycarbonate lenses. These lenses are becoming more popular as the technology improves. There are even varying levels of high index available too!

A COMPARISON OF DIFFERENT LENS MATERIALS

LENS CHARACTERISTIC	GLASS	CR-39 PLASTIC	POLYCARBONATE PLASTIC	HIGH-INDEX PLASTIC
Weight	Heavy	Light	Very light	Very light
Impact Resistance	Fair	Good	Excellent	Good
Tintability	Fair	Excellent	Good	Good
UV Protection	Excellent (inherent ability)	Poor (but can be treated)	Excellent (inherent ability)	Poor (but can be treated)
Scratch Resistance	Excellent	Fair	Fair	Fair
Thickness per Diopter	Thick	Thicker	Very thin	Thinnest
Available as Photochromic Lens?	Yes	Yes	Yes	Yes
Suitable for Rimless Frames?	No	Yes, in lower prescriptions; no, in higher prescriptions	Yes	Yes

The chief *disadvantage* of CR-39, polycarbonate, and high-index plastics is that they scratch more easily than glass. However, as briefly mentioned above, a scratch-resistant coating can be applied to plastic lenses to reduce their susceptibility. Scratch-resistant coatings are very effective (and getting better), but they do not approximate the hardness of glass when it comes to scratches. With a minimal amount of care to your lenses though, they should not scratch under normal wearing conditions.

Traditional Glass

Glass lenses are still available and do have certain advantages. If you have a mild prescription and a frame that is not very large, the weight of the lenses may not be a problem. They are more scratch-resistant than plastic, and they have an inherent ability to block out UV light. There is also a new version of

glass that simulates some of the properties of high-index plastic, forming thinner, lighter glass lenses that are scratch-resistant.

There's more to consider, however. Ordinary tinting does not work as well in glass as in plastic lenses. The tint can't be changed if you change your mind about the color, and in the higher prescriptions it isn't as uniform in glass as it is in plastic. The main problem with glass lenses, in addition to their weight, is that they can splinter when broken and seriously injure your eyes. Today's glass lenses are tempered (required by Federal law) to minimize splintering, but they are still not as safe as plastic or polycarbonate lenses. I do not recommend glass lenses when playing sports.

By the way, both glass and plastic lenses that react to light and automatically darken as the surrounding light gets brighter are available. So, when you move from indoors to a sunny outdoor environment, you can have automatic protection. Such glass lenses are termed *photochromic lenses*. Plastic lenses that react to light are called *Transitions lenses*. Transitions lenses can change, but they do not get as dark as glass photochromic lenses. Yet the technology continues to advance in this area as well, so newer versions of this lens work better.

So, which is the best lens for you? If you just need to wear glasses occasionally for reading and you have a tendency to toss them around carelessly, glass is the best way to go. If you wear glasses on a full-time basis but your prescription is not very high, CR-39 plastic will do nicely. If your prescription is very high or you're in a high-risk environment for breakage, polycarbonate or high-index plastic is for you. For kids, who are always tough on glasses, polycarbonate is recommended, since it's the safest way to go. Glass will certainly last longer and not become as badly scratched, but polycarbonate is a much safer choice. For a quick comparison of glass, CR-39, polycarbonate, and high-index lenses, see the table below.

EYEGLASS LENS COATINGS

Have you ever noticed how in photographs of people wearing glasses, you can see their lenses but not their eyes? That's because of the reflection of the room lights or sunlight off the front surface of the lens. This occurs because only 92 percent of light passes through a lens; 8 percent bounces off the surface. An anti-reflective lens coating can take care of this problem.

The coating has some distinct advantages. With an anti-reflective coating on the lens, over 99 percent of the light can pass through, with less than 1 percent deflected. Other people can now see the wearer's eyes through the lenses, and the lenses almost seem to "disappear."

Some consider this a major cosmetic advantage, especially if they wear a high prescription; high prescriptions occasionally cause rings of reflected light to be visible in the lens. Moreover, people who drive at night appreciate the coating because it eliminates the glare from oncoming headlights. It has one disadvantage, however—it tends to smudge. So, this coating requires special cleaning and handling. Luckily, newer technology is now available to provide a smudge-proof surface that, moreover, doesn't peel off.

Lenses can also be treated with coatings that block UV light, coatings for scratch-resistance, and tinted coatings. Sunglasses can even be treated with a mirror coating, which does darken the lens a little but is mostly done for the way it looks. Importantly, the photochromic process is not a coating; the material is integrated into the lens matrix.

Having your lenses coated will add to the price of your glasses, but it will add to the value of them as well. Discuss the different lens coatings with your eyecare professional. Find out what's available and which products best suit your needs.

EYEGLASS FRAMES

We have spent a good deal of time on eyeglass lenses—types; materials; and coatings. But we won't get very far with those lenses if we don't put them into a frame. That step brings a whole new set of options. Frames, too, are available in various materials. In addition, they come in various levels of quality and, of course, various styles. Reading through this section will help you make a much more informed decision when you are selecting frames.

Frame Materials

Most eyeglass frames are made of some version of plastic, metal, or nylon. However, researchers are hard at work trying to come up with new materials for frames. In this section, we'll discuss what's available, and the pros and cons that come with your options.

Plastic Frames

The traditional plastic frame is made from a material called zyl (pronounced "zile"). Zyl has the unique property of being easily bent into a particular shape when heated and then holding that shape when cooled. This is critical when adjusting frames to fit thousands of different faces. Zyl is also available in a variety of translucent and opaque colors. It is the most popular material for eyeglass frames.

Carbon fiber is made by adding carbon powder to plastic, which gives the material the strength of metal and the weight of plastic. Carbon-fiber frames are very durable and also manage to hold their shape very well. The color choices are numerous, but all carbon-fiber frames are opaque.

Cellulose propionate is an inexpensive plastic that is usually used for cheap sunglass frames. It is highly breakable, difficult to adjust, and difficult to color completely. This material is mostly used for drug-store reading glasses and sunglasses.

Ultimately, plastics are still popular for fashionable frames. Each type of plastic has its own advantages, and each can be used to enhance your appearance.

Metal Frames

Although many metal frames are gold-colored, it is rare to find real gold in eyeglass frames today. For years, eyewear manufacturers have used a process called *electroplating* to create a gold look on the metal. Most of today's frames are still made using this process.

Aluminum offers a high strength-to-weight ratio—it is light in weight, yet strong. This metal is resistant to corrosion, and it can be treated to take on a variety of colors. However, since it cannot be soldered or welded easily, the design possibilities are limited, and screws and rivets must be used to connect the frame sections.

Beryllium is a metal that was developed by the National Aeronautics and Space Administration (NASA). It is strong, lightweight, and resilient. Because of its high cost, however, it is often combined with other metals, such as copper, to make frames.

Stainless steel is actually 67-percent iron and 18-percent chrome. It is very resistant to corrosion, and frames can be made thin because of its springiness. However, it does not hold adjustments well or allow for easy soldering repair. In addition, it is slightly brittle.

Titanium is a metal that has a high tensile strength, is ultra-light in weight, has impressive durability even when thin, and has excellent corrosion resistance. It is easy to adjust. Yet titanium is difficult to weld or solder, and it is extremely expensive. Titanium-composite frames have the amazing ability to return to their original shape regardless of how much they are bent out of shape. The frames can literally be twisted around on themselves and then return to their original form. This is why titanium is referred to as "memory" metal. These frames are becoming much more popular.

Metal frames have excellent qualities and

offer a high-class look. However, beware of metals that are too inexpensive, since they usually lack durability and may turn green with age. Identify your specific needs, and only then make a choice on the type of metal that would work best for you.

Nylon Frames

Nylon is used mostly in the manufacturing of sports and safety glasses. The frames are unbreakable when new, but lose moisture and become brittle with age. So, nylon frames should not be considered a long-term investment.

Polyamide is a blend of nylons. It features durability, reduced weight, flexibility, scratch-resistance, a non-irritating surface, and the ability to hold translucent colors. Polyamide does, however, lose its adjustment if heated.

Are you overwhelmed by the number of choices? Whether your answer is "yes" or "no," we can't stop here. There's more to consider.

Appropriate Frames for Your Specific Face and Lifestyle

Have you ever heard the saying: "Boys don't make passes at girls who wear glasses"? This saying is so out of date now that you may never even have heard it. Eyeglass frames have gotten much more attractive over the past twenty years, and today are even considered an enhancement, much like makeup and jewelry. To choose eyeglass frames, go to a reputable optical shop and plan to spend some time there. Look for quality and style, not just price.

Quality Issues

Selecting quality eyewear is like picking out fine jewelry. Unless you know exactly what you're looking for and how to judge it, you may be fooled into paying for something you're not getting. Certainly not all frames are alike.

Fashion designers have created quite a stir in the eyeglass-frame world in the past few years. The optical industry is suddenly a part of the fashion scene. Most designers have some knowledge of what goes into products that bear their names. However, some just sell their names, handing total control over to manufacturers, who are then free to use the least expensive manufacturing methods. It's best to examine a frame carefully and to ask the optician to tell you about its durability and other characteristics.

The quality of a frame is evident in the material used, the workmanship, the attention to detail, and the integrity of the hinges and nose pads. Examine a frame as you would a piece of jewelry to see if the quality stands out. You may want to compare a few different frames to get a sense of what represents quality workmanship. Also, check any warranties that come with the frame. Good frames are warranted for at least a year or two.

In general, expect to pay about $95 to $150 for a high-quality plastic frame, and $175 to $225, or more, for a high-quality metal frame. Rimless frames usually run a bit more. In 2018, an "average" pair of glasses (single vision lenses and frame) cost $376. Quality, however, is worth the price. A frame that won't crack, chip, peel, tarnish, or corrode is valuable and a pleasure to own. As with any purchase, you most often get what you pay for.

Style Concerns

Styles change in frames as they do in clothes, cars, makeup, and just about anything else we use to adorn ourselves. There are basic styles that have been around for years and will be here for years to come. And there are styles that make a statement, albeit for a short period of time. Picking the right frame for your face shape, skin tone, hair color, makeup, clothing, and lifestyle takes some expertise. Try to find a trustworthy optician who has experience, knowledge, and taste in eyewear. Word-of-mouth referrals are a good source. If you see someone who has good-looking glasses, find out where that person purchased them.

Here are some tips to help you select the right frame for you. First, determine your face shape. To do this, pull your hair away from your face, look in a mirror, and outline your face on the mirror with lipstick. (This is a bit messy, but it works.) Once you know the shape of your face, you can choose the general shape of your eyeglasses. The general rule is that your eyewear shape should contrast with your face shape. "Choosing a Frame for Your Face" on page 365 gives specific advice for the seven different face shapes. Some additional fashion tips to consider are listed below:

- If you have a long nose or wide-set eyes, look for a thick, darkly colored bridge that rests low on the nose.

- If you have close-set eyes, look for a high, thin, lightly colored bridge or a thin frame shape.

- If you have a short face or a wide face, look for a highly placed temple.

- If you have a full hairstyle around your face, look for a thin, light frame.

- If you have minimal or sleek hair around your face, look for a bold frame.

- The top of the frame should be at or just below the eyebrow line.

- Your eyes should be close to the center of the lens area.

Back in the 1960s, "granny glasses" were all the rage. These were rimless frames that were barely noticeable. They simply had two *temples*—the part that goes from the lens to your ear—and a nosepiece bridge, which were held to the lenses with a few screws. Any shape lenses could be used, though the small round ones were the most popular.

Granny glasses are harder to come by these days, but they can still be found. Their main disadvantage is that holes must be drilled into the lenses, and the screws used to attach the frame pieces to the lenses often loosen. Drilling a hole in a lens can cause it to crack. If you have rimless glasses, be careful when handling them, especially when putting them on, taking them off, and cleaning them. Only some types of plastic lenses can be used for rimless glasses, since glass would break if a hole were to be drilled into it.

If you like the idea of rimless glasses but not the holes in the lenses, what about the nearly rimless option? Frames that have an upper rim but just thin nylon cords to support the bottoms of the lenses are called *rimlon* frames. The cords are positioned in grooves cut into the edges of the lenses. Rimlon frames have many advantages. They are light in weight, are not very noticeable on the face, and yet are durable

CHOOSING A FRAME FOR YOUR FACE

Take the following pointers into consideration when you are selecting a frame. First, however, you must determine your particular face shape.

Oval Face

Description: An oval face is considered to be a "well-balanced" face. The top half balances the bottom half. Frame: An oval face can wear just about anything, as long as the frame is in proportion to the face.

Round Face

Description: A round face has a large, curved forehead and a rounded chin. The face looks "full," with very few angles. Frame: Angular or geometric frames give better contours to a round face.

Heart-Shaped Face

Description: The forehead is the widest part of the heart-shaped face. Then the face narrows, and the chin is slightly pointed. Frame: Try a frame with straight top lines and rounded sides, such as "aviator" or "butterfly" shapes.

Rectangular Face

Description: The rectangular face is long and narrow with a square-ish chin. Frame: Frames with a strong top bar and round bottom lines are a good choice.

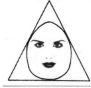

Triangular Face

Description: The triangular face has a narrow forehead, but is full around the cheeks and chin. Frame: A heart-shaped frame is best. Square frames, aviator frames with a straight top, or wire frames that are rimless on the bottom can also work well.

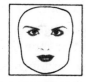

Square Face

Description: The square face has a wide forehead and a wide cheek and chin area. The jaw is angular. Frame: Oval or round frames add soft lines to a square face.

Diamond-Shaped Face

Description: The diamond-shaped face has a small forehead, a wide temple area, and a small chin area. Frame: A butterfly-shaped frame is best. You can also try a square frame.

This chart is courtesy of You! Are Something Beautiful, *La Habra, CA.*

if they are of good quality. They also have disadvantages, though. The nylon cords stretch with time, so the lenses can pop out (replacing the cord is easy, however); the edges of the lenses are exposed and can chip; and the higher prescriptions look very obvious. High-index lenses work well with these types of frames.

The Process of Choosing Frames for Children

Choosing frames for children takes special effort and care. Try to make it fun, not frustrating. Approach the process in a way that makes your child want to wear and enjoy the glasses. While you will feel compelled to contribute your opinions, let the child make the final choice to assure that he is happy with the final pair. That way, he will be more likely to use his glasses as instructed by the doctor.

Children's frames need to be durable. The glasses will likely be on and off a dozen times per day, so they should be able to withstand wear and tear. Many kids' frames have spring hinges on the temples. When the temples are bent outward, they just spring back to the proper position. (These hinges are becoming popular for adults, too.) To make staying on the child's face easier, some frames have cable temples, which wrap around the ears. Cable temples are especially good for smaller children.

For infants and toddlers, patience is the key to fitting glasses. Let the baby play with the glasses first so that he can become familiar with them and want to keep them. Have the baby put the glasses on, and don't worry if they're upside down. Make a game out of it—on and off, on and off, a few times. Encourage the baby to enjoy the experience.

Older kids want frames that are "cool," and those frames are often the same ones that adults have. Smaller versions of the more popular adult frames are big sellers for kids. Many are adapted to children's sizes by building up the nosepiece bridge to fit the smaller face. Brighter colors are used because children's clothes are brighter. Many designers have come out with specific lines of frames for children.

Treat your older child with respect, and discuss the different features of each frame and whether the frame is good for his needs. Your optician should be able to advise you here. The optician should make sure that the bridge of the frame fits the child's nose correctly, since children's skin is softer and more sensitive to pressure. The temples should be adjusted so that there is no excessive pressure behind the ears. Comfort is a function of the weight and tension of the glasses being distributed as evenly as possible. Expect a growing child's frame to fit for about a year. Don't buy a frame that is too big and expect the child to grow into it.

When you and your child pick up the finished glasses, have your child first look at the glasses. Let him put the glasses on himself and look through them. (If your child is an infant or toddler, you will probably need to play the on-and-off game again.) At this point, the optician can advise your child and make adjustments to the frame. The optician should also explain how to clean and care for the glasses and give your child a glasses case, stressing the importance of keeping the glasses in the case when they are not being worn. Bring your child back in a week or two for an adjustment. Your child can then tell the optician about wearing the glasses, and the optician can reinforce how well the child is doing.

The prices of children's frames shouldn't be quite as high as the prices of adult frames, but don't skimp on quality to save a few dollars. In general, children's frames should sell for about $75 to $100. Occasionally you'll see special offers that combine both frame and lenses together as a package price. The keys to a successful frame for children are function, fit, and comfort. And don't forget that it is critical for children who wear corrective lenses to have their vision checked every year.

Prescription Considerations

When choosing a frame, the type and kind of prescription may make a difference. The next section of this chapter will explore how to read and understand an eyeglass prescription. For now, here are a few considerations when it comes to putting that prescription into frames.

Do you have a multifocal lens prescription? If you are wearing a progressive lens (PAL), the eye size of the frames should be somewhat "deeper" (vertically) to assure that all areas of vision are clear. However, newer technology allows narrower frames to be used. And do you have a significantly high—often called "strong"—prescription? If your prescription is rather high, the lenses may become relatively thick. So, you may want to consider a frame with a smaller eye size. However, thanks to the newer high-index lenses, the lenses can be thinner, so this might not be as much of a bother as it once was. Also, with a high correction you will likely want to stay away from rimless frames, which show the entire edge of the lens. Stick to a plastic or thicker metal frame.

Don't forget to consider how and where you wear your glasses. Are you an athlete? Do you work with chemicals? If safety is a concern, the right frame is essential. Specific safety frames are available to assure proper eye protection in all hazardous environments.

Take some time to choose the right frame for you. Don't limit yourself to ten minutes to find a frame that you might wear for a year or two. Remember that people will see your eyeglass frame before they see your face, so think about the image you want to project. Consider this: Most people have at least six pairs of shoes and only one pair of glasses, but how often do other people first look at your shoes?

THE EYEGLASS PRESCRIPTION

If you have ever had a prescription for eyeglasses, you may have noticed that it looked rather confusing. Whatever happened to 20/20? As you may remember from our discussion about 20/20 vision in "The Eyes and the Visual System" (see page 7), visual acuity can be determined by reading special charts. A prescription for glasses, though, cannot. Look at Figures 3.7 and 3.8, and I'll explain how to read a prescription so that you can judge how your eyes are doing when you look at one. Note that this section refers to an eyeglass, not a contact lens, prescription—they are very different!

The basic prescription is broken down into two general categories—distance vision and near vision. In the illustrations at left, you see the abbreviations "OD" and "OS." These, respectively, stand for *oculus dexter*, the Latin term for "right eye," and *oculus sinister*, the Latin term for "left eye." Some prescription forms more straightforwardly say "right" and "left," or "R" and "L."

The first column on the left, labeled "Sphere," is for indicating the basic power of the lenses. If the numbers in this column are preceded by minus signs, the prescription is for minus lenses, which correct for nearsightedness. If the numbers are preceded by plus signs, the prescription is for plus lenses, which correct for farsightedness. (It is possible to be farsighted in one eye and nearsighted in the other, although this is uncommon.) The unit of measurement is the *diopter,* which gives the refractive power of the lens. The larger the number is, the greater is the requested correction. A typical prescription for a mildly nearsighted patient would be about –0.25 to –1.50 diopters; –1.75 to –3.00 diopters would be a moderate prescription; –3.25 to –6.00 diopters would be for a significant correction; and over –6.00 diopters would be a severe prescription. For farsightedness, up to about +1.50 diopters would be considered a mild prescription; +1.50 to +3.50 diopters would be a moderate prescription; +3.50 to +4.50 diopters would correct for significant farsightedness; and over +4.50 diopters would be assigned for severe farsightedness.

FOR MR. JOHN DOE EXAM DATE

℞		SPHERE	CYLINDER	AXIS	PRISM	BASE
DIST.	OD	-1.00	-0.75	180	—	—
	OS	-2.25	-1.25	75	—	—
NEAR	OD					
	OS					

PD 64/60 SPECIAL INSTRUCTIONS

O.D.

FIGURE 3.7 **An Eyeglass Prescription to Correct Nearsightedness and Astigmatism.**

FOR MS. JANE DOE EXAM DATE

℞		SPHERE	CYLINDER	AXIS	PRISM	BASE
DIST.	OD	+1.50	—	—	—	—
	OS	+0.50	-0.50	90	—	—
NEAR	OD					
	OS					

PD 64/60 SPECIAL INSTRUCTIONS

O.D.

FIGURE 3.8 **An Eyeglass Prescription to Correct Farsightedness and Astigmatism.**

In the nearsighted prescription illustrated in Figure 3.7, the patient needs a distance correction of –1.00 diopters in his right eye and –2.25 diopters in his left. Here's a pop quiz: Which of this patient's eyes is worse—the left or the right? Would his right eye be considered mildly, moderately, or significantly nearsighted? What about his left eye?

In the prescription illustrated in Figure 3.8, the patient is farsighted. Their right eye needs a distance correction of +1.50 diopters, and the left eye needs a correction of +0.50 diopters. Is he mildly, moderately, or significantly farsighted in his right eye? What about in his left eye? A similar prescription might be written for a presbyopic patient.

The second and third columns on both prescriptions are labeled "Cylinder" and "Axis." They are for indicating the amount and the direction of any astigmatism. Picture the cornea of a normal eye as being shaped like a basketball (a sphere) and that of an astigmatic eye as more like a football (a squashed sphere). The "Cylinder" column gives the amount of correction the astigmatic eye needs. It is expressed in diopters with a plus or minus sign. The "Axis" column gives the direction of the astigmatism—that is, which way the "football" is turned. This is expressed in degrees between 1 and 180. The prescription illustrated for the nearsighted patient shows astigmatism in both eyes. The farsighted patient needs correction for astigmatism only in the left eye. Changes in the degree of nearsightedness and farsightedness are common over time. Astigmatism normally remains about the same in adulthood, although minor changes may occur after the age of sixty.

The fourth column on both prescriptions is headed "Prism." A prism correction bends light and may be prescribed for special binocular vision problems. It is less commonly used in prescriptions. The final column, entitled "Base," refers to whether the base of the prism in the lens should point up, down, in, or out.

The "PD" at the bottom of the form is short for "pupillary distance," the distance between the patient's pupils. It is usually written using two numbers, as in the illustrations. These figures express the distance between the pupils when looking at a distant object and when looking at a near object. These distances are measured in millimeters and don't change during adulthood.

In most states, eyeglass prescriptions expire after one year, although in some, they remain good for two years. You should have your eyes checked at least once a year anyway!

INSTRUCTIONS ON HOW TO CARE FOR YOUR GLASSES

Taking care of glasses doesn't take much time or effort, but a little care can go a long way. When you first get your glasses, make sure that someone who knows what they are doing adjusts them. There is nothing more annoying than having your glasses hurt behind your ears or slip down your nose while you're reading.

To check the fit of your glasses, look down at the floor with the glasses on and shake your head firmly. The glasses shouldn't slip at all. Sometimes it takes a few days before glasses that are too tight start hurting. Don't get discouraged if it takes two or three return visits to the optician to get a proper fit.

Many opticians and pharmacies sell little eyeglass-repair kits. These kits are okay, but a word of caution is necessary. The screwdrivers are small, and it doesn't take much to strip the head of a tiny screw or to "inject" yourself with the tiny screwdriver. The best thing to do is to take your glasses back to your optician every three months or so for a tightening and "tune-up." If you take them back to the shop where you bought them, you should not be charged for this service. Sometimes optical shops offer this complimentary service as a public relations promotion.

How about daily care? Well, you should always wet plastic lenses before wiping them. If you don't, the dirt on the lens may scratch the surface. I recommend using a one-to-one mixture of glass cleaner and water. Dry the lenses with a soft cotton cloth, not with paper tissues. Lenses with an anti-reflective coating must be cleaned with a special cleaning agent, which you most likely can buy from your optician. To clean your frames, soak the glasses in detergent overnight.

Even with good care, lenses generally need to be replaced about every one to two years. Frames usually have to be replaced about every two years. Take good care of your glasses, and they'll take good care of your vision.

CONCLUSION

With the popularity of "refractive surgery" today (see page 371), you might get the impression that eyeglasses will eventually be obsolete. Well, don't count on it! There is nothing wrong with wearing glasses if they help you to see or to correct any type of eye malfunction. And many people are using them as a fashion statement—just look at all of the designers who are getting into the act! In addition to correcting vision problems, your eyeglasses should work for your particular lifestyle and fashion tastes. So take time to find the right eyeglass material and frames, not to mention the right eyecare professional.

ORTHOKERATOLOGY

In the 1960s, when hard contact lenses were first being fitted, doctors discovered that the lenses caused a slight change in the shape of the cornea. They also noted that this flattening of the cornea caused a reduction in the degree of nearsightedness. Patients would take their contacts off and be able to see much better for the remainder of the day. However, by the next day their vision was poor again and the contacts were put on so that they could regain clear distance vision. Over the course of the following decade, these observations led to the development of a therapeutic treatment called *orthokeratology*, which is explored in the following section.

THE EFFECTIVENESS OF ORTHOKERATOLOGY

By the early 1970s, a group of optometrists were discussing what they believed was happening to the corneas of contact lens wearers. They called the process *orthokeratology* (or-tho-care-ah-TOL-oh-gee), from the Greek words *orthos*, which means "straight," and *kerato*, which pertains to the cornea. They saw this process of "straightening" the cornea with contact lenses as similar to straightening the teeth with dental braces, and they started to do it therapeutically. Special lenses were devised, and cases were carefully studied.

ARE YOU A CANDIDATE FOR ORTHOKERATOLOGY?

Anyone who has to wear eyeglasses or contact lenses for several hours a day can appreciate a technique that, for some, offers 20/20 vision after a week of treatment. Orthokeratology—or ortho-k, as it is sometimes called—isn't for everyone, though. To be a candidate, you must have a fairly low degree of myopia, or nearsightedness (ideally, -4.00 diopters or less) and a low degree of astigmatism, as well. Although ortho-k can work for people of any age, those under forty generally experience the best results.

More research has since been conducted, and now there are documented cases of contact lenses actually reducing nearsightedness to the point of complete correction. This process used to take anywhere from twelve to eighteen months, depending on the degree of nearsightedness. With new lens designs and materials, however, it now can take as little as one week to achieve the same effect.

The lenses now used for orthokeratology are made of a material similar to that used for the rigid gas permeable lenses prescribed for standard vision correction, but they transmit enough oxygen so that they can be worn overnight. The most popular of the orthokeratology programs is called Corneal Refractive Therapy (CRT). Approved in 2002, the program allows the doctor to fit contact lenses to the patient to be put on just before bedtime. The lenses are then removed upon awakening and the patient will notice that her distance vision is clearer. This process is continued on a nightly basis, and clear (20/20) vision usually results within a week. CRT is designed only for treatment of low-to-moderate amounts of nearsightedness and slight amounts of astigmatism, not for treatment of farsightedness. There are other newer versions of this type of program as well, so ask your eyecare professional if she has been trained to perform this procedure.

THE POSSIBLE SHORTCOMINGS OF ORTHOKERATOLOGY

Are there any cautions or downsides to orthokeratology? Well, CRT can cost up to four times more than using standard rigid gas permeable lenses because the program requires several visits to the optometrist and utilizes a complicated lens design. The program is effective as long as the lenses are consistently worn, but if the lenses are removed for an extended period of time, the eye will return to its original shape and refractive error (or very close to it). So the effects of CRT are reversible, lasting only as long as the lenses are used. Finally, as touched upon earlier, CRT is limited to low or moderate amounts of myopia and will work with only minor amounts of astigmatism, as well.

CONCLUSION

Considering the information presented in these pages, does orthokeratology sound interesting to you? If so, contact the Orthokeratology Academy of America for help in locating a doctor in your area who specializes in the procedure. For the address and other contact information of the society, see page 415 of the Resource Organizations section.

REFRACTIVE SURGERY

Refraction is the changing of the path of light. In the optical arts, refraction refers to how the light enters the eye and comes to a focus on the retina. Light starts to refract toward the retina as soon as it enters the eye. In nearsightedness, however, the light refracts in a way that causes it to focus in front of the retina when looking at a distant image. In farsightedness, the light is focused in back of the retina. In astigmatism, because the cornea is shaped like a barrel instead of a sphere, the light is focused at two different points around the retina and cannot be reconciled without assistance.

Methods of surgery to correct refraction problems have been developed. Since about 80 percent of the eye's refractive power comes from the front part of the cornea, refractive surgery consists of altering the shape of the cornea to cause the light rays to refract properly and focus directly on the retina. When successful, it can dramatically reduce or eliminate your need for glasses or contact lenses. However, as with all surgeries, you should not jump in without complete information on the surgical procedure, the healing process, and the long-term effects. Here's the scoop on the latest in refractive surgery.

TYPES OF REFRACTIVE SURGERY

The more widely practiced types of refractive surgery include the following: photorefractive keratectomy (PRK), laser-assisted intrastromal keratomileusis (LASIK), conductive keratoplasty (CK), and small incision lenticular extraction (SMILE). In addition, an intracorneal ring (ICR) is currently used for special circumstances—mostly keratoconus. All of the procedures involve changing the shape of the cornea or changing the focusing power of the lens inside the eye so that light entering the eye comes to a focus more accurately.

One recent addition to the list of surgeries is refractive lens exchange (RLE), which is the placement of a multifocal intraocular lens. This is especially useful for people who have myopia that is greater than -12.00, are over forty-five years old, and have presbyopia. The procedure replaces the eye's normal (or healthy) crystalline lens with a multifocal lens.

The process is similar to what surgeons are doing with cataract surgery, except a clear lens is removed instead of one that is clouded. (For more on cataract surgery, see page 335.)

Another new solution for refractive problems is an intraocular contact lens. In this case, an artificial lens is placed in front of the existing natural lens. However, this procedure creates many side effects, so it is rarely used.

For a quick comparison of the most popular procedures, see the table on page 373. The next few pages present more in-depth material on a number of the techniques just mentioned so that you will have a clearer idea of what these procedures entail.

Photorefractive Keratectomy (PRK)

Photorefractive keratectomy is a computer-assisted surgical technique that uses an excimer (EX-im-er) laser to correct refractive errors. In October 1995, the FDA approved the first excimer laser system for use in this procedure. In PRK, the cornea is reshaped using the energy from the light emitted by the laser. Specifically, the laser produces an ultraviolet beam of light and emits it in pulses. Each pulse delicately removes microscopic layers of tissue from the cornea. A computer that is pre-set to your particular needs controls the laser.

After the procedure, healing may take several weeks, although usually vision is good and no eye discomfort is experienced after the first week. For the first few days, a contact lens is used to bandage the eye. Drops are applied to the eye for several weeks to help reduce the inflammation. To date, more than 1,000,000 people in forty countries have had PRK. Many refractive surgeons prefer the PRK procedure because there is no "flap" created,

COMPARISON OF THE THREE MOST POPULAR TYPES OF REFRACTIVE SURGERY

CHARACTERISTIC	PHOTOREFRACTIVE KERATECTOMY (PRK)	LASER-ASSISTED INTRASTROMAL KERATOMILEUSIS (LASIK)	CONDUCTIVE KERATOPLASTY (CK)
Range of Correction (in diopters)	−1.00 to −10.00 D.	−3.00 to −10.00 D.	+0.50 to +2.00 D.
Duration of Procedure	5 minutes.	20 minutes.	3 minutes.
Risk of Complications*	Very low.	Low.	Low.
General Physical Recovery Time (to return to work)	3 days.	1 day (usually).	1 day (usually).
Visual Recovery Time (visual acuity)	1 to 2 weeks.	1 week.	1 week.
Side Effects Immediately After Surgery	Irritation; watering; sometimes burning for about 3 to 4 days.	Scratchy sensation.	Discomfort and/or foreign-body sensation; glare; halos; over-correction; tearing.
When Second Eye Can Be Treated	Same day, if desired.	Same day, if desired.	Usually performed on one eye only.

While overall complication rate is low, when complications do occur they can cause serious loss of vision, especially with LASIK.

as is done with LASIK. When LASIK has side effects, they are typically related to the flap. In addition, because the tissue of the eye being operated on is "connective" tissue, any person with a disease that affects connective tissue—such as lupus or rheumatoid arthritis—should not have the procedure performed.

Laser-Assisted Intrastromal Keratomileusis (LASIK)

Laser-assisted intrastromal keratomileusis is the most popular of all refractive procedures. In LASIK, a superficial layer of the cornea or "flap" of tissue is cut from the cornea and lifted up. Then, the laser evaporates the tissues under it. It is a procedure that combines the use of the excimer laser from PRK with the creation of a corneal flap from ALK.

LASIK has traditionally been used more than PRK and has been commonly used since the late 1990s. To date, the procedure has been performed on several million patients in the United States and millions more worldwide. In fact, LASIK is the most commonly performed refractive procedure by eye surgeons around the world. ALK and PRK, the two procedures that make up LASIK, have been approved by the FDA. However, some of the risks associated with LASIK (and not with PRK) are post-surgical dry eyes; a wrinkling of the surgical flap; induced astigmatism; instability of the flap; growth of cells under the flap (which is a serious complication); and greater difficulty in treating infections.

While the LASIK flap traditionally has been made using the microkeratome (small blade used to cut the cornea), a new procedure has become popular. It is known as Intralase, and uses a bladeless way of creating the flap. When this newer procedure is used, the surgery is sometimes called "All-Laser LASIK" or "Bladeless LASIK." There are some positive aspects to performing the procedure in this manner, but the biggest advantage is that the flap itself has a cleaner edge and thus will fit back more precisely. The main drawback is that it is a more expensive procedure.

You may have heard of a type of LASIK called "wave-front." This refers to a way of measuring the refractive error of the eye in more ways than just nearsightedness, farsightedness, or astigmatism. The technique was developed by the same physicists who invented complicated optics for telescopes—optics that allowed images to be focused with more detail. The techniques of those physicists have been adapted to the lasers used in eye surgery to assist in refining the correction process. Wave-front procedures may eventually become the state-of-the-art in laser surgery, but the cost of the procedure will be higher. In many patients they may yield improved vision compared to standard PRK or LASIK.

Conductive Keratoplasty

Conductive keratoplasty, also called NearVision CK, can change how the eye focuses light by reshaping the cornea to make it steeper. CK uses radio waves, instead of a laser or scalpel, to bring near vision back into focus. It is performed using a small probe, thinner than a strand of human hair, that releases radio waves. The probe is applied in a circular pattern on the outer cornea to shrink small areas of collagen (corneal tissue). This circular shrinkage pattern creates a constrictive band

(like the tightening of a belt), increasing the overall curvature of the cornea. The procedure, which takes less than three minutes, is done in-office with only eye drop anesthesia.

CK is most often performed on one eye to achieve a monovision effect. Some people who have had CK have experienced side effects that have impaired their vision for a few days after the procedure. Some side effects include the following: discomfort and/or foreign body sensation; glare; halos; over-correction (addition of too much power); and tearing. Although these risks are relatively rare, they should be taken into consideration by anyone who is thinking about having the procedure done. Moreover, recent trials have noted that the effect of CK is temporary.

The majority of patients who have the CK procedure do end up being able to read without glasses. However, depending on your age and the type of refractive disorder you have, you may need additional vision treatment—such as surgery, reading glasses, or bifocals—as well, at some point. This is because your eyes continue to change as you age.

Small Incision Lenticle Extraction (SMILE)

As the newer lasers became more sophisticated, they were found to be able to cut into some layers of the eye without disturbing other layers. Small incision lenticle extraction, or SMILE, is the newest and most recently FDA-approved laser vision-correction procedure. The main procedural difference between a SMILE procedure and LASIK or PRK is that an excimer laser is not used. Instead, a femtosecond laser cuts a tiny keyhole incision in a patient's cornea, where the lenticule (a small piece of corneal tissue) is then removed. This helps to reshape the cornea and improve vision, thus incorporating the benefits of both LASIK and PRK.

Currently, SMILE can correct vision only for those with low to moderate levels of myopia (nearsightedness). If your prescription does not fall under this category, SMILE is not currently the best option for you. SMILE also has the advantage of being an option for those who were not good LASIK candidates due to thin corneas. Similar to PRK, no flap is created with SMILE, which allows for more of the outer corneal layer to remain intact. Because of this, SMILE is safer than LASIK for patients that are at risk for trauma to the head or eye (e.g., boxers) because of its greater corneal stability. In addition, there is evidence that SMILE is a better option for candidates predisposed to chronic dry eye, as studies show that fewer corneal nerves are cut than with a LASIK flap.

SMILE has been performed over half a million times around the world. During its clinical trials, SMILE has exhibited fast visual recovery with minimal post-operative discomfort. The visual recovery from a SMILE procedure is almost as fast as that of LASIK but much faster than a PRK procedure.

WHAT SHOULD YOU EXPECT DURING AND AFTER SURGERY?

The next couple of paragraphs will give you a better idea of the physical experience of refractive surgery and the surgery's ocular results. Because the recovery experience differs from person to person, we shouldn't spend time on very specific reactions. But many people want to know what general symptoms and vision changes occur within the first couple of weeks. Let's consider just two of the refractive surgery procedures—PRK and LASIK—so that you can get a basic idea of what to expect.

Immediate Postoperative Experience

Refractive surgery is typically performed on an outpatient basis with a topical (eye drop) anesthetic. Immediately after the surgery, you can expect certain symptoms and outcomes. The expectations will change according to what type of procedure you have chosen.

The postoperative discomfort of PRK is generally more significant than what follows LASIK. So, your doctor may prescribe a soft contact lens that functions as a bandage and eases the discomfort, as well as eye drops that reduce the inflammation. Infection is also a risk during the first two to three days following the procedure, but you will be given antibiotic eye drops and told which activities to avoid in order to minimize this risk. Most doctors recommend that you stay home from work for a few days, but after that, you can resume your normal activities.

The risk of postoperative pain for LASIK surgery is somewhat lower than it is for PRK. You may just feel a scratchy sensation. Your visual recovery may be faster than it is with PRK. In fact, you may be able to return to work as early as the day after surgery.

The Days and Weeks that Follow

The amount of time it takes the vision to stabilize after refractive surgery varies from days to months, since the healing process differs from patient to patient. However, most people can expect some general results. Of course, these differ according to the procedure chosen, too.

Let's first discuss PRK. If you have mild to moderate nearsightedness, the chances are excellent that you will end up with 20/20 vision from PRK. On day one, your vision will likely be in the range of 20/40 to 20/80; days two to four, you should expect between 20/40 to 20/200; and for days four and five, anticipate your vision to be 20/30 to 20/80. You should be able to drive by the fifth or sixth day after surgery, and have excellently clear vision within two to four weeks after the procedure.

The most common complaints after undergoing PRK are a hazy sensation and halos around lights. For some patients, it may take from weeks to months to reach optimal vision after PRK, often depending on the initial lens prescription. Several newer medications have reduced this time significantly.

If you select LASIK, you will likely have minimal discomfort and may return to work sooner. However, if there is a problem with the procedure, it most often occurs with the flap that is created during the procedure. (Please note that long-term "flap" problems do not occur with PRK.) If the procedure needs a "touch-up" or a further procedure, this flap can be simply lifted up for as long as a year after the original procedure was performed. While this might be a good thing, it also has some disturbing potential consequences. After the procedure, you will be given eye drops to reduce the swelling and an antibiotic to reduce the risk of infection. Any minimal discomfort for the first few days should be easily resolved

with an aspirin-type medication. Within a week, you'll feel close to normal.

Regarding LASIK, if you are under-corrected or over-corrected, or if your vision regresses over time, your doctor may suggest further surgery to improve the result. However, many patients require only a single procedure. Note that one significant result can be dry eyes, which is a result of cutting the nerves that enter the cornea. There is a likelihood of dry eyes for at least six months, and sometimes indefinitely.

Like all three procedures, SMILE produces an excellent refractive outcome that rewards patients with wonderful eyesight and freedom from glasses and contacts. Studies show that visual outcomes from SMILE, LASIK, and PRK are virtually identical. There is some data that implies that SMILE may have a lower retreatment (enhancement or touch-up procedure) rate than LASIK or PRK.

Again, these expectations are general guidelines, and your experience may be different. Be sure to fully discuss the expected results with your doctor before you commit to and undergo a refractive surgery procedure. It is also helpful to talk to individuals who have had the type of surgery you are considering, just to get a few firsthand reports.

IS REFRACTIVE SURGERY RIGHT FOR YOU?

With the help of your eye doctor, and after careful consideration of your particular lifestyle, healing tendencies, and life circumstances, you should be able to determine whether you are a good candidate for refractive surgery and which procedure is best suited to your visual requirements. But in general, there are certain conditions that are contraindicated for refractive surgery. You are most likely not a candidate for the surgery if you:

- are under eighteen years of age
- have uncontrolled vascular disease
- have active autoimmune or collagen vascular diseases, such as lupus, scleroderma, or rheumatoid arthritis
- use immunosuppressive drugs
- have severe dry eye symptoms
- demonstrate signs of keratoconus
- are pregnant or nursing
- have a residual, recurrent, or active eye disease
- have unstable or uncontrolled diabetes
- have progressive myopia or hyperopia
- have uncontrolled glaucoma
- have had previous herpes infections of the eye

If you are still at the stage at which you are deciding whether refractive surgery is a good idea for you, the first step you should take is to get a complete eye examination and discuss the possibilities with your doctor. Besides determining your refractive error, your doctor will also check that you have no disease or corneal irregularity that could complicate a refractive surgery procedure. The doctor should also ask you questions about your lifestyle and occupation, and discuss your needs and wishes. This is when you should ask your doctor any questions you may have. Below are sample questions that you might want to cover with your eye doctor:

- Am I a good candidate for refractive surgery?
- Which procedure would be best for me?
- What are the risks of the surgery?
- What are the side effects?
- How long will the side effects last?
- How long will it take my eyes to fully heal?
- If the results are less than I had hoped for, what can be done?

Both optometrists and ophthalmologists are qualified to discuss refractive surgery and the different procedures currently being used. They also should be able to answer all of your questions in a satisfying way. Many optometrists work with a particular ophthalmologist, and the team may manage your case together. Certainly, be cautious of offices that herd in dozens of patients at once for group presentations. They will most likely offer the least personalized care. You should also be skeptical of doctors who think everyone is a refractive surgical candidate, regardless of visual needs.

CONCLUSION

Refractive surgery is an individual decision. Your particular refractive problem, as well as your goals, the expected outcome of surgery, your tolerance for discomfort and side effects, and even your lifestyle and occupation, are among the factors that you and your doctor should take into consideration when discussing the possibility of surgery for you. Refractive surgery is not for everyone—but it just might be a great solution for you.

SUNGLASSES

Sunglasses are a specific type of eyewear for a specific purpose. They should be chosen carefully because they alter the light that reaches your eyes. In this section, we'll take a look at the different properties of sunglasses and what you should look for in a quality pair.

PROTECTING YOUR EYES WITH SUNGLASSES

Sunglasses have traditionally been worn for comfort in bright sunlight and for style. Now, research has added protection from harmful light rays to the list. So, wearing sunglasses when outdoors is really part of a healthy lifestyle routine. If you wear glasses, you don't need to settle for those clip-on lenses that are not likely to fit your glasses—or your fashion tastes—well. Any eyeglass prescription can be made in a tinted lens for use in bright sunlight. If you don't wear glasses, you should get a pair of *good quality* nonprescription sunglasses.

Protection from Ultraviolet Light

Ultraviolet (UV) light—also called ultraviolet radiation—is light that is not visible to the human eye because it is below the visible spectrum in wavelength. However, it is above the visible spectrum in wave frequency, another way of measuring light, which is why it is called *ultra*violet, meaning "above violet." UV light rays come from the sun, and some of them reach the earth and our eyes. These rays are responsible for sunburn, skin cancer,

and snow blindness, and may contribute to the formation of cataracts. (For a discussion of cataracts, see page 177.) UV light may also have a hand in the formation of a pinguecula, a yellowish spot on the front of the eye. Although having a pinguecula is not a serious condition, an irritated spot can be uncomfortable and is easily inflamed by excessive wind, dust, sun, or smoke. (For more information on pinguecula, see page 301.)

More specifically, UV light has a wavelength of between 286 and 400 nanometers (the smaller the number, the higher the frequency, and the more energy in the radiation). It can be further divided into subsections: UVC light has a wavelength that is less than 286 nanometers; UVB light has a wavelength of between 286 and 320 nanometers; and UVA light has a wavelength of between 320 and 400 nanometers. UVC light is not normally considered a threat because much of it is blocked out by the earth's atmosphere before it reaches us.

Most commercial, "off-the-rack" sunglasses for sale in pharmacies and drug stores offer little to no UV protection. In fact, the lenses in these kinds of sunglasses may actually cause your eyes to absorb *more* UV light than they normally would. This is because your pupils dilate when you wear sunglasses. If the sunglasses don't filter out UV light, more UV light will enter your eyes than it would if you weren't wearing sunglasses at all and your pupils were constricted just the usual amount! And even if a manufacturer claims that a pair of sunglasses offers "100-percent

UV protection," the optical quality of off-the-rack sunglasses is often poor.

Glass lenses block about 98 percent of UV light, and CR-39 and high-index lenses can be treated to also offer good UV protection. The newer polycarbonate lenses offer 100-percent protection against UV light. Thus, you have a number of options. For a complete discussion of these types of lenses, see "Eyeglass Lens Materials" on page 359.

Protection from Blue Light

Blue light has a wavelength of between 400 and 500 nanometers, and it is perceivable by the eye. It is considered less dangerous than ultraviolet light, but, according to recent evidence, it may be responsible for damage to the eye's retina. Most UV light is absorbed by the lens of the eye, where it may eventually cause a cataract to develop, while blue light goes through the lens and is absorbed by the retina. Some studies suggest that this might be one cause for macular degeneration. (See "Macular Degeneration" on page 273).

Because blue light scatters more than other colors (which is why the sky appears blue), it also causes glare on sunny days. Thus "blue-blocker" sunglasses have become popular. Amber and brown sunglass lenses block blue light, improving the contrast in your vision and reducing the glare, as well as protecting your retina from long-term exposure to blue light. However, as previously suggested, protection and optical quality are two different properties in sunglasses and both should be present for the best results. So, if you're paying only $10 for a pair of sunglasses, you're definitely not getting a quality product.

Also recall that there is a marketing campaign to have blue light blocked for users of computer displays. As noted previously, you'd have to spend over thirteen hours in front of a computer screen to equal just fifteen minutes in the sun. If you want to prevent blue light damage to the retina, include a full spectrum of colors in your diet. However, blue-light protection is more critical in sunglasses than it is in computer glasses.

Protection from Infrared Light

Infrared light, with a wavelength of more than 700 nanometers, is also not visible to the human eye. Its wavelength is longer than what we can perceive. However, its wave frequency is less than what we can perceive, so it is called *infra*red, which means "less than red." The cornea absorbs most of the infrared light, but the lens also absorbs some.

This type of light produces heat and is more intense at high altitudes and around bodies of water. It is also produced by the kind of flame used in glass blowing and welding. Therefore, high-altitude skiers, boaters, and some glass blowers and welders are at risk for infrared damage, which can cause cataracts after repeated exposure over a number of years. Some high-quality sunglasses block infrared light, but most sunglasses do not.

Now you are familiar with the various types of light that can cause damage to your eyes. And you are well aware of the fact that cheap sunglasses almost always don't provide full protection. Let's take this discussion a little further and learn how to rate sunglasses so that you choose the best product for your needs.

CONSIDERING POLARIZING LENSES

Light normally travels in a diverging direction from its source, like ripples in water after a pebble breaks the surface. The waves travel in all directions and are considered "non-polarized." When light is polarized, it is limited to just one direction of vibration. A good analogy is to think of holding one end of a rope through a picket fence. If you are rotating the rope in a large circular motion, that represents non-polarized light waves. However, the rope section on the other side of the fence will only be moving in the up-and-down direction (due to the pickets in the fence), so that side will be polarized.

People who spend time around water know the value of polarizing lenses. These lenses polarize light—that is, they prevent it from scattering and causing glare. Polarizing lenses are made from crystals that are aligned in such a way that they change the orientation of light rays. This allows the blockage of glare, especially that off the surface of water.

The best polarizing lenses are made of glass, but some good-quality plastic polarizing lenses are also available. Polarizing sunglasses are not necessarily more expensive than other sunglasses, but having the lenses of your prescription sunglasses polarized will add to their total cost. Most polarized lenses come in gray or brown, but they can also come in yellow, orange, amber or blue. Everyone would benefit from having polarized sunglasses, but those who spend time around water would especially benefit.

Currently, most LCD displays (cockpit displays, LCD clocks, digital watches, credit card machines, etc.) use polarizing technology in their units. This polarization, combined with polarized lens sunglasses, will serve to completely block an image. This is because of the direction of the polarizing filters. In order to see through a polarized sunglass lens onto a polarized digital display, simply rotate your head left or right (ear toward the shoulder) and the image will appear! Polarizing sunglasses are great, but it's important to know their limitations in today's technology.

CHOOSING LENS COLORS

The color that you choose for the lenses of your sunglasses is a matter of personal preference. However, most experts agree that gray, green, brown, and amber are the lens colors that reduce glare the best. Gray lenses are neutral, transmitting all the colors evenly, so you see all of the colors as they are. Green lenses resemble your natural color sensitivity and allow a maximum amount of useful light to reach your eyes. (The human eye is more sensitive to the colors in the yellow/green part of the spectrum than in the other parts, so it "tunes in" better to those colors.) Brown and amber lenses have the advantage of blocking out blue light.

Photochromic lenses, such as Corning's Photogray, have been around for about seventy years now and continue to be very popular. These lenses automatically darken to a gray or brown color when the surrounding light becomes brighter, and they lighten as it becomes darker. The color change takes about a minute to complete. Photochromic lenses will not become completely dark while you're driving because the windshield of the car will block out some of the UV light.

The original photochromic process could be used only with glass lenses, but Transitions lenses, which are plastic, are becoming quite popular. Transitions lenses do become lighter indoors than photochromic glass lenses, and the newer technology allows them to become darker outdoors. However, depending on how dark you prefer your sunglasses, they may not become dark enough for your liking. Both glass and plastic photochromic lenses are of excellent quality, and the color-change process never wears out. Prescription eyeglass wearers like these lenses a lot because they can wear them all the time rather than having to switch to sunglasses when they go out into the sun.

ASSESSING SUNGLASS QUALITY

Think back to your last purchase of sunglasses. What aspects of the sunglasses that you tried on were most important to you? What was your priority—cosmetic appeal, the fit of the frame, or eye health? The following sections reveal what you *should* be analyzing as you look for a pair of sunglasses.

The Quality of the Lenses

Many people choose their sunglasses based on how well the frame fits and how the glasses look, rather than on the quality of the lenses. That's unfortunate, because there are a number of things to consider. Off-the-rack sunglasses are likely to have lenses made of a type of plastic called cellulose acetate. This plastic is usually stamped out into a lens shape and inserted into a frame. The lenses often warp

and distort the light passing through them, which can cause headaches. Considering their low-cost materials and the low-cost labor used to make them, these "fun glasses" sell for between $5 and $15. This low price has led to the unfortunate notion that sunglasses should be cheap and can be easily replaced when lost or broken. I often hear people say they want cheap sunglasses because they're "just for the beach"—but the beach is where quality sunglasses are needed the most for protection!

Quality sunglasses are a different story. They are made of optically ground plastic, usually CR-39, or glass. Lenses that are optically ground have true curves, substantial "body" that helps to maintain their shape, and clear optics. Plastic lenses can be tinted any color, as well as bleached of color if you change your mind later and want to use them as regular glasses. Glass lenses can be tinted, but not bleached.

Glass lenses are almost always optically ground, so they work well as sunglasses. Many of the more popular brands of sunglasses are glass. Good sunglasses are made in one of two ways: the color can be incorporated directly into the lens, or a tinted coating can be applied to the front, back, or both surfaces of the lens. The only disadvantage of the coating method is that the coating can be scratched off accidentally. With proper care, however, either type of tinted lens works well.

The Amount of UV Light Protection

The FDA has approved a voluntary labeling system to assist consumers in judging the UV-light protection offered by sunglasses. It has adopted three categories of lenses. First is the "cosmetic" lens category. These sunglasses are largely "just for looks"; they are fashion accessories. Such sunglasses block out 70 percent of UVB light, 20 percent of UVA light, and 60 percent of visible light. The second-category lenses are the general-purpose lenses for activities such as boating and hiking. They block out 95 percent of UVB light, 60 percent of UVA light, and 60 to 92 percent of visible light. The third and final category is special-purpose lenses, which are for activities such as skiing, mountain climbing, and sunning. They block out 99 percent of UVB light, 60 percent of UVA light, and 97 percent of visible light.

Look for the UV-light rating on your next pair of sunglasses. Also, many optical shops can measure the amount of UV transmission through a lens with a special meter. However, keep in mind that even the best UV-light protection is no guarantee of good optical quality in a sunglass lens.

The Fit of the Frames

While the lenses are the most important part of a pair of sunglasses, you also need to pay attention to the frame. The frames of off-the-rack sunglasses usually can't be tightened or properly adjusted. Unfortunately, many people don't have high standards when it comes to the fit of a pair of sunglasses; the basic requirement is that the sunglasses don't fall off their face when tried on. But the frames used for good sunglasses are of similar quality to those used for prescription glasses. They can be adjusted to fit properly, and they will hold their adjustment. Where fit is concerned, you definitely get what you pay for!

Clearly, there is a science to sunglasses. If you have fallen into the trap of thinking that sunglasses are an item that you pick up at the local drug or department store in order to complete your summer ensemble, I hope this section has convinced you that you should expect a lot more from your lenses. Wearing quality sunglasses is an important part of proper eye care. Regarding your approach to sun exposure and your eyes, the decisions you make now will be affecting you for many years to come.

BUYING SUNGLASSES FOR CHILDREN

Most people know that UV light can severely damage your skin, and so they use sunscreen, especially on their children. (Side note: spray-on sunscreens are terrible for several reasons.) Yet parents are far less likely to protect their children's eyes with sunglasses. And far fewer people understand that extended exposure to sunlight in childhood can lead to cataracts and age-related macular degeneration in adulthood.

It is very important for you to purchase sunglasses for children who are under your care. When doing so, try to follow these guidelines:

• Start early. Beginning in infancy, children should wear sunglasses. While that may sound unusual, there is a good rationale behind this suggestion. Because their intraocular lenses aren't fully developed to block light, youngsters' eyes are especially vulnerable to UV-light damage. In addition, wearing sunglasses will help children get used to wearing frames, so as they get older, those children will not be likely to pull off their sunglasses so often.

● Don't buy toy sunglasses; buy real ones with UV-light protection. Shatterproof polycarbonate lenses that don't pop out of the frames are the best.

● Lenses should block 75 to 90 percent of light. Put the pair of sunglasses on the child and look at her eyes. If you can see the child's eyes, the lenses are likely not dark enough.

● The lenses shouldn't change the colors that the child sees. Neutral gray lenses are recommended because they do not distort color vision.

● The lenses should block peripheral UV radiation. The glasses should be large enough to extend out to the sides to block peripheral rays.

● The lenses should carry an ultraviolet-protection sticker. The American Optometric Association Seal of Acceptance means that the sunglasses block 99 to 100 percent of UV radiation.

We must convince ourselves that sunglasses should not be something that becomes a part of life only once the teenage years hit. A lot of future eye trouble can be avoided by teaching a child the importance of using sunglasses. If you take all of the above-listed factors into consideration when purchasing sunglasses for a child, then you should end up with a pair of sunglasses that is very effective.

CONCLUSION

Don't let price be your primary consideration when choosing sunglasses. Evaluate your specific sunglass needs. For example, do you need them for the beach, motorcycle or bike riding, or driving a car? What lens material best suits your lifestyle? How much UV protection is necessary? Choose a store that carries a variety of eyewear and eyecare options and that is convenient so that you can go in for adjustments or repairs periodically. In fact, when you enter such a store, first confirm that there is someone on the premises who can adjust glasses. In addition, try on several styles, and check for fair pricing. As with most things, you do get what you pay for in sunglasses.

SYNTONICS

Syntonics (sin-TAHN-iks), which is also known as optometric phototherapy, has been used clinically for over eighty years in the field of optometry. It is the branch of ocular science that deals with the application of selected visible-light frequencies through the eyes. Syntonics has been utilized with continued success in the treatment of a range of visual dysfunctions, including strabismus, lazy eye, accommodative insufficiency, convergence insufficiency, and vision-related learning disorders, as well as the visual consequences of traumatic brain injury. Let's learn a little more about this type of therapy.

THE HISTORY BEHIND SYNTONICS

Through most of history, the role of light in human function has been limited chiefly to the process of seeing. Early pioneers of the effects of light on health found that colored lights applied to the skin could have a nonintrusive curative effect on bodily ailments. Then, at the turn of the twentieth century, it first became known that light entering the eyes not only serves vision, but also travels to other important brain regions. It was believed that applying certain frequencies of light by way of the eyes could restore balance within the body's regulatory centers, thereby directly affecting the source of visual dysfunctions. This balance is referred to as *syntony* (*SIN-ton-ee*). And the prescribing of specific light applications to the eyes for therapeutic reasons became known as syntonics.

A phototherapy treatment plan may span a period of one to two months and require three to five sessions per week. A series of twenty phototherapy sessions of twenty minutes each may be prescribed to begin a vision therapy program, or phototherapy may be implemented concurrently with other vision therapy techniques. (For more information on vision therapy in general, see the section below.) Although syntonics is rarely used in isolation from other procedures, in some cases, along with a lens prescription, it may be enough to solve the visual complaint.

SUPPORT FOR SYNTONICS

As so often happens with therapies that are not considered mainstream, positive clinical

---

WHAT CAN BE TREATED WITH SYNTONICS?

Syntonics—or optometric phototherapy, as it is sometimes called—is the branch of ocular science that deals with the use of selected light frequencies. The following are some of the conditions that have been found to respond favorably to the use of syntonics:

- Blurred vision
- Double vision
- Reduced peripheral vision
- Strabismus (poor eye alignment)
- Amblyopia (lazy eye)
- Convergence problems
- Visually related headaches
- Dyslexia
- Brain injury
- Seasonal affective disorder (SAD)

---

experience with syntonics has preceded any validating research. Many doctors feel that this therapy is not "accepted" by the healthcare community and therefore do not include it in part of their treatment protocols. Researchers and other professionals are still a step away from understanding the clinical methods and practice of light stimulation, which syntonists—those professionals who practice syntonic procedures—have used with positive results for over half of a century.

However, the interest in phototherapy has increased in recent years. Research has shown that color changes the interaction and timing in the visual-processing system, and this may be one of the reasons why a stronger interest in syntonics has developed. Another may be the use of approaches such as the Irlen method, which uses color overlays and tinted eyeglass lenses to help improve reading. (For more information on the Irlen method, see page 36.)

One other development that supports the validity of phototherapy is the discovery of a condition now known as seasonal affective disorder (SAD). This is a condition of psychological depression that usually occurs during the winter months, when the daylight hours are short. Between 1992 and 1994, more than 5,000 articles were published in the medical literature describing light's effect on physiology. Roughly 1,100 studies used color, and nearly 800 dealt with experimental phototherapy. It is now widely accepted that the natural light of the sun is more beneficial to the human system than artificial light. In addition, it is now common to find full-spectrum lighting in indoor environments, especially classrooms. While this might be related to vitamin D levels (vitamin D is created in the body by the sun's rays on the skin),there is likely a connection between the full-spectrum of sunlight and positive effects in the body.

CONCLUSION

Although many people are unfamiliar with the field of syntonics, the College of Syntonic Optometry was established in 1933. It continues to be dedicated to research on the therapeutic application of light to the visual system. Might you consider this type of vision therapy? To find a professional trained in syntonics, contact the College of Syntonic Optometry. (See page 417 of Resource Organizations for contact information.)

VISION THERAPY

Some people just want to go to their doctor, get a prescription to remedy whatever ails them, and be on their way. However, a growing number of people are interested in playing a more active role in their health care and in learning how to take care of themselves. For these people, a program of vision therapy is the perfect prescription when it comes to certain needs. Vision therapy is a program of techniques and other activities designed to reduce stress, guide the development of the visual system, improve the visual skills, and enhance visual performance.

THOSE WHO WOULD BENEFIT FROM VISION THERAPY

Chances are that, because you have decided to read this book, you are very interested in taking on an active role in your own eye health care. But could your eyes actually benefit from vision therapy techniques? Well, that depends on what kind of eye problems you have. Answer the following questions to help you decide whether vision therapy is something that is worthwhile for you to pursue.

• Is your vision, near or distance, ever blurry, even for a few seconds?

- Do you ever see double?

- Do you lose your place while reading?

- Do your eyes feel tired if you read for an hour or more?

- Do you get a headache toward the end of the day, especially around your forehead or temples?

- Do your friends see things before you can bring them into focus?

- Do you do a lot of close work on the job, and then go home and use a computer?

- Does squinting improve your eyesight?

- Do you need stronger glasses every year or two?

If you answered "yes" to any of these questions, you may find vision therapy to be of help to you. So now what? Before you read up on the history of vision therapy and the various techniques available to you, consider another way to assess how much your eyes need some therapeutic attention.

Tomorrow morning, take a good look at your eyes in the bathroom mirror immediately after you get up (yes, before your cup of coffee!). Try to describe to yourself how your eyes look, and then try to describe how your body feels. Be specific. After you eat breakfast and take a shower, but before you leave for work, take another close look at your eyes. Do you see any difference? How does the rest of your body feel? After work, look at your eyes once again and see if they had a "hard day at the office" too. Basically, you are looking for signs of stress, strain, and fatigue, all of which can show up in your eyes.

Your eyes do a lot of work in an average day and can get stressed just like any other body part. Thinking about the above questions and taking a close look at your eyes from time to time can help you get to know your eyes better. Techniques to relax the eyes and improve the vision can help your eyes work better.

THE HISTORY BEHIND VISION THERAPY

The idea of vision therapy dates back at least as far as the 1920s. However, today's vision therapy—which is sometimes called optometric vision therapy—is quite different from the programs of the past. The following paragraphs trace the history of this approach to eye health care.

The Bates Method

In the 1920s, a New York ophthalmologist named William H. Bates developed a theory that stress and eyestrain are the primary causes of all vision problems. He reasoned—though not entirely scientifically by today's standards—that reducing stress on the eyes would reduce refractive errors, and he developed a program of relaxation techniques in line with his theory. Dr. Bates advised his patients never to stare or look directly at objects, but rather to look "through" them. He also advised against prolonged fixation of the eyes in one position, and recommended doing techniques such as the following: "swinging," which consists of shifting your weight from foot to foot while scanning a room; "sunning," which involves closing your eyes, turning toward the sun, and rolling your head back and forth; and "palming," which involves closing your eyes and holding the palms of your hands over them to create complete darkness.

Dr. Bates appreciated the connection

between the mind, brain, and eyes. He also said that memory and visual perception are linked. And the doctor wasn't entirely wrong. Stress certainly does influence vision, and there is a close connection between the eyes and the brain. His techniques probably did help people to relax their eyes, but his explorations (and lack of solid research) didn't go far enough and didn't effectively treat most vision problems. Yet today, optometric vision therapists still use some of Dr. Bates's techniques. In fact, the palming and head rolling techniques that are presented on page 395 are based on Dr. Bates's techniques.

Modern Optometric Vision Therapy

Modern vision therapy was first practiced in the 1930s by Dr. A.M. Skeffington, an American optometrist, and is still being refined. Today, it is practiced primarily by optometrists who specialize in vision therapy. Optometric vision therapy combines a series of office visits with exercises done at home. "Exercise," in this case, does not refer to aerobic exercise or strength training, but rather to activities designed to improve binocular coordination and eye-brain coordination. When you practice vision exercises—or vision techniques, as I prefer to call them—you won't strengthen your eye muscles, for they're already strong enough, but you will improve the efficiency and smoothness of the muscles that control your eye movements and the focusing of your eyes' lenses. You'll also improve the connections between your eyes and your brain, and between your two eyes.

The office visits for vision therapy, which may take several months to complete, are generally thirty to sixty minutes in length and held two to three times per week. In the office,

lenses, prisms, and techniques involving light and pictures are used to encourage the eyes to work differently from the way in which they have been working. Some optometrists also try to improve vision by stimulating the visual system with different flashes of color. (See "Syntonics" on page 383.) The homework consists of techniques intended to improve vision, but without much equipment.

True optometric vision therapy is more than just a group of techniques. It is an individualized program of progressively arranged conditions of learning for the development of a more efficient and effective visual system. It can be used to improve nearsightedness, farsightedness, presbyopia, visual discomfort, learning difficulties, strabismus, lazy eye, slow reading, poor reading comprehension, poor visual perception, poor sports performance, and job-related visual disabilities. What it does *not* do is treat conditions such as attention deficit/hyperactive disorder and dyslexia. However, it might provide some help to individuals with those conditions if deficient visual abilities are involved. Some of the visual skills that optometric vision therapy seeks to improve are listed below.

- Tracking—the ability to follow a moving object, such as a ball in flight or vehicles in traffic, smoothly and accurately with both eyes.

- Fixation—the ability to quickly and accurately locate and inspect with both eyes a series of stationary objects, one after another, such as the words in a sentence while reading.

- Accommodation—the ability to look quickly from far to near and vice versa, such as from the dashboard to the cars on the street, or from the chalkboard to a book, without blurriness.

- Depth perception—the ability to judge the relative distances of objects, and to see and move accurately within a three-dimensional space, such as when parking a car.

- Peripheral vision—the ability to monitor and interpret what is happening around you while attending to a specific task with your central vision; the ability to use visual information perceived from a large area.

- Binocular coordination—the ability to use both eyes together, smoothly, equally, simultaneously, and accurately. This includes the ability to converge the eyes, aiming them toward each other to look at a near object, and to relax the convergence, moving the eyes away from each other to refocus on a distant object.

- Hand-eye coordination—the ability to use the hands and eyes together in a synchronized manner so that a task such as hitting a ball can be performed with efficiency.

- Attention maintenance—the ability to continue doing a particular skill or activity with ease and without interfering with the performance of other skills.

- Near-vision acuity—the ability to clearly see, inspect, identify, and interpret objects at near distances (within 20 feet of the eyes).

- Distance-vision acuity—the ability to clearly see, inspect, identify, and interpret objects at a distance (more than 20 feet away from the eyes).

- Visualization—the ability to form mental images in the "mind's eye" and retain them for future recall or for synthesis into new mental images beyond the current or past experiences.

- Relaxation—the ability to relax the eyes

and the visual system. This is important for preventing and treating eyestrain.

There are two professional organizations that support doctors who do vision therapy. They are the Optometric Extension Program Foundation (OEPF) and the College of Vision Development (COVD). Refer to the appendix titled Resource Organizations for contact information regarding these two groups. Many times a doctor who advertises in the phone book will put the "FCOVD" (Fellow of the COVD) letters behind her name, so that would be a good indicator of a vision therapy doctor. But even in the absence of a *complete* vision therapy program, vision therapy techniques can help to improve the visual skills listed above. So continue to read this section for the "how-to" on several techniques.

VISION THERAPY TECHNIQUES

So are you ready to learn about specific techniques? Following are some you can do at home. It's usually best to do these techniques early in the day, before your eyes are too tired. Don't try to do all of the techniques every day. Instead, spread them out over the course of a few days. Note which of the techniques are the most difficult for you, then concentrate on those particular ones for several weeks, and see what improvements you can make in your vision.

Please note that these are general techniques that are often a part of a cursory at-home vision therapy program. They may or may not be appropriate for your particular visual condition. Only an optometric examination can determine if they can be helpful to your situation.

Accommodative Rock

The accommodative rock helps to improve the eyes' ability to change focus and see clearly at near and at distance. Accommodation is the process by which the eyes change focus, and it is probably the most important and most often performed function of the eyes. The ability to focus decreases with age, but adequate focusing ability can be maintained for longer periods of time with techniques such as this one. To do the accommodative rock, follow the steps listed below.

1. Fasten several large letters, such as a banner newspaper headline, to a wall, and stand back 20 feet. If necessary, use your glasses to see the letters clearly.

2. Take a group of small letters, such as the body of a newspaper article, and hold them in one hand.

3. Cover one of your eyes with your free hand, keeping the eye itself open, and bring the small print as close to your face as you can while still being able to see it clearly. Stop.

4. Look at the large letters on the wall again. Are they clear?

5. Continuing to hold the small print at the same distance, look at it again. Is it clear?

6. Repeat steps 4 and 5 for a few minutes, until you can see both the distance and near letters easily. The accommodation should take only a second.

7. Try the technique with the other eye.

8. Repeat the entire exercise, with the small letters held 1 inch closer.

I suggest that you do this technique for five minutes with each eye at least twice per day. Preferably, finish both sessions before evening tiredness sets in. You can also try this technique throughout the day, whenever you find yourself with a near and a distant object on which to focus—for example, a wall clock and your wristwatch.

Rotations

Rotations increase the eyes' tracking ability and help your capacity to pay attention to an activity. Smooth eye movements are basic to good vision. You'll need an empty pie pan and a marble for this technique. To do rotations, follow the steps listed below.

1. Put the marble in the pie pan, and hold the pie pan about 16 inches from your eyes.

2. Tilt the pie tin so that the marble rolls around the edge at a steady pace. Follow the marble with your eyes only; do not move your head.

3. Repeat step 2, rolling the marble around the edge of the pie pan in the opposite direction.

Do this technique for two minutes in each direction, once per day. You'll become dizzy if you keep the marble going in the same direction for more than two minutes. If possible, have a friend watch your eyes to see how smoothly they move.

Alphabet Fixations

Alphabet fixations improve the ability to center the eyes—that is, to fixate them—on an object in an instant. Fixation is one of the skills used in reading. This technique also helps with near-vision acuity. To do alphabet fixations, follow the steps listed below.

1. Cut two strips of paper. Type or clearly print the alphabet in a vertical direction on each strip.

2. Hold the strips about 18 inches from your face and a bit farther apart than shoulder width.

3. Call out the letters in alphabetical order, making sure to read each letter off a strip before calling out its name. Alternate between the strips, reading the "a" from one strip, the "b" from the second, the "c" from the first strip again, and so on. Keep your head absolutely still as you do this.

4. Spell words using the strips, again reading the letters before calling them out and alternating between the two strips as in step 3. For example, spell the word "boy" by taking the "b" from the left-hand strip, the "o" from the right-hand strip, and the "y" from the left-hand strip again. Your speed should increase with practice.

Do this technique for five minutes, once per day. It sounds more complicated than it actually is. You will find that the technique flows rather easily once it is put into practice.

An alternative (and more technologically advanced) way to do this technique is with a unit called "Eye Yoga." The EYE YOGA headset immediately provides an "active recovery" response, targeting the direct source of the discomfort—the intra & outer muscles. This offers them relief by encouraging them to relax and stretch out of the contracted hold, increasing blood flow and nutrients to these areas and improving the user's physical and mental focus. This leaves the eye area feeling rejuvenated and refreshed. The unique aspect of this unit is that, while still encouraging eye tracking and movements at a close distance, it also has a "magic window" that allows long-distance viewing as a part of the program. Thus, in addition to its routines, it allows the user to perform a process similar to the "accommodative rock," as previously discussed. The maker of the heasdset has recently released a new version called "Eye Yoga 20-20-20 Pro," which features some advanced technology. You can find the company's contact information in the Resource Suppliers on page 410.

Monocular Fixations

The monocular (one-eyed) fixation technique enhances the ability to fixate with one eye at a time. This particular technique is also designed to improve hand-eye coordination. You'll need a string, a small ring (such as a wedding band or a key ring), and a knitting needle or long pencil. To do monocular fixations, follow the steps presented below:

1. Tie the string to the ring and hang the string (from a doorway, for example) so that the ring is at eye level. Stand about 2 feet away from the ring.

2. Hold the knitting needle or pencil in your right hand, cover your left eye, step forward on your right foot, and try to put the knitting needle or pencil through the ring without touching it. Try this several times.

3. Return to the original standing position, 2 feet away from the ring.

4. Move the knitting needle or pencil to your left hand, cover your right eye, step forward on your left foot, and try to put the knitting needle or pencil through the ring again without touching it.

After mastering the technique using a stationary ring, repeat the technique but with a swinging ring. This is great practice for the skills used in many sports. Do this technique for five minutes with each eye, once per day.

Wall Fixations

Wall fixations improve your ability to fixate and your peripheral vision at the same time. You'll need eight white 3-by-5-inch index cards, a felt-tipped marker, a blank wall, a book, and maybe some gentle music. To do wall fixations, follow the steps listed below.

1. Number the index cards from one to eight, one number per card. Using the felt-tipped marker and a bold stroke, position each number in the center of the card and make it 2 inches tall. Fasten the cards in a haphazard order to a blank wall in an 8-foot square shape. (See Figure 3.9 below.)

2. Stand about 6 feet from the wall, facing the center of the card pattern. Put a book on your head to keep your head steady, and cover one eye.

3. Starting with the "1" card, shift your eyes from card to card in numerical order. Keep your head very still and look directly at each number, being aware of the other numbers in your peripheral vision.

4. Repeat steps 2 and 3 first with the other eye, then with both eyes together.

Do this technique for two minutes with each eye, then for two minutes with both eyes, once per day. When you become adept at shifting your eyes from card to card, move closer to the wall. Continue to move closer as your skill improves. As you move closer to the wall, your eye movements will need to become more extreme. If you wish, do this technique to gentle music to help keep your eye movements smooth and steady. The EYE YOGA headset is also valuable to replace this technique.

Marsden Ball

The Marsden ball technique is a great activity for improving tracking and fixation, as well as hand-eye coordination and attention maintenance. You'll need a rubber ball about 4 inches in diameter, some strong thread or string, and a ballpoint pen. To do the Marsden ball technique, follow the steps listed below.

FIGURE 3.9 **Sample Set-Up for Wall Fixations.**

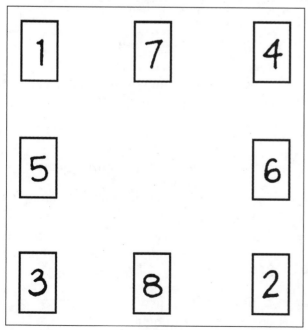

1. Write letters randomly all over the ball with the ballpoint pen.

2. Attach the thread or string securely to the ball, and suspend the ball so that it can swing freely. A doorway offers an especially good place to hang the ball.

3. Cover one of your eyes, give the ball a slight push, and try to touch one letter at a time, calling out the letter at you do so. Keep your head as still as possible.

4. Repeat step 2 with the other eye.

Do this technique for two minutes with each eye, once per day. As mentioned above, the Marsden ball technique effects improvement in a number of areas, so practicing it is time well spent.

Deep Blink

The deep blink is designed to improve your ability to accommodate and the acuity of your distance vision. It's also a relaxation technique. Note that if you feel dizzy or faint at any time while performing the technique, stop and rest. You'll need a blank wall, a chair, and some large letters, such as a banner newspaper headline. To do the deep blink, follow the steps listed below.

1. Fasten the large letters to the wall, and remove your glasses or contacts. Stand a few feet from the letters and gradually move back until the letters start to blur. Position the chair at that point.

2. Sit in the chair in a relaxed posture. Take a deep breath, and let it out slowly. Repeat this a few times until you feel relaxed.

3. Take a deep breath and hold it. With your breath held, close your eyes, clench your fists, and tighten the muscles in your whole body—legs, arms, stomach, chest, neck, face, head, and eyes. Keep your muscles tightened for about five seconds.

4. At the end of the five seconds, snap your hands and eyes open, exhale quickly through your mouth, and relax your entire body. Breathe slowly, and look at the letters, blinking gently as necessary. Stay very relaxed and try to look through, rather than at, the letters. After a second or two, the letters should become clear. (If you feel dizzy or faint after tightening and relaxing your muscles, omit this part. Just take slow, deep breaths, and practice looking through the letters on the wall.)

5. If the letters remained clear, push your chair about a foot back from the wall, and repeat steps 3 and 4. Continue moving your chair back to see how far away you can sit from the letters and still keep them clear.

Do this technique at least once per day. You may be amazed to find that after a few weeks, you can sit quite a few feet farther back from where you started and still see those letters.

Brock String Technique

The Brock string technique helps to improve depth perception, peripheral vision, and binocular coordination. You'll need a piece of string that is 4 feet in length. To do the Brock string technique, follow the steps listed below.

1. Tie a knot in the middle of the string. Attach one end of the string to any object that is at

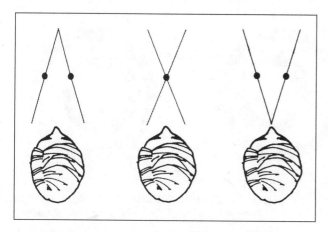

FIGURE 3.10 **An Illustration of the Brock String Technique.**

your eye level. (You can sit or stand for this technique.) Hold the string between your thumb and forefinger, stretch it taut, and hold it up against your nose.

2. Look at the far end of the string. You should see an A without the crossbar. You should see the knot in the middle of the string as two knots, one on each side of the A. (See Figure 3.10, above.)

3. Look at the knot in the string. It may take a few seconds, but you should be able to see an X pattern with one knot in the middle.

4. Shift your gaze back and forth from the A to the X pattern until the movement is smooth and requires little effort.

5. Move your gaze up the string, toward your nose. As you do this, you should find the center of the X moving up, too. When your gaze gets very close to your nose, the X should become a V, and the knot in the middle of the string should appear to be two knots, one on each side of the V, in your peripheral vision.

6. Shift your gaze from the A to the X to the V pattern until the movement is smooth and requires little effort.

7. Continue shifting your gaze, shortening the string, but keeping the knot centered.

Do this technique for five minutes, once per day. Again, the instructions may sound complicated. However, once you set up and start practicing the technique, the steps will flow easily.

Convergence Stimulation

Convergence is the aiming of the eyes toward one another as you look at near objects. This skill is critical for all near-point activities, such as reading. Convergence stimulation helps to develop binocular coordination, of which convergence is one aspect, and good depth perception. It also improves attention maintenance. You'll need Figure 3.11 on page 394 and a pencil. To do convergence stimulation, follow the steps listed below.

1. Hold the illustration at your normal reading distance and focus your eyes on it. If necessary, wear your glasses or contact lenses. You should see two sets of concentric circles.

2. Position the point of the pencil in between the two sets of concentric circles and focus on it, remaining at your normal reading distance.

3. Move the pencil slowly toward your eyes, leaving the illustration where it is. Keep focusing on the point of the pencil, but be aware of the circles beyond it as you do. You should begin to see three, rather than two, sets of concentric circles when the pencil is approximately 6 inches from your eyes. The set in

the middle—the one that's not really there—should appear as a three-dimensional figure, farther away from you than the larger ones and resembling a cup or flower pot. Keep the pencil still, and keep looking at it. Your eyes should feel as if they're crossing; they're actually just pulling in toward each other.

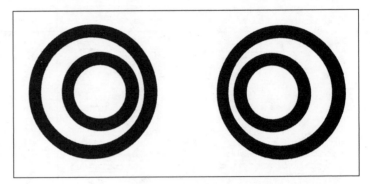

FIGURE 3.11 **Illustration for Use With Convergence Stimulation and Convergence Relaxation.**

4. Relax your focus and look away from the illustration for a second or two, then look back at the illustration and see if you can regain the image described in step 3. This may take some practice.

5. Repeat step 4 until it is easy to maintain and hold the center image.

Do this technique for several minutes every day. Alternate it with convergence relaxation, the next technique. Convergence stimulation and convergence relaxation exercise the same set of eye muscles, but pull them in different directions. If one of the techniques is much easier for you than the other, concentrate on the one that's more difficult until you can do it as easily as the other one.

Convergence Relaxation

Convergence relaxation is the opposite of convergence. It's the ability of the eyes to relax—that is, to diverge from their converged position—as they focus on a distant object. Excessive near-point work can cause the eyes to have trouble relaxing, so practicing convergence relaxation is good for breaking up your day if you do a lot of reading or computer

work. The technique helps with binocular coordination, depth perception, and attention maintenance. You'll once again need Figure 3.11 below, plus a blank wall. To practice convergence relaxation, follow the steps listed below.

1. Stand at least 10 feet away from the blank wall and focus your eyes on it.

2. Slowly bring Figure 3.11 into your line of sight at your normal reading distance, but keep your eyes focused on the wall. You can hold the illustration just above the point on the wall where your eyes are focused. You should see three sets of concentric circles, just as you did in the convergence stimulation technique. But this time, while the center set of circles should still seem to be three-dimensional, it should also appear to be closer to you than the outside circles and resemble upside-down cups or flower pots. The other sets of circles, which will be in your peripheral vision, may appear this way, too.

3. Relax your focus and look away from the illustration for a second or two, then look back at the illustration and see if you can regain the image. This may take some practice.

4. Repeat step 3 until it is easy to maintain and hold the center image.

Do this technique for several minutes every day. Alternate it with convergence stimulation, the previous technique. As suggested above, work more diligently on the technique that is more difficult for you.

Palming

Palming is a relaxation technique that can be performed between other techniques and throughout the day. It allows you to relax your mind and your eyes; you don't focus on anything but blackness. It can also increase your visualization skills. Palming is adapted from the Bates method. To do palming, follow the steps listed below.

1. Close your eyes and cover them with your hands. Keep your palms over, but not touching, your eyelids. Your fingers should overlap near your hairline, and you should have enough room to breathe easily. Rest your elbows on a table. All you should see is complete blackness. If you see flashes of light, just let them go and allow the blackness to return. You can either continue to focus on the blackness, or you can now start to visualize a relaxing scene of your own choosing.

2. Take a deep breath and feel the muscles around your eyes completely relax. Breathe deeply and slowly eight times.

Perform this technique as needed, at least eight times per day. It is preferable to perform palming before you start an intense near-point task, such as reading or computer work. You might find that it is quite meditative!

Head Rolling

Head rolling is another relaxation technique based on the Bates method. It increases the blood flow, which increases the flow of life-maintaining oxygen to the brain and eyes. It also feels good! To do head rolling, follow the steps listed below.

1. While seated, gently drop your head forward, reaching your chin toward your chest.

2. Slowly roll your head around from one shoulder to the other, making a complete circle. Keep your shoulders level and maintain regular breathing. Make two or three complete revolutions with your head.

3. Repeat step 2, rolling your head in the other direction.

Use this technique first thing in the morning, and again later in the afternoon for a relaxation break. It is also good to use this technique as a short break from computer work. Its added benefit of calming the mind makes it a general health-enhancing practice.

Remember, these are general vision therapy techniques that can provide a solid foundation for good visual habits. To remedy a specific visual deficiency, you will need to visit an eye-care professional who can properly evaluate and prescribe the appropriate techniques. If any of these techniques are extremely difficult to do, you may have a visual dysfunction that is subtle but should nevertheless be evaluated. So, when did you have your last eye examination?

CONCLUSION

Vision therapy is a program that helps to "fine tune" the visual system. It is not a "cure-all" and will not help you to throw away your glasses from lack of use. So don't be fooled by exaggerated claims from some infomercial. Remember, if it seems too good to be true, it likely is! That being said, a qualified eyecare professional who works with vision therapy can assist you or your child in using the eyes clearly and comfortably for all of your educational and work demands.

Glossary

accommodation. The ability of the eye to adjust its focus for near vision, distance vision, and all points in-between.

accommodative insufficiency. The loss of ability to focus on an object to the degree expected for one's age. This condition can occur only in people under 40 years of age. See also *presbyopia.*

acuity. See *visual acuity.*

acupressure. An ancient Chinese medical practice that involves the use of finger pressure to stimulate specific points in the body that assist in healing. See also *acupuncture.*

acupuncture. An ancient Chinese medical practice that involves the use of extremely fine needles to stimulate specific points in the body that assist in healing. See also *acupressure.*

aftercataract. See *secondary cataract.*

albinism. A genetic condition in which all the normal pigmentation in the body is absent.

amblyopia. See *lazy eye.*

amino acid. One of the chemical substances that are the building blocks of protein.

Amsler grid. A grid-pattern chart that is used to detect central visual field defects.

anisocoria. A difference in the size of one pupil as compared with the other.

anisometropia. A difference in the refractive error of one eye as compared with the other.

antihistamine. A type of medication used to suppress allergic reactions. Antihistamines can cause increased pressure in the eyes, and should not be used by people who have glaucoma.

antioxidant. A substance that blocks oxidation reactions in the body, some of which can lead to cellular dysfunction and destruction. The antioxidant nutrients include beta-carotene, vitamin C, vitamin E, and selenium. Other antioxidants are the amino acid glutathione, and the enzymes superoxide dismutase (SOD), peroxidase, and catalase.

anti-reflective lens coating. A coating that is applied to an eyeglass lens to allow the passage of more light through the lens, and to decrease the scattering of light from the surface of the lens.

aqueous fluid. See *aqueous humor.*

aqueous humor. A watery fluid that surrounds the iris and lens in the front part of the eye and provides some nutrition to the adjoining parts of the eye. Also called the aqueous fluid.

arcus senilis. A condition where the peripheral area of the cornea turns a whitish discoloration; this condition eventually forms a circle around the entire peripheral area of the cornea.

artificial intraocular lens. An artificial lens that

is often inserted during cataract surgery to take over the focusing that the eye's own lens can no longer do. Some lenses are now available in multifocal designs. See also *lens.*

astigmatism. A condition in which the cornea is shaped more like the side of a barrel than the side of a ball, causing the light passing through it to be spread over a diffuse area of the retina rather than focused into a single point; a refractive error. See also *emmetropia; farsightedness; nearsightedness; presbyopia; refractive error.*

atherosclerosis. A condition in which fats are deposited in the body's arteries. It is associated with high blood pressure, high blood levels of cholesterol and triglycerides, obesity, smoking, diabetes, stress, family history of atherosclerosis, physical inactivity, and the male sex.

Bates method. A system of techniques devised by Dr. William Bates to improve eyesight. Dr. Bates theorized that stress is the cause of most vision problems, and that relaxation is the cure.

beta-carotene. A nutrient related to vitamin A that is used by the body to manufacture vitamin A. Beta-carotene is an excellent antioxidant.

bifocal contact lens. A contact lens that compensates for presbyopia by correcting both distance and near vision. See also *contact lens.*

bifocal lens. A corrective lens that contains two segments—one for distance viewing and one for near viewing. See also *lens; trifocal lens.*

binocular. Two-eyed.

binocular coordination. The ability to use both eyes in a smooth, efficient manner.

biofeedback. A technique for controlling autonomic (normally uncontrollable) body functions. It involves learning to respond to a signal, such as a tone, when changes occur in the pulse, blood pressure, or other autonomic body function.

bioflavonoids. A diverse group of compounds found in most plants, including fruits and vegetables. They can act as antioxidants, immune-system regulators, and anti-inflammatory agents.

blepharitis. A condition in which the eyelid is chronically inflamed.

blepharospasm. An involuntary contraction of the eyelid muscles.

blink reflex. A reflex in which the eyes automatically close in response to the sudden movement of an object toward them.

bloodshot eyes. An increase in the amount of blood flowing into the blood vessels on the surface of the eye; most often associated with a bacterial, virus or allergic reaction. See also *pinkeye.*

blue light. Light with a wavelength of between 400 and 500 nanometers. It can cause damage to the retina.

blue-blocker sunglasses. Sunglasses with lenses that block out blue light.

board certification. In medicine, a designation indicating that a practitioner has met standards above and beyond those required for a license to practice, and has passed a specialty examination in a particular field, such as ophthalmology.

carotene. A yellow pigment present in some plants and animals. It is abundant in yellow vegetables such as carrots, squash, and corn, and is convertible to vitamin A in the human liver.

cataract. A condition in which the lens inside the eye loses its transparency and begins to become opaque, eventually preventing light from reaching the retina. See also *congenital cataract; glass blower's cataract; secondary cataract; senile cataract.*

central serous retinopathy. A condition in which there is swelling of the macular area of the retina, causing a distortion in central vision.

central vision. The direct, line-of-sight vision. Also called the macular vison. See also *peripheral vision; visual field.*

chalazion. A condition in which the duct of one of the meibomian glands in the eyelid becomes plugged, resulting in inflammation. Also called a meibomian cyst. See also *stye.*

choroid. A layer between the retina and sclera, consisting primarily of blood vessels that provide nourishment to the retina.

closed-angle glaucoma. See *narrow-angle glaucoma.*

collagen. A fibrous protein found in the connective tissues in the skin, bones, ligaments, and cartilage.

color deficiency. A condition in which a person is missing either a certain type of color cone in the retina or has cones that are deficient in the ability to process color signals. Most people who are labeled colorblind are actually color deficient. See also *colorblindness.*

color receptors. See *cones.*

colorblindness. Strictly speaking, a complete absence of color vision. The condition is extremely rare. See also *color deficiency.*

complete protein. Dietary protein that contains the full complement of amino acids, especially the eight that the body cannot produce on its own. See also *protein.*

complex carbohydrate. A carbohydrate that includes fiber, which slows the release of sugar from the carbohydrate into the bloodstream and provides dietary fiber as well. The sources of complex carbohydrates include whole grains, fruits, and vegetables. See also *simple carbohydrate.*

computer vision syndrome. The complex of eye and vision problems associated with near work that are experienced during or after computer work.

cones. The specialized, cone-shaped cells in the retina of the eye. They are responsible for color vision. Also called color receptors. See also *photoreceptors; rods.*

congenital cataract. A cataract that is present at birth. See also *cataract.*

conjunctiva. A clear mucous membrane that covers both the sclera and the insides of the eyelids, and contains glands that moisten the front of the eyeball.

conjunctivitis. See *pinkeye.*

contact lens. An artificial lens that rests on the cornea of the eye, and corrects for refractive errors. See also *bifocal contact lens; daily-wear contact lens; disposable contact lens; extended-wear contact lens; flexible-wear contact lens; gas-permeable contact lens; hard contact lens; lens; rigid gas-permeable contact lens.*

convergence. The moving of the two eyes toward each other. This normally happens when the eyes change focus from distance to near.

convergence excess. A condition in which the eyes turn in toward one another too much when viewing a near object.

convergence insufficiency. A condition in which the line of sight of both eyes don't turn in far enough when viewing a near object.

cornea. The outermost, transparent part of the outer protective layer of the eye. Its bulging curvature is responsible for most of the refraction that occurs in the eye.

corneal abrasion. A small cut or scrape on the front surface of the cornea.

corneal neovascularization. A condition in which there is a growth of new blood vessels into the cornea. It most often is due to the over-wearing of contact lenses.

corneal ulcer. A loss of tissue in the cornea due to a progressive erosion or loss of cells.

CR-39. A type of plastic material used to make eyeglass lenses.

cross-eyed. Having an eye that turns inward toward the nose while the other eye looks straight ahead. See also *strabismus; wall-eyed.*

cytomegalovirus. A common virus of the herpes family that can cause disease in infants and in persons with compromised immune systems.

daily-wear contact lens. A contact lens designed to be worn on a full-time basis, but not overnight. See also *contact lens.*

depth perception. The ability to perceive size and distance relationships among objects in space.

deuteranopia. A defect in the perception of the color green. See also *protanopia.*

developmental optometry. The specialty of optometry that pertains to the visual development of children through adulthood. Developmental optometrists commonly treat visual-perception difficulties, strabismus, and other vision-related disabilities.

diabetes mellitus. A disorder of carbohydrate metabolism in which the body is unable to use glucose (sugar) properly. It is usually caused by a lack of the hormone insulin or an inability to utilize insulin.

diabetic retinopathy. A disorder of the blood vessels in the retina stemming from diabetes. It is one of the leading causes of blindness in the United States.

diopter (d). A unit of measurement used to describe the focusing power of a lens.

diplopia. See *double vison.*

directionality. The ability to distinguish right from left on another person or object without reference to your own body.

disposable contact lens. A contact lens designed to be discarded after the prescribed wearing time, which is usually between one to two weeks or quarterly. See also *contact lens.*

distance vision. The vision used to see objects twenty or more feet away. See also *intermediate vision; near vision.*

doll's-eye reflex. A reflex in which a baby's eyes continue to look at a certain person as his or her head is slowly turned or nodded back and forth.

double vision. The condition of seeing double. Also called diplopia.

drooping eyelids. A condition in which the eyelids (usually the upper lid) lag down or pull away from the eye due to loss of muscle tone.

dry eye disease. A condition in which the tear film of the eye is deficient or evaporates too quickly.

dyslexia. An inability to read and understand written language despite having normal intelligence.

dystonia. A neurological movement disorder in which sustained muscle contractions cause twisting and repetitive movements or abnormal postures.

edema. Swelling that results from an accumulation of fluid.

emmetropia. The condition of the optically normal eye. When light passes through the cornea, it comes to a focus directly on the retina. See also *astigmatism; farsightedness; nearsightedness; presbyopia; refractive error.*

enzyme. A type of protein that is capable of inducing chemical changes in other substances without being changed itself.

extended-wear contact lens. A contact lens designed to be kept in overnight for several days. See also *contact lens.*

extracapsular cataract extraction. A technique used in cataract surgery in which the cataract-covered lens is removed, but the capsule surrounding the lens is left intact. See also *intracapsular cataract extraction.*

extract. A concentrated essence, such as of an herb, made by leaching the active properties using either alcohol or water. See also *infusion; tincture.*

extraocular. Outside the eyeball. Used to describe the muscles that move the eyeball. See also *intraocular.*

eye pressure. See *intraocular pressure.*

eyestrain. A condition exhibiting nonspecific symptoms such as fatigue, red eyes, eyestrain, pain in or around the eyes, blurred vision, headache, and occasional double vision.

farsightedness. A condition in which the eye is too short or the cornea too flat, causing the light passing through the cornea to come to a focus behind the retina when viewing a distant object; a refractive error. The farsighted person can see distant objects clearly, but sees near objects as blurry. Also called hyperopia. See also *astigmatism; emmetropia; nearsightedness; presbyopia; refractive error.*

figure-ground discrimination. The ability to distinguish an object from its background. Some optical illusions are interesting because it is not clear which part is the figure and which is the ground.

fine motor. Referring to the small muscles of the body, such as those of the fingers. See also *gross motor.*

flexible-wear contact lens. A contact lens designed to be either taken out each night or left in overnight according to the wearer's wishes. See also *contact lens.*

floaters. Small bits of protein or cells within the vitreous of the eye. They vary in size and shape, and are occasionally visible as specks before the eyes.

focusing flexibility. The ability of the eye to easily change its focusing power from distance to near to distance again.

form perception. The ability to perceive the shapes of objects, including those of words on a page.

gas-permeable contact lens. A contact lens made of a material that allows the passage of oxygen and carbon dioxide. See also *contact lens.*

giant papillary conjunctivitis. A condition in which the inside surface of the upper eyelid creates large bumps most often due to physical irritation from contact lenses.

glass blower's cataract. A cataract that results from constant exposure to infrared light. It is found in glass blowers who work without eye protection. See also *cataract.*

glaucoma. A condition in which the pressure within the eye is increased, causing compression of the retina and optic nerve, as well as a reduction in the blood flow to the eye. If untreated, it can lead to blindness. See also *narrow-angle glaucoma; open-angle glaucoma.*

glucose. A sugar that is formed in the body during digestion. It is essential to the chemistry of the body.

Graves' disease. An autoimmune disease. It most commonly affects the thyroid, causing it to grow to twice its size or more (goiter) and be overactive, with related symptoms such as weight loss, frequent defecation, disturbed sleep, and irritability. It can also affect the eyes, causing bulging eyes (exophthalmos).

gross motor. Referring to the large muscles of the body, such as those of the legs, arms, trunk, and head. See also *fine motor.*

hand-eye coordination. The ability to use the eyes and hands together to accomplish a task.

hard contact lens. A rigid plastic contact lens that does not allow the passage of oxygen or carbon dioxide. See also *contact lens.*

hemoglobin. The iron-containing pigment in red blood cells. Its function is to carry oxygen from the lungs to the rest of the body.

hemorrhage. Profuse or abnormal bleeding.

herpes viruses. A group of viruses, including herpes simplex and herpes zoster, that can infect the eyes, mouth, genitals, and other parts of the body.

hydrophilic. Literally means "water-loving." It is used to describe a type of plastic utilized in making soft contact lenses.

hyperopia. See *farsightedness.*

hypertensive retinopathy. A condition associated with high blood pressure that eventually creates an inflammatory condition of the retina.

hyphema. A condition in which blood has collected in the anterior chamber of the eye.

infection. A condition in which the body is invaded by an organism that multiplies and produces injurious effects.

inflammation. The response of the body to an injury. It usually involves swelling, redness, heat, pain, and impaired functioning of the affected area.

infrared light. Light with a wavelength of more than 700 nanometers, which puts it above the range of the human visual spectrum. Also called infrared radiation.

infrared radiation. See *infrared light.*

infusion. A preparation made by steeping herbs in hot water; tea. See also extract; tincture.

intermediate vision. The vision used to see objects at roughly arm's length away. See also *distance vision; near vision.*

international unit (IU). A unit of potency based on an accepted international standard. Vitamins A and E, among other supplements, are usually measured in international units.

intracapsular cataract extraction. A technique used in cataract surgery in which both the cataract-covered lens and the capsule surrounding it are removed. See also *extracapsular cataract extraction.*

intraocular. Inside the eyeball. Used to describe the eye muscles that control focusing, as well as the eye's lens and other structures. See also *extraocular.*

intraocular lens, artificial. See *artificial intraocular lens.*

intraocular pressure. The pressure within the eyeball. An increased level of intraocular pressure is known as glaucoma. Also called eye pressure.

iris. The colored portion of the eye that surrounds the pupil. Its expansion decreases the amount of light entering the eye through the pupil, and its contraction increases the amount of light.

iritis. A condition in which the iris is inflamed.

Irlen lenses. Colored lenses developed by Dr. Helen Irlen that help some people with a certain form of dyslexia to read with more ease and comprehension.

keratoconus. A condition in which the cornea has a conelike bulge.

keratomileusis. A surgical procedure in which an outer layer of the cornea is removed, reshaped, and then sewn back in a effort to reshape the cornea and correct for a refractive error.

lacrimal gland. A gland located just above the eyeball that produces tears to wet the eye.

laser. A device that emits intense heat and power at close range. It is used in surgery and some diagnostic procedures. Its name is an acronym for "Light Amplification by Stimulated Emission of Radiation."

laser-assisted intrastromal keratomileusis (LASIK). A surgical procedure in which a microkeratome is used to make a flap in the cornea and a laser is then used to remove a wedge from the cornea in an effort to reshape the cornea and correct for a refractive error.

laterality. The ability to distinguish right from left on another person or object with reference to your own body.

lattice degeneration. A condition of thinning of the peripheral retina that can lead to a detachment, most often associated with extreme amounts of myopia.

lazy eye. A condition in which a healthy eye cannot achieve 20/20 vision with any corrective device. It usually results from the brain suppressing the vision in that eye to avoid seeing two different images from the two eyes. Also called amblyopia.

legal blindness. See *low vision.*

lens. The resilient, transparent structure in the eye that focuses light on the retina by changing the curvature of its front surface. It is located near the front of the eye, directly behind the pupil. Also, a transparent device that corrects for

refractive errors by causing light to be focused on the retina of the eye. It includes eyeglass lenses, contact lenses, and the artificial intraocular lenses that are implanted after cataract surgery. See also *artificial intraocular lens; bifocal lens; contact lens; trifocal lens.*

light sensitivity. A condition in which the eyes are extremely sensitive to light. Also called *photophobia.*

low vision. A condition is which the best visual acuity, with correction, is less than 20/200 or the visual field extends less than 20 degrees in each direction from the point where the attention is focused. Also called legal blindness.

macula. The central area of the retina that is used for direct, central vision. In humans, it has only cones, no rods.

macular degeneration. Irreversible and progressive damage to the macular portion of the retina, resulting in a gradual loss of fine, or reading, vision. It is a leading cause of blindness in the United States, and is usually associated with aging.

macular vision. See *central vision.*

meibomian cyst. See *chalazion.*

meibomian gland. A sebaceous gland within the structure of the eyelid that secretes an oily substance that lubricates the edge of the eyelid and helps to prevent tears from evaporating. Each eyelid has twenty to thirty meibomian glands.

metabolic rate. The rate at which the body carries out its metabolic functions.

metabolism. The entire complex of physical and chemical processes necessary to sustain life. It includes the breaking down of certain substances (such as foods) to release energy, and the synthesis of others (such as proteins) for the growth and repair of tissues.

migraine headache. A type of headache that is severe and frequently involves just one side of the head. It may last for several days, and may be associated with nausea, distorted vision, and the appearance of flashes of light.

milligram (mg). A unit of measurement equivalent to one one-thousandth of a gram. It is used to measure weight.

mineral. An inorganic substance that occurs in nature. Some minerals, such as iron and calcium, are essential to the proper functioning of the human body.

minus lens. A lens that decreases the focusing power of the light passing through it, causing the light to focus farther back, on the retina. It is used to correct for nearsightedness. See also *lens; nearsightedness; plus lens.*

monovision. A technique in which one contact lens is prescribed for distance vision and the other is prescribed for near vision. It is used an as alternative to bifocal contact lenses.

motor development. Pertaining to the development of the muscles and their coordination.

multiple sclerosis. An inflammatory disease of the central nervous system. It can cause visual disturbances because it often affects both the optic nerve and the nerves that control the muscles of the eyes.

myopia. See *nearsightedness.*

nanometer (nm). A unit of measurement equal to one one-billionth of a meter. It is used to measure the wavelength of light.

narrow-angle glaucoma. A form of glaucoma in which the drainage channel for the eye fluids is blocked. Also called closed-angle glaucoma. See also *glaucoma; open-angle glaucoma.*

nasal side. The side closest to the nose, as opposed to the ear. It is used to describe the location of structures in the eye and other parts of the face. See also *temporal side.*

near vision. The vision used to see objects sixteen inches away or closer. See also *distance vision; intermediate vision.*

nearsightedness. A condition in which the eye is too long, the cornea too steeply curved, or the lens unable to relax, causing the light passing through the cornea to come to a focus in front of the retina when viewing a distant object; a refractive error. The nearsighted person can see near objects clearly, but sees distant objects as blurry. Also called myopia. See also *astigmatism; emmetropia; farsightedness; presbyopia; refractive error.*

night blindness. A loss of the ability to see at night. Also called nyctalopia.

nystagmus. A form of involuntary eye movement. It is characterized by alternating smooth pursuit in one direction and quick movement in the other direction.

oculomotor. Referring to the movement of the eyeball.

occupational progressive lens. An eyeglass lens designed with no lined areas to allow clear vision at the near and intermediate viewing distances. See also *progressive lens.*

open-angle glaucoma. A form of glaucoma in which there is sufficient space for the eye fluids to drain, yet the pressure in the eye is still increased. See also *glaucoma; narrow-angle glaucoma.*

ophthalmologist. A medical doctor who specializes in eye diseases and eye surgery. See also *optician; optometrist.*

ophthalmoscope. An instrument with a mirror and light system that is used to view the interior of the eye, especially the retina, optic nerve, and choroid.

optic atrophy. A decline in blood flow to the optic nerve and eventual death of the nerve.

optic disk. The portion of the optic nerve that is formed by the gathering of all the transparent nerve fibers from the retina. The optic disk itself is not light-sensitive.

optic nerve. The bundle of fibers that carries the visual impulses from the retina to the brain.

optic neuritis. A condition of inflammation of the optic nerve.

optician. A licensed technician who makes and dispenses eyeglasses according to prescriptions from optometrists and ophthalmologists. In some states, opticians can also fit contact lenses. See also *ophthalmologist; optometrist.*

optometric vision therapy. A therapy program designed to realign and alter the functioning of the visual system. It includes techniques and other activities to reduce the visual stress, guide the development of the visual system, improve the visual skills, and enhance visual performance. Also called vision therapy.

optometrist. A licensed eyecare practitioner who examines and treats the eyes and visual system for refractive errors, eye-brain coordination problems, and signs of injury and disease. See also *ophthalmologist; optician.*

orbit. The area of the skull in which the eyeball and its associated parts are situated.

orthokeratology. A program of progressive contact lens fitting that gradually reduces the amount of nearsightedness and/or astigmatism.

palming. A technique use to relax the eyes; often part of a vision therapy program.

peripheral vision. The part of the visual field that is outside the direct line of vision; the side vision. See also *central vision; visual field.*

phacoemulsification. A technique employed in cataract surgery in which the eye's lens is disintegrated and then evacuated through a vacuum tube.

photochromic. Capable of changing color when exposed to ultraviolet light.

photochromic lens. An eyeglass lens that is capable of changing color when exposed to ultraviolet light.

photophobia. See *light sensitivity.*

photoreceptors. Sensory cells that are stimulated by light. In humans, they are the rods and cones of the retina. See also *cones; rods.*

pinguecula. A small, raised, yellowish area on the sclera, usually on the nasal side. It is a benign growth and does not grow onto the cornea.

pinkeye. An inflammation of the conjunctiva. It can be caused by an infection, allergy, or irritation. Also called conjunctivitis.

plus lens. A corrective lens that increases the focusing power of the light passing through it, causing the light to focus farther forward on the retina. It is used to correct for farsightedness and presbyopia. See also *farsightedness; lens; minus lens; presbyopia.*

polarizing lens. An eyeglass lens that reduces glare by decreasing the scattering of the incoming light rays.

polycarbonate. A type of plastic material used to make eyeglass lenses. It has a higher refractive index and more impact resistance than CR-39.

presbyopia. A condition in which the eye's lens has hardened and lost its focusing flexibility, causing difficulty with near vision; a refractive error. It usually occurs after the age of forty. See also *astigmatism; emmetropia; farsightedness; nearsightedness; refractive error.*

progressive addition lens (PAL). A type of multifocal corrective lens in which the transition from the distance segment to the intermediate segment and then to the near segment of the lens is gradual and uninterrupted. See also *lens; trifocal lens.*

protanopia. A defect in the perception of the color red. See also *deuteranopia.*

protein. A naturally occurring combination of amino acids that forms the basis of living cells. See also *complete protein.*

pterygium. A wing-shaped growth on the front of the eye, normally starting on the sclera on the nasal side and slowly growing over the cornea.

pupil. The round hole in the center of the iris through which light passes. It ordinarily appears black because very little light comes from the dark chamber behind it.

pupil reflex. A reflex in which the pupils constrict in response to light. Both pupils should constrict when a light is shined into either eye.

radial keratotomy. A surgical procedure in which radial cuts are made into the cornea in an effort to flatten it and correct for a refractive error.

recurrent corneal erosion. A condition in which the front layer of the cornea fails to heal following an abrasion or other trauma.

refraction. The bending of a light ray when it passes from one transparent medium into another of a different optical density. Also, the portion of a vision examination in which corrective lenses are used to sharpen the vision to within the normal limits.

refractive error. A condition in which the light passing through the cornea is refracted incorrectly and therefore does not come to a focus on the retina, causing blurred near and/or distance vision. See also *astigmatism; emmetropia; farsightedness; nearsightedness; presbyopia.*

refractive surgery. A surgical procedure to alter the refractive state of the eye.

refractor. An instrument used for diagnosing refractive errors.

resolving power. The ability to distinguish two points from each other at a given distance. It is a measure of visual acuity.

retina. The inner lining of most of the back chamber of the eye. It contains layers of nerve cells that are sensitive to light.

retinal detachment. A condition in which the inner layer of the retina detaches from the outer layer. If it is detected early and treated promptly with surgery, it can be corrected and the vision can be restored.

retinitis pigmentosa. A condition in which the retina begins to deteriorate at around the age of ten, leading to night blindness, then loss of the peripheral vision, and finally blindness. It is a progressive congenital disease with no cure.

rhodopsin. A light-sensitive pigment present in the rod cells of the retina. It is responsible for the transformation of light energy into nerve energy. Also called *visual purple.*

riboflavin. See *vitamin B$_2$.*

rigid gas-permeable contact lens. The modern version of a hard contact lens. A rigid lens allows the passage of oxygen and carbon dioxide. See also *contact lens.*

rods. The straight, thin cells in the retina of the eye. They contain rhodopsin and are responsible for night vision and vision in dim light. See also *cones; photoreceptors.*

sclera. The tough, white, fibrous outer protective layer of the eye.

scotopic sensitivity syndrome (SSS). A condition in which night vision is used at all times, which can lead to visual distortions and difficulty reading. It was first described by researcher Helen Irlen in the 1980s.

seasonal affective disorder (SAD). A condition marked by mental depression during the winter months. It is thought to be related to the lack of sunlight.

secondary cataract. The development of an opacity of the eye's lens capsule after cateract removal. Also called aftercataract. See also *cataract*.

seeing. The process of receiving light through the eyes and transmitting visual impulses to the brain for interpretation. See also *vision*.

senile cataract. A cataract that develops in the later years of life. See also *cataract*.

simple carbohydrate. A simple sugar, such as glucose or lactose (milk sugar), that is rapidly absorbed into the bloodstream. See also *complex carbohydrate*.

Sjögren's syndrome. An autoimmune disorder in which the body's defense system attacks and destroys the glands that produce tears and saliva.

slit lamp. A specialized microscope using a narrow slit of light and high magnification. It is used to examine the exterior portions of the eye.

Snellen chart. A chart imprinted with rows of black letters, with the letters graduating in size from the smallest on the bottom row to the largest on the top row. It was developed by Dutch ophthalmologist Herman Snellen (1834–1908), and is used for testing visual acuity.

soft contact lens. A contact lens made of a comfortable soft plastic with a high water content. See also *contact lens*.

strabismus. A condition in which the two eyes do not align properly while looking at a single object. One eye turns away (out, in, up, or down) from the point of regard. See also *cross-eyed; wall-eyed*.

stroke. the rapidly developing loss of brain function(s) due to a disturbance in the blood supply to the brain.

stye. A condition in which the hair follicle of an eyelash becomes infected, resulting in inflammation, redness, and soreness. See also *chalazion*.

subconjunctival hemorrhage. Bleeding from broken blood vessels under the conjunctiva. It appears as a red spot on the white sclera. Though it looks alarming, it usually resolves without treatment.

suppression. The "tuning out" of the image of one eye when in conflict with the image of the other eye; occurs at the level of the brain.

syntonics. A system of healing using colored lights of specific wavelengths. Also called color therapy.

temporal lobes. Areas of the brain located on both sides of the head surrounding the ears. The temporal lobes process auditory and some visual information.

temporal side. The side closest to the ear, as opposed to the nose. It is used to describe the location of structures in the eye and other parts of the face. See also *nasal side*.

thyroid gland. A gland located in the neck that produces thyroid hormone.

thyroid hormone. The substances produced by the thyroid gland that play a role in the regulation of the metabolism. An overabundance of thyroid hormone is associated with damage to the eyes.

tincture. A concentrated essence, such as of an herb, made by extracting and concentrating the active properties using alcohol. See also *extract; infusion.*

tonometer. An instrument that measures the pressure in the eye. It is used to screen for glaucoma.

toric contact lens. A contact lens designed to treat astigmatism. See also *contact lens.*

tracking. The ability to follow a moving target.

trifocal lens. A corrective lens that contains three segments—one for distance viewing, one for intermediate viewing, and one for near viewing. See also *bifocal lens.*

tunnel vision. The loss of peripheral, or side, vision while maintaining central vision.

20/20 vision. The visual acuity in the optically normal human eye. The term comes from the ability to read a specific row of letters or other symbols on a chart such as the Snellen chart from a distance of 20 feet. Deviations from the norm are expressed as, for example, 20/30, which indicates the ability to read at 20 feet what an optically normal person can read at 30 feet.

ultraviolet (UV) light. Light with a wavelength of less than 400 nanometers, which puts it below the range of the human visual spectrum.

vision. The entire visual process of receiving light through the eyes, the eyes transmitting visual impulses to the brain, and the brain interpreting the various aspects of the impulses and initiating the body's response to them.

vision therapy. See *optometric vision therapy.*

visual acuity. The acuteness or keenness of vision; the ability to discriminate the fine details of objects. The normal visual acuity is 20/20. Also called acuity.

visual field. The entire area that can be seen without shifting the position of the eyes. It includes the central and peripheral vision. See also *central vision; peripheral vision.*

visual impulse. The sensation caused by light striking a photoreceptor. The sensation is then transmitted to the brain by nerves.

visual memory. The ability to remember objects and other information based on having perceived them visually.

visual purple. See *rhodopsin.*

visualization. The ability to form a mental image of an object that is not actually present.

vitamin. An essential organic compound necessary for human metabolism but not manufactured by the human body. Vitamins must be taken in wholly or partly from nutrient sources.

vitreous humor. A clear, jellylike substance that fills the posterior (back) chamber of the eye and serves as a support structure for the retina.

wall-eyed. Having an eye that turns outward toward the ear while the other eye looks straight ahead. See also *cross-eyed; strabismus.*

Recommended Suppliers

The following list of suppliers is included so that you can find and use the supplements and remedies that are recommended within this book. It is not intended to be an exhaustive list of all possible sources of the suggested products. Rather, I have listed these companies because I have found their products to be of good quality. Following these companies is a list of organizations that may provide additional information regarding various eye issues. Please be aware that the addresses, phone numbers, and other contact information are subject to change.

HERBAL PRODUCTS

Dragon Herbs
321 Santa Monica Blvd
Santa Monica, CA 90401
888-558-6642
www.dragonherbs.com
Curated by master herbalist Ron Teeguarden, Dragon Herbs features a number of herbal products designed to encourage good health.

Herbs, Etc.
1340 Rufina Circle
Santa Fe, NM 87501
800-634-3727
www.herbsetc.com
Herbs, Etc. offers bulk herbs, herbal remedies, and supplements.

Herb-Pharm
PO Box 116
William, OR 97544
503-846-6262
http://herb-pharm.com
Most of this company's herbs are grown on their own certified organic farm. After hand-harvesting, the herbs are transported to a manu-facturing facility, where full-spectrum liquid herbal extracts are made along with herbal capsule products.

Nature's Way Products, Inc.
825 Challenger Drive
Green Bay, WI 54311
800-962-8873
www.naturesway.com
Their products include any kind of herbal or vitamin available on the market.

Wind River Herbs
PO Box 1462
Thayne, WY 83127
307-883-7070
800-903-4372
www.windriverherbs.com
Wind River Herbs' products include herbal formula blends, single herb extracts, body care products, and herbal teas.

Zand Immunity
222 S Main Street
Salt Lake City, UT 84115
800-643-7251
www.zandimmunity.com
ZAND embraces Traditional Chinese Medicine principles by developing formulas that address the whole body, not just the primary illness.

HOMEOPATHIC REMEDIES

Boiron
4 Campus Boulevard, Building A
Newtown Square, PA 19073
800-BOIRON-1
www.boironusa.com
Boiron offers eye-related products to treat disorders such as dry eye, chalazion, irritated eyes, strained eyes, styes, and more.

Hahnemann Labs
San Rafael, CA 94901
415-451-6978
888-427-6422
www.hahnemannlabs.com
Hahnemann Labs' products include a full array of homeopathic remedies for professionals and consumers.

Homeopathic Educational Services
812C Camelia St.
Berkeley, CA 94710
(510) 649-0294
www.homeopathic.com
Homeopathic Educational Services' products include books, articles, and homeopathic remedies.

Natural Ophthalmics
PO Box 1510
Dillon, CO 80435
877-220-9710
www.natoph.com

Their products include homeopathic eye drops to be distributed by eyecare professionals.

Newton Homeopathic Laboratories, Inc.
2360 Rockaway Industrial Boulevard
Conyers, GA 30207
800-448-7256
770-922-2644
www.newtonlabs.net
Newton makes easy-to-use homeopathic formulas that promote health and wellness for the entire family, pets included.

Standard Homeopathic Company
PO Box 61067
204-210 West 131st Street
Los Angeles, CA 90061
800-624-9659
www.hylands.com
Their products include a full range of homeopathic remedies.

LIGHTING AND EQUIPMENT

Eye Yoga 20-20-20 Pro
https://eyeyoga.com.au
The eye yoga headset is a vision therapy tool that immediately provides an "active recovery" response, targeting the direct source of the discomfort—the intra & outer muscles. Thus, offering relief by encouraging them to stretch and relax.

GE Lighting
Nela Park
1975 Noble Road
East Cleveland, OH 44112
800-435-4448
www.gelighting.com
Products of this leading innovator in progressive lighting are used for commercial and residential purposes.

Lumiram Electric Corporation
707 Executive Blvd., Ste. 1A
Valley Cottage, NY 10989
800-354-1044
www.lumiram.com
Lumiram is a leading manufacturer of full-spectrum natural light products, including Chromalux light bulbs.

NUTRITIONAL SUPPLEMENTS

Bausch + Lomb
400 Somerset Corporate Blvd.
Bridgewater, NJ 08807
800-553-5340
www.bausch.com
B+L is an industry leader in eyecare products, including contact lenses, solutions, pharmaceutical eye drops, nutritional supplements and more.

GlaxoSmithKline Corporation
800-245-1040
www.emergenc.com
This company is the maker of Emergen-C brand dietary supplements.

EnChroma
510-497-0048
https://enchroma.com
Eyeglasses to improve color perception. Available through eyecare professionals.

EyePromise
716-I Crown Industrial Ct.
Chesterfield, MO 63005
866-833-2800
www.eyepromise.com
EyePromise provides scientifically supported eye vitamins for people looking to support their eye and overall health with critical vitamins, minerals, and antioxidants that may be missing from their daily diet.

Fortifeye Vitamins
3101 SW College Road #205
Ocala, FL 34474
866-503-9746
www.fortifeye.com
Fortifeye provides patients with the highest-quality, science-based nutritional supplements for eye and total body health.

Health Thru Nutrition
30 New York Ave.
Westbury, NY 11590
866-319-6299
www.htnnaturally.com
The mission of HTN is to empower people to live healthier lives by providing superior quality nutrition products and serving as a trusted source of nutrition information.

Longevinex
Resveratrol Partners LLC
4425 S. Jones Blvd., Suite 1
Las Vegas, NV 89103
866-405-4000
www.longevinex.com
Longevinex has taken the Resveratrol molecule and designed a version of it that is effective as a mimic of a calorie-reduced diet. This allows the body to heal. All the raw materials are tested for quality and the final product is retested in the same manner.

Nordic Naturals, Inc.
94 Hangar Way
Watsonville, CA 95076
831-724-6200 x3
800-662-2544 x3
www.nordic.com
Nordic Naturals offers a complete line of fish oil products.

Rainbow Light Nutritional Systems
Rainbow Light
211 W. Pettigrew Street
Durham, NC 27701
800-475-1890
www.rainbowlight.com
This company is the creator of a food-based line of supplements for superior digestibility and increased energy support.

Wakunaga of America
23501 Madero
Mission Viejo, CA 92691
949-855-2776
800-421-2998

https://kyolic.com
This company plays a unique role in promoting public health worldwide through the research, development, manufacturing, and marketing of high-quality medicinal herbs.

Vista Advanced
15207 N. 75th Street, Suite 104
Scottsdale, AZ 85260
866-999-1497
www.vistaotc.com
VISTA offers an innovative approach to help people achieve the outcomes they desire. The company is committed to real-life results and superior treatment outcomes so people can live their best life.

Resource Organizations

The following organizations can answer questions, provide referrals, and tell you how to find more information on the subject about which you are interested. Some organizations provide literature or offer classes and workshops that will help you broaden your understanding of their areas of specialty. Others provide services and technology designed for people with specific vision problems. Feel free to contact these groups by mail or phone, or to visit their information-packed websites.

BLINDNESS AND LOW VISION

American Council of the Blind, Inc.
2200 Wilson Boulevard, Suite 650
Arlington, VA 22201
202-467-5081
800-424-8666
www.acb.org

The American Council of the Blind, founded in 1961, is the nation's leading membership organization of blind and visually impaired people. It endeavors to improve the lives of the blind and visually impaired through its efforts to represent them effectively, enhance educational and rehabilitative services for them, and better educate the public to promote better understanding about blindness and low vision.

American Foundation for the Blind
11 Penn Plaza, Suite 300
New York, NY 10001
212-502-7600
www.afb.org

The American Foundation for the Blind (AFB) is a national nonprofit organization that works to enhance the lives of people with vision loss in several ways: making the latest technologies more available to those with vision loss; providing better information to those who serve and work with the visually impaired; and connecting people with vision loss and their families with helpful resources that can help to improve the daily quality of living.

Association for the Education and Rehabilitation
  of the Blind and Visually Impaired
1703 North Beauregard Street, Suite 440
Alexandria, VA 22311
877-492-2708
703-671-4500
www.aerbvi.org

AER aims to support professionals who work with and for people with visual impairments in the areas of education and rehabilitation. It offers development opportunities, publications, and public advocacy.

Foundation Fighting Blindness
11435 Cronhill Drive
Owings Mills, MD 21117
800-683-5555
www.blindness.org
This foundation "drives the research" on retinitis pigmentosa (RP), macular degeneration, and the entire spectrum of retinal degenerative diseases.

National Association for the Visually Handicapped
NAVH New York
22 West 21st Street, 6th Floor
New York, NY 10010
212-889-3141
https://www.nchpad.org
NAVH helps the visually challenged with the psychological effects of their impairments and offers low vision services, visual aids, and training.

National Federation of the Blind
1800 Johnson Street
Baltimore, MD 21230
410-659-9314
www.nfb.org
The NFB improves blind people's lives through advocacy, education, research, technology, and programs encouraging independence and self-confidence.

Prevent Blindness America
211 West Wacker Drive, Suite 1700
Chicago, IL 60606
800-331-2020
www.preventblindness.org
This is the nation's leading volunteer organization for eye health and safety.

Research to Prevent Blindness, Inc.
645 Madison Avenue, Floor 21
New York, NY 10022
212-752-4333
800-621-0026
www.rpbusa.org

Research to Prevent Blindness is the leading voluntary health organization supporting eye research directed at the prevention, treatment, or eradication of all diseases that threaten vision.

Trace Research & Development Center
University of Wisconsin-Madison
2107 Engineering Centers Building
1550 Engineering Drive
Madison, WI 53706
608-262-6966
https://minds.wisconsin.edu/handle/1793/6747
The Trace Research & Development Center is a part of the College of Engineering, University of Wisconsin-Madison. It works to improve access to the latest information and telecommunication technologies.

DYSLEXIA AND LEARNING DISABILITIES

American Speech-Language-Hearing Association
2200 Research Boulevard
Rockville, MD 20850-3289
301-296-5700
www.asha.org
The American Speech-Language-Hearing Association is a large professional, scientific, and credentialing association. Members and affiliates include speech-language pathologists, audiologists, and speech, language, and hearing scientists in the United States and internationally.

International Dyslexia Association
40 York Road, 4th Floor
Baltimore, MD 21204
410-296-0232
www.interdys.org
This nonprofit organization offers information, referrals, training, and support to professionals and families regarding the effects of and treatment of dyslexia.

Irlen Institute for Perceptual and Learning
  Disabilities
Irlen Institute International Headquarters
5380 Village Road
Long Beach, CA 90808
800-55-IRLEN
www.irlen.com

The Irlen Method is a non-invasive, patented technology that uses colored overlays and filters to improve the brain's ability to process visual information.

HERBAL THERAPY

Institute for Traditional Medicine (ITM)
2017 SE Hawthorne Boulevard
Portland, OR 97214
503-233-4907
www.itmonline.org

This nonprofit organization explains the nature of traditional medicine and shows how it can be used currently to help those who seek it.

Oriental Healing Arts Institute
2005 Palo Verde Avenue, Suite 274
Long Beach, CA 90815
949-587-1238
www.ohaibooks.org

The Oriental Healing Arts Institute (OHAI) is a nonprofit educational organization. It is affiliated with the Brion Research Institute of Taiwan, a research institute for Oriental medicine in Asia.

OPTOMETRIC VISION THERAPY

College of Optometrists in Vision Development
  (COVD)
215 West Garfield Road, Suite 200
Aurora, OH 44202
888-268-3770
330-995-0718
www.covd.org

COVD advocates for comprehensive vision care, promoting a developmental and behavioral approach. It certifies professional competency in vision therapy, serves as an informational and educational resource, and advances research and clinical care in vision development and therapy.

Optometric Extension Program (OEP) Foundation,
  Inc.
Optometric Extension Program Foundation
1921 East Carnegie Avenue, Suite 3-L
Santa Ana, CA 92705
949-250-8070
www.oepf.org

OEP is an international organization that gathers and distributes information on vision and the visual process with the intention of advancing the discipline of optometry. Their goal it to effect progress through research and education on vision, the visual process, and clinical care.

ORTHOKERATOLOGY

Orthokeratology Academy of America
2853 East New York Avenue, Suite B
Aurora, IL 60502
866-851-9922
www.okglobal.org

The Orthokeratology Academy of America was founded to forward the science of this therapeutic treatment through workshops, courses, and other programs. The website offers a "Find an Ortho-K Doctor" service for interested patients.

SPECIFIC CONDITIONS

American Diabetes Association
ATTN: National Call Center
1701 North Beauregard Street
Alexandria, VA 22311
1-800-DIABETES
www.diabetes.org

The American Diabetes Association funds research to prevent cure and manage diabetes; delivers services to hundreds of communities; provides objective and credible information; and gives voice to those denied their rights because of diabetes.

Benign Essential Research Foundation
PO Box 12468
Beaumont, TX 77726
409-832-0788
www.blepharospasm.org
This foundation offers information on and support groups concerning blepharospasm.

The Glaucoma Foundation
80 Maiden Lane, Suite 1206
. New York, NY 10038
212-285-0080
https://glaucomafoundation.org
The Glaucoma Foundation is a not-for-profit organization. It is committed to leading the fight against glaucoma and to identifying new treatments and cures.

National Keratoconus Foundation (NKCF)
6222 Wilshire Boulevard, Suite 260
Los Angeles, CA 90048
310-623-4466
www.nkcf.org
The NKCF is a nonprofit organization dedicated to increasing keratoconus awareness and research. It offers a wealth of resources, including information guides, referrals, and outreach programs.

National Multiple Sclerosis Society
205 East 42nd Street
New York, NY 10017
212-986-3240
www.nationalmssociety.org
The National MS Society is a collective group with many chapters. Its members are committed to making progress in the research and treatment of MS.

The National Organization for Albinism
and Hypopigmentation (NOAH)
PO Box 959
East Hampstead, NH 03826
800-473-2310 (US and Canada)
603-887-2310
www.albinism.org
NOAH is a U.S.-based nonprofit organization that offers information and support to people with albinism, their families, and the professionals who work with them. NOAH is operated by volunteers and is funded primarily by dues and contributions of its members.

Retinitis Pigmentosa Foundation
RP International
PO Box 900
Woodland Hills, CA 91365
818-992-0500
www.rpinternational.org
RP International offers facilities for demonstrating the latest in visual aids for the partially sighted.

MISCELLANEOUS

American Academy of Ophthalmology
PO Box 7424
San Francisco, CA 94120
415-561-8500
www.aao.org
The American Academy of Ophthalmology is the largest national membership association of ophthalmologists, medical doctors, and osteopathic doctors who provide comprehensive eye care, including medical and surgical care.

American Academy of Optometry (AAO)
6110 Executive Boulevard, Suite 506
Rockville, MD 20852
301-984-1441
www.aaopt.org
The AAO aims to ensure excellence in optometric practice by fostering research and spreading information on vision science at its annual meeting.

American Optometric Association
243 North Lindbergh Boulevard
St. Louis, MO 63141
314-991-4100
www.aoa.org

The American Optometric Association represents approximately 36,000 doctors of optometry, optometry students, and paraoptometric assistants and technicians.

College of Syntonic Optometry
2052 W. Morales Drive
Pueblo West, CO 81007
719-547-8177
877-559-0541
www.syntonicphototherapy.com

The College of Syntonic Optometry promotes functional and rehabilitative vision therapy. Its website offers a "Practitioners Search" feature.

Corporate Vision Consulting
842 Arden Drive
Encinitas, CA 92024
800-383-1202
760-944-1200
www.cvconsulting.com

Corporate Vision Consulting is dedicated to assisting you in comfortably using a computer without straining your eyes. This includes customized eye exams and software, such as the Eye-CEE System for Computer Users.

Eye Bank Association of America, Inc.
  (EBAA)
1015 18th Street, NW, Suite 1010
Washington, DC 20036
202-775-4999
www.restoresight.org

The EBAA's Medical Advisory Board develops standards related to the recovery, preservation, storage, and distribution of eye tissue for transplantation and research, as determined by the ophthalmological medical community.

Ocular Wellness & Nutrition Society (OWNS)
PO Box 63
Cheyenne, WY 82003
307-264-2878
866-703-7229

The mission of the Ocular Wellness & Nutrition Society (OWNS) is to provide leadership, education, advice, and guidance to eye care and other health care professionals and consumers regarding the role of nutritional support as it relates to vision and eye health.

Index

WHAT YOU MUST KNOW ABOUT DRY EYE

How to Prevent, Stop, or Reverse Dry Eye Disease

Jeffrey Anshel, OD

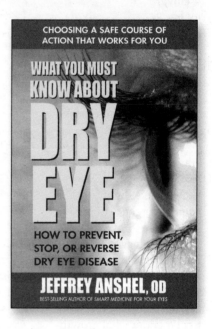

While the condition known as *dry eye* may sound like a minor problem, it can cause tremendous discomfort, even pain. Worse, this disorder can lead to eye fatigue, blurred vision, and difficulty driving, especially at night. In a healthy eye, lubricating tears continuously bathe the cornea—the dome-shaped outer surface of the eye. These tears provide a layer of liquid protection from the environment while nourishing the cells, keeping the eyes comfortable, and helping the eyes function properly. But when the glands near the eyes fail to produce tears of adequate quality or quantity, dry eye syndrome occurs.

Written by optometrist Jeffrey Anshel, *What You Must Know About Dry Eye* is divided into two parts. Part One begins by explaining the anatomy of the eye and how it works. It then focuses on dry eye—what the condition is, what causes it, how it impacts vision, and how it is diagnosed. In Part Two, the author examines a full range of treatments. First, he looks at conventional therapies, from over-the-counter artificial tears to prescription drugs. He then guides the reader in using smart nutrition and a proven supplement plan to relieve dry eye while making the eyes healthier, more comfortable, and able to see more clearly.

If you are one of the millions of people who suffer from dry eye, you know that this disorder can affect both your feeling of well-being and your ability to function in the world. *What You Must Know About Dry Eye* tells you how to relieve this common condition while improving and safeguarding your vision.

$16.95 US • 144 pages • 6 x 9-inch paperback • ISBN 978-0-7570-0479-7

WHAT YOU MUST KNOW ABOUT EYESTRAIN

Jeffrey Anshel, OD

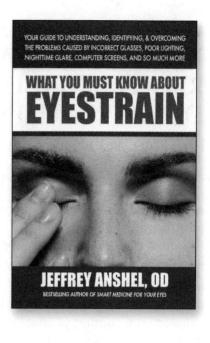

Do you often find yourself rubbing your eyes? After working on a display screen or reading a book, do you wind up having a headache? Do you seem to have problems focusing your vision, with or without glasses? If the answer to any of these questions is yes, you may be suffering from eyestrain. Your vision is one of your most important senses, and by not recognizing the signs of eyestrain, you are leaving yourself subject to a host of problems, including:

- Headaches
- Blurred vision
- Eye pain
- Dry eye
- Excessive tearing
- Excessive blinking
- Double vision
- Eye fatigue
- Heavy eyes
- Burning sensation
- Difficulty focusing
- Poor night vision
- Neck & shoulder pain
- Poor visual acuity
- Bloodshot eyes

The good news is that there is no reason to suffer from these common and annoying symptoms. Noted optometrist and bestselling author Jeffrey Anshel, OD, has written a guide to understanding and eliminating all of them. Written in plain English, *What You Must Know About Eyestrain* provides you with the up-to-date information required to identify the source of the problem—whether it is your display screen, inadequate lighting, poor nutrition, or merely the process of aging—and take the necessary steps to resolve it.

If you are one of the millions of people suffering from eyestrain, you will discover that, with few exceptions, most of the solutions to this problem are both simple and relatively inexpensive to achieve. With a copy of *What You Must Know About Eyestrain* in hand, you will be able to see your way to comfortable vision.

$16.95 US • 192 pages • 6 x 9-inch paperback • ISBN 978-0-7570-0501-5

WHAT YOU MUST KNOW ABOUT AGE-RELATED MACULAR DEGENERATION

How You Can Prevent, Stop, or Reverse AMD

Jeffrey Anshel, OD, and Laura Stevens, M.Sci

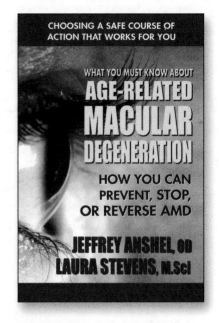

Age-related macular degeneration—AMD—is the most commonly diagnosed eye disorder in people over fifty. Well over two million Americans have been told they have AMD, and that number is expected to grow substantially. While this is a frightening statistic, over the last several years, medical researchers have shown that a number of effective treatments can slow, stop, and even reverse the progress of AMD. Now, best-selling authors Dr. Jeffrey Anshel and Laura Stevens, who herself has been diagnosed with this condition, have joined forces to produce an up-to-date guide to what you need to know to combat and even prevent AMD.

The book is divided into four parts. Part One explains how the eye works and how AMD develops, in both its wet and its dry forms. It then looks at the most common risk factors and explains how each of these factors negatively affects the structures of the eye. In Part Two, the authors look at the specific nutrients that affect the various cells of the eye. Included is a discussion of AREDS—the National Eye Institute's study that showed which supplements help protect the eye from disease. Part Three offers an additional weapon against AMD. It explains why diet matters and offers advice on selecting foods that promote eye health while eliminating those that do the most damage. Part Four provides practical suggestions and easy-to-follow tips on how to incorporate this valuable information into your life.

If AMD runs in your family or you have been diagnosed with this potentially life-altering condition, it is important to know that there is not only hope, but a real path to a better, healthier life. Knowledge is power, and the more you know, the more likely you are to avoid the consequences of AMD. Let *What You Must Know About Age-Related Macular Degeneration* help you safeguard one of your most precious gifts—eyesight.

$17.95 US • 288 pages • 6 x 9-inch paperback • ISBN 978-0-7570-0449-0

WHAT YOU MUST KNOW ABOUT FOOD AND SUPPLEMENTS FOR OPTIMAL VISION CARE

A Practical Guide to Supplements, Diet, and Lifestyle for Peak Ocular Health

Jeffrey Anshel, OD

As children, we were told to eat our carrots if we wanted good eyesight. Carrots contain beta-carotene, which the body can convert into vitamin A—a necessary nutrient for optimal vision. For most of us, that's where our knowledge of vitamins and eye health stops. Over the last twenty years, many studies have demonstrated that certain foods and natural supplements can play a major role in the treatment of eye problems. From the best-selling author of *Smart Medicine for Your Eyes* comes a new, concise guide to these powerful substances.

What You Must Know About Food and Supplements for Optimal Vision Care is divided into three parts. Part One is an overview of nutritional principles. This section explores the function of nutrients that benefit not only the visual system but also the entire body. Part Two provides a list of common eye disorders and includes a brief discussion of each condition, supplying handy charts that detail the nutritional, herbal, and homeopathic treatments that may be used to alleviate each disorder. Part Three offers further guidance by presenting dietary approaches to eye health and providing important information on the interaction of various foods and medications.

By eating mindfully and choosing supplements wisely, there is much you can do to support eye health. In this helpful and easy-to-use resource, Dr. Anshel provides you with a wealth of information on the most effective natural products and foods available to promote optimal vision.

$16.95 US • 176 pages • 6 x 9-inch paperback • ISBN 978-0-7570-0410-0

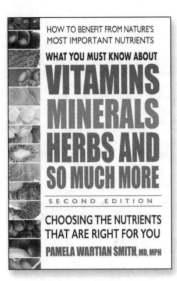

$16.95 • 512 Pages
6 x 9-inch paperback
ISBN 978-0-7570-0471-1

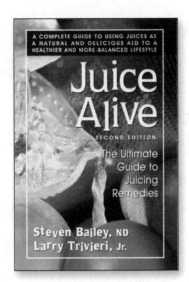

$14.95 • 288 Pages
6 x 9-inch paperback
ISBN 978-0-7570-0266-3

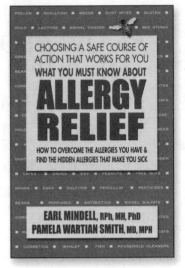

$17.95 • 288 Pages
6 x 9-inch paperback
ISBN 978-0-7570-0437-7

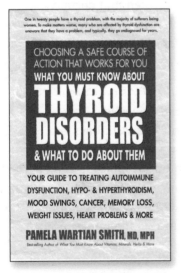

$16.95 • 224 Pages
6 x 9-inch paperback
ISBN 978-0-7570-0424-7

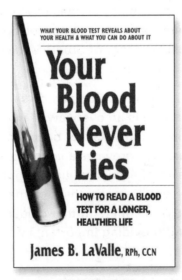

$16.95 • 368 Pages
6 x 9-inch paperback
ISBN 978-0-7570-0350-9

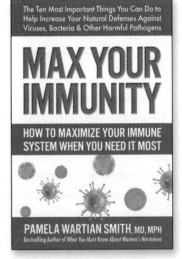

$16.95 • 280 Pages
6 x 9-inch paperback
ISBN 978-0-7570-0512-1

**For more information about our books,
visit our website at www.squareonepublishers.com**